# ALZHEIMER'S DISEASE - CHALLENGES FOR THE FUTURE

Edited by **Inga Zerr**

**Alzheimer's Disease - Challenges for the Future**
http://dx.doi.org/10.5772/58663
Edited by Inga Zerr

**Contributors**

Sibel Cevizci, Aysegul Uludag, Ahmet Uludag, Jianshe Wei, Cheryl Wellington, Sophie Stukas, Iva Kulic, Shahab Zareyan, Jose Fernandez-Checa, Elena Posse De Chaves, Yoshiya Oda, Genaro Ortiz, Alfredo Celis de la Rosa, Miguel A Macías-Islas, Fermín Pacheco-Moisés, Irma E Velázquez-Brizuela, L Javier Flores-Alvarado, Erica Daniela González-Renovato, Luis Figuera, Angelica Sánchez-López, Dhea Nuño-Penilla, Lorenzo Sánchez-Romero, Mario Mireles-Ramírez, J Luis Flores-Alvarado, Jean-Christophe Bier, Sandra De Breucker, Carlo Salustri, Rosanna Squitti, Mariacristina Siotto, Serena Bucossi, Franc Llorens, Rita Moretti, Jose Luna-Muñoz, Luis Oskar Soto-Rojas, Fidel De La Cruz, Miguel Angel Ontiveros-Torres, Amparo Viramontes-Pintos, Maria del Carmen Cardenas-Aguayo, Marco Meraz-Ríos, Citlaltepec Salinas-Lara, Benjamín Florán-Garduño, Susan van Hooren, Wim Waterink

**Published by InTech**

Janeza Trdine 9, 51000 Rijeka, Croatia



**Publishing Process Manager** Iva Lipovic

**Technical Editor** InTech DTP team

**Cover** InTech Design team

First published June, 2015

Printed in Croatia

Additional hard copies can be obtained from orders@intechopen.com

Alzheimer's Disease - Challenges for the Future, Edited by Inga Zerr

p. cm.

ISBN 978-953-51-2137-4

For EU product safety concerns:
IN TECH d.o.o., Prolaz Marije Krucifikse Kozulić 3, 51000 Rijeka, Croatia,
info@intechopen.com or visit our website at intechopen.com.

# Meet the editor

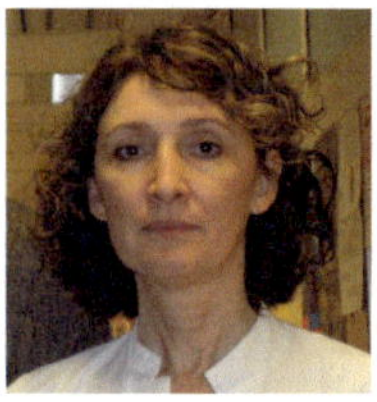

Inga Zerr is Chair of the Clinical Dementia Center at the Department of Neurology, University Medical School, Georg August University Göttingen. With over 220 original publications her current research interest is focused on understanding of the molecular basis of disease heterogeneity in Alzheimer´s disease and definition of predictors for disease progression in AD.

# Contents

**Preface IX**

**Section 1 Epidemiology and Molecular Pathology 1**

Chapter 1 **Epidemiology of Alzheimer's Disease with the Projection of Falls Among the Aged Population 3**
Aysegul Uludag, Sibel Cevizci and Ahmet Uludag

Chapter 2 **The Cascade of Oxidative Stress and Tau Protein Autophagic Dysfunction in Alzheimer's Disease 27**
Zhenzhen Liu, Peifu Li, Jiannan Wu, Yi Wang, Ping Li, Xinxin Hou, Qingling Zhang, Nannan Wei, Zhiquan Zhao, Huimin Liang and Jianshe Wei

Chapter 3 **Neuroinflammation and Alteration of the Blood-Brain Barrier in Alzheimer´s Disease 47**
Luis Oskar Soto-Rojas, Fidel de la Cruz-López, Miguel Angel Ontiveros Torres, Amparo Viramontes-Pintos, María del Carmen Cárdenas-Aguayo, Marco A. Meraz-Ríos, Citlaltepetl Salinas-Lara, Benjamín Florán-Garduño and José Luna-Muñoz

Chapter 4 **Metals Involvement in Alzheimer's Disease — A Patho-Genetic View 73**
Carlo Salustri, Mariacristina Siotto, Serena Bucossi and Rosanna Squitti

**Section 2 The Role of Lipids and Cholesterol 97**

Chapter 5 **Lipids and Lipoproteins in Alzheimer's Disease 99**
Sophie Stukas, Iva Kulic, Shahab Zareyan and Cheryl L. Wellington

Chapter 6 **Free Cholesterol — A Double-Edge Sword in Alzheimer Disease 141**
José C. Fernández-Checa

Chapter 7 **The Mevalonate Pathway in Alzheimer's Disease — Cholesterol and Non-Sterol Isoprenoids 167**
Amany Mohamed, Kevan Smith and Elena Posse de Chaves

**Section 3 Biomarkers 223**

Chapter 8 **Recent Progress in the Identification of Non-Invasive Biomarkers to Support the Diagnosis of Alzheimer's Disease in Clinical Practice and to Assist Human Clinical Trials 225**
Francois Bernier, Pavan Kumar, Yoshiaki Sato and Yoshiya Oda

Chapter 9 **New Frontiers in Alzheimer's Disease Diagnosis 257**
Franc Llorens, Sabine Nuhn, Christoph Peter, Inga Zerr and Katharina Stoeck

**Section 4 Clinical Aspects 295**

Chapter 10 **Genetic, Biochemical and Histopathological Aspects of Familiar Alzheimer's Disease 297**
Genaro Gabriel Ortiz, Fermín P. Pacheco-Moisés, Erika D. González-Renovato, Luis Figuera, Miguel A. Macías-Islas, Mario Mireles-Ramírez, L. Javier Flores-Alvarado, Angélica Sánchez-López, Dhea G. Nuño-Penilla, Irma E. Velázquez- Brizuela, Juan P. Sánchez-Luna and Alfredo Célis de la Rosa

Chapter 11 **Gait Pathway in Subcortical Vascular Dementia and in Alzheimer's Disease 325**
Rita Moretti, Arianna Sartori, Beatrice Baso and Silvia Gazzin

Chapter 12 **The Alzheimer's Patient in the Emergency Department — Specificities of Care 339**
De Breucker Sandra, Pepersack Thierry and Bier Jean-Christophe

Chapter 13 **Uncontrolled Sexual Behaviour in Dementia 353**
Susan van Hooren and Wim Waterink

# Preface

This book addresses many facets of Alzheimer´s disease, from epidemiology and clinical management of the patients to new approaches to understand the disease pathology. Currently discussed pathways are highlighted and discussed. The collection covers actual topics of interest for basic researchers and clinicians and provides insights in the complex problems in Alzheimer´s disease.

**Inga Zerr, MD**
Clinical Dementia Center
Department of Neurology
University Medical School
Georg August University Göttingen
Germany

Section 1

# Epidemiology and Molecular Pathology

# Chapter 1

# Epidemiology of Alzheimer's Disease with the Projection of Falls Among the Aged Population

Aysegul Uludag, Sibel Cevizci and Ahmet Uludag

Additional information is available at the end of the chapter

http://dx.doi.org/10.5772/59876

## 1. Introduction

With aging, the loss of the ability to adapt to environmental factors in progressive decline occurs. Particularly in North European countries, the elderly population continues to gradually increase. Currently, in developing countries with a high youth population,it has been mentioned that the size of epidemiology in the aging population revealed a more realistic projection. The aging population is rapidly increasing. Of the 600 million elderly (60 years and over) that are living,the ratio will increase by 25% in the next 25 years, and the population of over 65 years old is expected to increase by 88% in the world. Most of the older population is found in developed countries than that are indicated. In this projection, the determination of health policies for the elderly necessarily becomes a first priority.

The old age period needs to be examined in physical, psychological, and social aspects. While physical changes occur in a chronological order, psychological perception changes are observed in learning, psychomotor, and personality characteristics. In the aspect of social perspective, the people live in many limitations [1]. The elderly population suffer with the following: approximately 8.0% have serious cognitive problems; 20% have chronic diseases, vision problems, and hearing loss; and 33% live with a limitation on movements [2].

Dementia is defined as one of the biggest problems faced by the elderly population. It is an overall term for diseases and conditions characterized by a decline in memory or other thinking skills that affects a person's ability to perform daily activities. According to DSM V criteria, dementia can be defined as a major and mild neurocognitive disorders. In epidemiological data, 24.2 million people live with dementia at that time, with 4.6 million new cases arising every year [3]. Dementia increases with age, especially over the age of 65 which are 1.5 times more often seen. Many conditions may cause dementia. However, the Alzheimer's disease (AD) is one of the reasons of the dementia that estimates 60-80%.

Alzheimer's disease is defined as a progressive loss of the cognitive function. This function loss history starts with the loss of memory and function, and eventually to all the intellectual activities of daily living and leads to premature death. Beta-amyloid plaques, neurofibrillary tangles, and neurodegeneration are the hallmark pathologic characteristics of AD [4]. To establish a diagnosis of AD with the onset of symptoms that can be done, in fact, already started the beginning of the 20 year before. Etiology has not been fully clarified, but the underlying causes are genetics, age, family history, the Apolipoprotein E-ε4 gene (APOE-ε4), mild cognitive impairment, education level, traumatic brain injury, and cardiovascular risk factors [5].

Alzheimer's disease causes slowly progressive irreversible cognitive destruction with the loss of performing even the daily activities. In particular, the most common problems encountered in this process is falling. Falls in patients have clinically more severe chronic process and present additional morbidity while mortality is increases. Alzheimer’s disease has approximately 2 times higher risk for falling [6,7]. For patients with dementia, when they fall, they are three times more likely to have broken hips. Hip fracture further increase the death rate of AD patients [8]. In AD patients, increased risk of falling remains less understood. In studies, cerebral white matter lesions may relate to cognition and postural balance [9-10].

In this chapter, the epidemiology of Alzheimer’s Disease with etiologic factors will be discussed, and with this projection, the risk and importance of falls in these patients will also be tackled.

## 2. The aging population

With aging, loss of the ability to adapt to environmental factors in progressive decline and aging population is rapidly increasing. Of 600 million elderly (60 years and over) that are living, the ratio will increase by 25% in the next 25 years, and the 65+ population is expected to increase by 88% in the world. Most of the older population is found in developed countries than that are indicated. In the year of 2056, 29.5% of Canadians, which is roughly 10.5 million people, are expected to be above 65 years of age [11]. Approximately 8% of the elderly population live with serious cognitive problems, while 20% have chronic diseases, vision problems, and hearing loss, while the another 33% live with limitation of movements [2,12].

While the geriatric population increases, the incidence of chronic diseases also increases. In particular, there are many physiological changes that occur in the geriatric period. The most prominent of these occur in the skeletal system. With aging, bone resorption decreases and senile osteoporosis occurs. In women, the menopause accelerated osteoporosis, and it threatens both male and female with aging. In addition to this change in the geriatric period, gastrointestinal system changes occur that reduce appetite and prevent the absorption of nutrients. This process in the geriatric period affects both the dementia process as well as increase the risk of co-morbidity.

There are also social aspects of geriatric patients with the same changes. The most prominent of these is related to the loss of spouse or loss of family members. Work situations, such as separation or lack of income increases, results to social problems in the elderly.

Today, in developed countries live alone in geriatric period stood out, with the rise of industrialization. In developing countries geriatrics are also dwindling along with family members. This facilitates the social isolation occuring in the aging population that live on their own.

One of the most significant changes experienced by the geriatric age group is also a change in mental health. Especially due to social isolation or existing health problems, mood disorders in the geriatric population is emerging. At the inital stage of dementia in people with mood changes, it is difficult to recognize the coexistence of disorder or delay.

## 3. The aging population and falls

In the elderly, physiologically changes and many chronic diseases occur, and the geriatric population also experience comorbidity problems. Falling is one of the major problems causing the increasing comorbidities and mortality rates. Falls, in the geriatric population, is the fifth leading cause of mortality [13]. Every year, geriatric patients aged 65 years and over is reduced by 30%, and for patients over 85 years of age, by 50%. Each year, 30-50% of falls are in nursing homes and 40% of those individuals fall again [14].

In the study from South Asia, it was found that the incidence of falls in China was 6-31%, while in Japan, it was 20% [15-17]. According to the WHO report, the rate of hospital admission caused by falls was found to be 1.6 to 3.0 per 10,000 population for people at the aged 60 years and over in Australia, Canada, the United Kingdom of Great Britain, and Northern Ireland (UK) [15]. Forty percent of all injury deaths are caused by falls [18]. Populations have various fall fatality rate for people aged 65 years and over: in the USA, 36.8 per 100,000 population; in Canada, 9.4; in Finland, 55.4 for people aged 50 and over [19-21]. Figure 1 indicates fatal falls by age group and gender [15,22]. Fatal fall rates increase with age for both gender, and the highest rate is seen at the age of 85 years and over. It has been found that men reported poorer health and a greater number of underlying conditions than women. These include increasing hip fracture and the risk of mortality [23].

Although population ageing is a triumph of humanity related to the extension of life-span, it brings back some challenges for societies [24]. The absolute number of people aged 60 years and over is expected to increase from 688 million in 2006 to 2 billion by 2050. For the first time, the population of aged people will be greater than the population of children under the 14 years of age [15]. In addition, being predisposed to falls and its serious consequences is fastest growing at the age of 80 and over. Figure 2 shows the population pyramid in 2005 and 2025 [15]. This figure shows that the percentage of older population is growing in parallel with a decreasing percentage of the younger population. The triangular shape of the 2005 population pyramid will transform into the more cylinder-like form in 2025 [15].

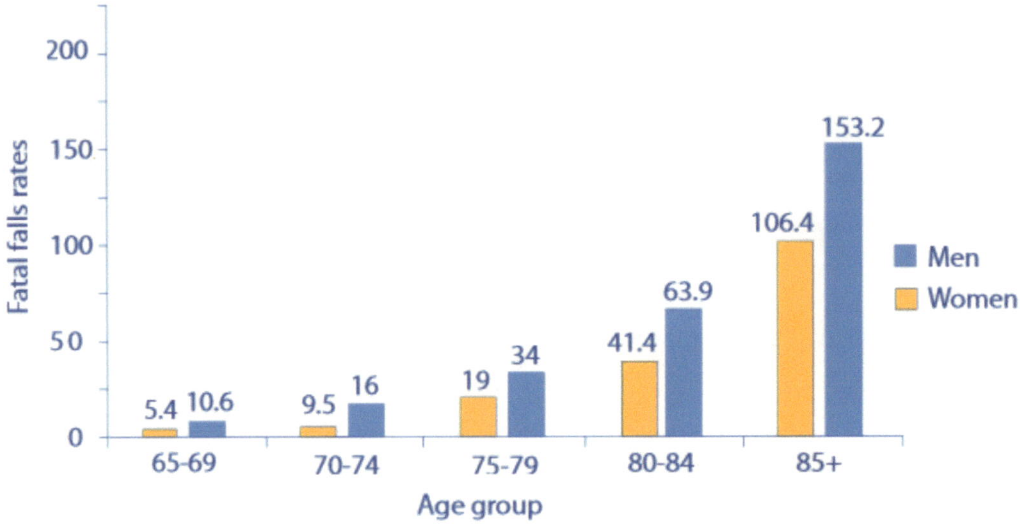


**Figure 1.** Fatal fall rates by age and sex group[15,22].

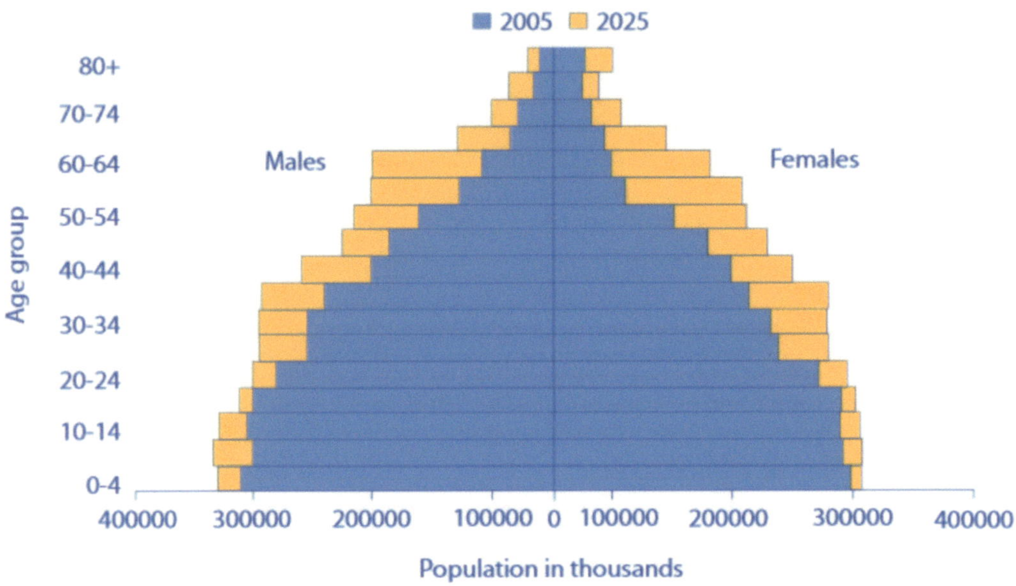


**Figure 2.** Global population pyramid in 2005 and 2025 [15,25].

The prevention of falls is a considerable challenge for the ageing population. The number of falls increase in magnitude as the number of aged people increase in many populations throughout the world [15]. Falls increase with age because of biological change. Consequently, the number of people aged 80 years and over will trigger a substantial increase of falls and injuries at an anxious rate. Actually, incidence of fall injuries have increased by 131% in the last three decades. The number of injuries caused by falls is predicted to be 100% higher in the year 2030 [15,21].

This applies to developing countries where ageing population is rapidly occurring and where close to 70% of the elderly population lives. To add, "the developed world that became richer before getting older, developing countries are getting older before becoming richer" [26].

The Ontorio working group linked the cause of the high incidence of falls to extrinsic and intrinsic risk factors. The intrinsic risk factors are the physical characteristics, demographics, and general health status of elders; e.g. psychosocial-demographic risks, medical risks and considered as risk and degree of dependency with activity levels. While the extrinsic factors are thought to be related to the physical and socio-economic environment; e.g. balance, slip hazards and vision hazard. [27].

Most falls result from a person's environment. The causes are, especially, the predisposing and precipitating factors of the person's environment. In most studies, about 25 to 45 percent of falls occur because of environmental hazards [28]. The other common causes are gait disturbance and muscle weakness. The risk factors of falls are dizziness, vertigo, drop attacks, postural hypotension, visual impairment, and syncope in patients. Lower extremity muscle weakness is a significant risk factor for falls because it increases the odds of falling fourfold. The other risk factors of falls are having fall history and gait or balance deficits which increases the risk threefold. Other high-risk situations for falls are the use of an assistive device, visual deficit, arthritis, impaired activities of daily living, depression, cognitive impairment, and age over 80 years. Studies reported that, medication increases the risk of falls, especially the use of four or more medications, which have been strongly associated with an increased risk of falls. In particular, the use of psychotropic medications, cardiac drugs including class 1A antiarrhythmic agents, digoxin, diuretics, and anticonvulsants have been implicated in increasing the risk of falls [29,30]. In a social perspective, falls are one of the most common geriatric syndromes because of the threat to the independence of older persons. Between 30 to 40 percent of community-dwelling adults older than 65 years fall each year, and the rates are higher for nursing home residents. Falls are associated with increased morbidity, mortality, and nursing home placement [31,32]. The other risk factors of falls are arthritis, depression and activities of daily living [33,34].

Falling due to fractures is very common in the geriatric population. In Canada, it is stated that a large 23,631 people 59 years and older were hospitalized due to femoral neck fractures. The most frequent cause of hospitalization for 65 years old and older is hip fracture. Femoral neck fractures with dependence in daily activities in patients older than 85 years also increases [35-40].

The American Academy of Family Practice offers a clinical assessment to determine the risk of fractures in the elderly. The risk groups are defined as the conditions shown in Table 1 below.

| Clinical Assessments and Interventions for Elderly at Risk for Falls* | |
|---|---|
| *Assessment and risk factor* | *Interventions* |
| Circumstances of previous falls | Changes in environment and activity to reduce the likelihood of recurrent falls |
| Medication use<br>High-risk medications<br>Four or more medications | Review and reduction of medications |
| Vision<br>Acuity < 20/60<br>Decreased depth perception<br>Decreased contrast sensitivity<br>Cataracts | Ample lighting without glare; avoidance of multifocal glasses while walking; referral to an ophthalmologist |
| Postural blood pressure; ≥ 20 mm Hg drop in systolic pressure, with or without symptoms, repeat immediately or after two minutes of standing | Diagnosis and treatment of underlying cause, if possible; review and reduction of medications; modification of salt restriction; adequate hydration; compensatory strategies; pressure stockings; pharmacologic therapy if the above strategies fail |
| Balance and gait<br>Patient's report or observation of unsteadiness<br>Impairment on brief assessment | Diagnosis and treatment of underlying cause, if possible; reduction of medications that impair balance; environmental interventions; referral to physical therapist for assistive devices and for gait and progressive balance training |
| Targeted neurologic examination<br>Impaired proprioception<br>Impaired cognition<br>Decreased muscle strength | Diagnosis and treatment of underlying cause, if possible; increase in proprioceptive input; reduction of medications that impede cognition; awareness on the part of caregivers of cognitive deficits; reduction of environmental risk factors; referral to physical therapist for gait, balance, and strength training |
| Targeted musculoskeletal examination: examination of legs and feet | Diagnosis and treatment of underlying cause, if possible; referral to physical therapist for strength, range-of-motion, and gait and balance training and for assistive devices; use of appropriate footwear; referral to podiatrist |
| Targeted cardiovascular examination<br>Syncope<br>Arrhythmia | Referral to cardiologist; carotid-sinus massage |
| Home hazard evaluation after hospital discharge | Removal of loose rugs and use of night lights, non-slip bath mats, and stair rails; other interventions as necessary |

**Table 1.** Clinical Assessments and Interventions for Older Persons at Risk for Falls

Tinetti ME. Clinical practice. Preventing falls in elderly persons. N Engl J Med 2003;348:45.

Health care services has provided the necessary preventive measures for fall-related fractures in the geriatric population. There are some precautions, in terms of extrinsic factors, that are also needed to be taken to prevent falls. In this regard, the US Preventive Task Force (USPSTF) offers suggestions to prevent fractures in elderly patients [41]. The USPSTF recommendations are given in Table 2 below.

| **Strength of Recommendations*** | |
|---|---|
| Key clinic Recommendations | Label |
| Home hazard assessment and modification is recommended for patients with a history of falls. | A |
| Exercise and physical therapy are recommended to prevent falls and injury from falls. | A |
| Patients should receive a multifactorial risk assessment and intervention because it is the most consistently effective strategy to prevent falls. | A |
| Evaluation of medications and withdrawal of medications that increase the risk of falling is recommended. | B |
| Dual-chamber pacemaker placement is recommended for selected patients with carotid sinus syndrome and syncope. | B |
| Hip protectors are recommended for patients at high risk of falling in an institutional setting. | B |
| Patients with a history of falls or with risk factors for falling should undergo a formal evaluation. | C |

* U.S. Preventive Services Task Force. Guide to clinical preventive services

**Table 2.** Recommendations and labels for preventing elderly people from falls

One of the most significant pathology in the geriatric age group is also dementia. The most common cause of dementia in the USA is Alzheimer's disease that has an annual health spending of 192 billion dollars. The cost for health expenditure has been based from a study but the social impact cannot be calculated [41].

## 4. Dementia in the aged population

The biggest problem is defined as dementia in the aged population. Dementia prevalence is estimated to amount to 24 million and predicted to quadruple by the year 2050 [41]. Dementia is defined as an overall term for diseases and conditions characterized by a decline in memory or other thinking skills that affects a person's ability to perform everyday activities. According to the DSM V criteria, dementia is defined in terms of major and mild neurocognitive disorders. In the epidemiological data, 24.2 million people lived with dementia at that time, with 4.6 million new cases arising every year [3]. In Canada; 2.0% of the population were diagnosed with dementia [11]. Dementia, increases with age, especially over the age of 65 years where it has been often seen by 1.5 times more.

Previous definitions of dementia have often included the requirement of a progressive and irreversible impairment. Dementia related so many things and can occur before or after the age of 65 [42].

Alzheimer's disease (AD) has been one of the top reasons of the dementia which estimates 60-80%. The etiology of Alzheimer's disease shows many reasons, although the exact etiologic factor could not be determined. The early-onset AD is referred to the existence of genetic factors associated with the etiology of APOE. While with the late onset AD, the etiological factors could not be determined [4].

## 5. Alzheimer's disease epidemiology

Alzheimer's disease is defined as a progressive loss of cognitive function. This function loss history starts with the loss of memory and function, and eventually to all the intellectual activities of daily living, and leads to processes that causes premature death. Beta-amyloid plaques, neurofibrillary tangles, and neurodegeneration are the hallmark pathologic characteristics of AD [4]. In fact, since 20 years ago, there were already initial steps to establish the diagnosis of AD with the onset of symptoms. Etiology has not been fully clarified, but the underlying causes are genetics, age, family history, the Apolipoprotein E-ε4 gene (APOE-ε4), mild cognitive impairment, education level, traumatic brain injury, and cardiovascular risk factors [5].

The prevalence of Alzheimer's disease, according to the countries' health-related database information from Holland, France, Italy, England and USA, is estimated at 3-7% [43].

Memory loss is the most pronounced behavioural abnormality, and is usually the first symptom in Alzheimer's disease. Memory is impaired for recent events, with relative preservation of remote memory. In the early stages of the disease, memory impairment may be an isolated dysfunction, followed in time by the development of impairments of attention, language function (defective word finding with otherwise fluent speech), visuospatial abilities (drawing, route finding), praxis (purposeful movements), calculations, visual, auditory and olfactory perception, problem-solving ability, and judgement. Patients with Alzheimer's disease have difficulty shifting their mental set from one task to another. Depression, personality changes, apathy, and irritability are also common features of the disease. Language abilities and social skills may be remarkably preserved, even in the later stages, and patients with well-established dementia may be able to maintain polite conversations with remarkable skill and thus appear to be intact to the casual observer. Paranoid delusions, illusions, and hallucinations are seen in a minority of patients, usually in the later stages. Up to half of the patients with Alzheimer's disease have limited awareness of their behavioural deficits. It should be emphasized that the behavioural features of this disease are highly variable from patient to patient: some patients may have preserved language function with impaired visuospatial abilities, while other patients at a similar stage in the overall disease process may show the reverse pattern of deficits. Motor function and urinary continence are usually not affected until later. This variability, or heterogeneity, in the behavioural manifestations of the disease is due to variations in the distribution of disease severity in brain regions. For example, patients with severe involvement of the left temporal and parietal cortex will have relatively more marked language dysfunction. The disease is progressive, with survival rates after an onset of 5 to 12 years duration [42,43].

As the elderly population in developed countries increases, it also can not be prevented to have an increase in the prevalence of Alzheimer's disease. This is due to the change in the direction of health policies. The unknown cause and limited treatment cause higher health expenditures and quite large losses in every perspective.

Alzheimer's Disease, has two types of progressive diseases. If the AD starts before 65 years of age, it is defined as early clinical onset. If it starts after 65 years of age, it is defined as late onset AD. Early-onset AD starts in middle age and is implicated in the etiology of genetic predisposition. Late-onset AD is the most commonly seen in the 70-80 age range, and after 65 years, there is a 2-fold increased risk of AD.

Some factors considered to be the etiology of Alzheimer's disease: age, genetics, family history, the Apolipoprotein E-ε4 gene (APOE-ε4), mild cognitive impairment, education level, traumatic brain injury, and cardiovascular risk factors.

**Age**: Age is associated with the increase in the prevalence of AD. After 65 years of age, it is known that a 2-fold increase likelihood of AD occurs every 5 years. When a person isover 85 years of age, the increased risk becomes 16-fold.

**Genetics:** There are many studies on this subject. There are some genes and polymorphisms that are genetically determined. These genes and polymorphisms are associated with the pathophysiology of white plaque in AD. Alzheimer's disease pathology in the brain is characterised by the presence of plaques of amyloid β peptides and intraneuronal tangles of hyperphosphorylated forms of microtubule-associated protein tau (MAPT) [44]. It is stated that in the studies of both componentscarry genetic forms of AD. Casual mutations in three genes have been identified in early-onset forms, establishing the central role of amyloid in Alzheimer's disease, which has become to be the most widely studied pathway since these discoveries [45-49]. Twin studies have observed that the transition rate is 80% [50].

In the absence of transitions in all AD patients with the same genes, it has been suggested that the environmental factors are related in the development of the disease. It has been genetically implicated, especially in the early onset of Alzheimer's disease with APOE ε4 allele presence. At the molecular level, especially in transition, Mendelian APP, PSEN1, and PSEN2 mutations were studied [45-49].

Mutations in PSEN1 and PSEN2 are also directly related to amyloid production; they impair the γ-secretase-mediated cleavage of APP, resulting in an increased ratio of amyloid β to amyloid β [51].

The results of the studies that show autosomal dominant Mendelian characteristics found that some genes were involved in the pathology of AD. The late-onset AD is also guilty of the changes in these genes. The genome-wide association and replication of these genes, additionally, have been reported for single nucleotide polymorphisms in or near CR1, PICALM, and BIN1[52]. Continued concerted efforts identified the association with single nucleotide polymorphisms especially in MS4A cluster, CD2AP, CD33, EPHA1, and ABCA7 [52-56].

**Apolipoprotein-ε4** (APOE ε4)

Apolipoprotein-ε4 allele is the best known factor for the late-onset and early-onset forms. The Alzheimer's disease risk is increased with having one ε4 allele roughly three-times and those with two ε4 alleles have a roughly 15-times-increased risk, compared with the most common genotype, APOE ε3ε3 [57].

Results of early studies suggested that this risk was greatest in patients who were 60–79 years of age at the onset, a notion confirmed by a study of more than 17,000 individuals with whom the risk of disease in APOE ε4ε4 carriers aged 60–69 years was as much as 35 times higher than that noted in APOE ε3ε3 carriers [58]. In APOE ε4 carriers, the lifetime risk of Alzheimer's disease (an estimate independent of APOE ε3ε3 and the actual probability of developing disease between birth and a given age) at age 85 years was estimated to be as high as 35% for female APOE ε3ε4 carriers and 68% for female APOE ε4ε4 carriers [59].

### 5.1. Cerebrovascular diseases

Hemorrhagic infarcts, vasculopathy or something which causes changes in white matter cause AD, however, the specific name for this cause or reason has not yet been identified. Infarcts can lead to losses in areas related to memory or due inflammation that occurs in AD [62,63].

### 5.2. Hypertension

In studies, the hypertension that especially occurs in middle aged people, could cause the onset AD. In many studies, vascular resistance of the resulting protein will lead to the extravasation of the blood-brain barrier and, thus, lead to damage in the cell structure, apoptosis, and damage in the brain. In addition, this may be considered as a cause of AD [62,63].

### 5.3. Type 2 Diabetes Mellitus

Type 2 DM is accused to be the cause of hyperinsulinemia in AD patients. Ensuring that the peripheral hyperinsulinemia down-regulates the insulin receptors in the brain, under physiological insulin needs provides a transition to the brain and leads to an increase in the IDE found mediated amyloid production [64,65].

### 5.4. Lipid disorders

Many studies considered cognitive impairment and AD are caused by lipid disorders, although there is no evidence to reveal exactly why. The reason for this is that genetics predisposition and apolipoprotein E, apolipoprotein J (APOJ, CLU), ATP-binding cassette subfamily A member 7 (ABCA7), and sortilin-related receptor (SORL1) are responsible etiology of AD and lipid metabolism [66-68].

### 5.5. Head injury

In the meta-analysis, it is particularly prevalent in people who underwent a traumatic brain injury with dementia [69-71]. Especially the men are more affected than the women. However, there are inconsistent evidences for head injuries increasing the risk of AD.

## 6. Alzheimer disease and risk of falls

The prevalence of falls in patients with mild to moderate dementia is at 42% [44]. Cognitive destruction of dementia patients have a worse prognosis than when they fall. In studies, falls are more frequently seen in patients with AD [45]. In the world, the geriatric age population is increasing and consequently the number of patients with AD is also increasing too meaning falls happen in the people in this group, which is a serious problem [44-47].

According to the CDC, every year people aged 65 and over fall [48-49]. Falls can cause fatal and nonfatal injuries, and can increase the risk of early death [50]. In fact, we know that falls are a preventable public health problem, especially for aging communities. In aging societies, Alzheimer diseases is another serious health problem, which is largely seen in developed countries. The death and injury rates that result from falls among older men and women have risen sharply over the past decade (Table 3). Aged people with Alzheimer's Disease are at a particularly high risk of falling. Problems with vision, perception, and balance increase as the Alzheimer's Disease advances, making the risk of a fall more likely [51].

| **Deaths** |
|---|
| *In 2011, about 22,900 older adults died from unintentional fall injuries.* |
| *Men are more likely than women to die from a fall. After taking age into account, the fall death rate in 2011 was 41% higher for men than for women.* |
| *Older whites are 2.7 times more likely to die from falls as their black counterparts.* |
| *Rates also differ by ethnicity. Older non-Hispanics have higher fatal fall rates than Hispanics.* |
| **Injuries** |
| *People age 75 and older who fall are four to five times more likely to be admitted to a long-term care facility for a year or longer, than those age 65 to 74.* |
| *Rates of fall-related fractures among older women are more than twice than those for men.* |
| *Over 95% of hip fractures are caused by falls. In 2010, there were 258,000 hip fractures and the rate for women was almost twice the rate for men (15).* |
| *White women have significantly higher hip fracture rates than black women.* |
| *Centers for Disease Control and Prevention, the National Center for Injury Prevention and Control. |

**Table 3.** Fall-related deaths and injuries*

The annual incidence of Alzheimer's disease patients that experience a fall in their age group is 60-80% of non-AD. Also AD patients are 3 times more likely to carry the risk of fall-related developments fraction [52-55].

Although not proven, there are already studies about the increasing frequency of falls in patients by De Groot et al., [9] and Maruyama et al., [10] that cerebral white matter lesions may relate to cognition and postural balance.

There is not known relation between falls and AD. But, changes in motor movements are thought to be related to the recently impaired cognitive function. It is not known whether changes in motor movement, or cognitive loss in AD and mild cognitive impairment had previously occurred [46-57]. Stark SL et al., [58] considered that motor movements are affected before than the cognitive impairment and is argued that the increase of brain amyloid levels increase the risk of falling.

Ogama N et al., [59] declared that AD patients with falls have higher white matter lesions (WML) than patients without falls. The posture and gait performance of the AD patients with falls were lower than patients without falls. It has been found that, the periventricular hyperintensity in frontal caps and occipital WMLs were strong predictors for falls, even after potential risk factors were considered. About the risk of dementia and AD patients, regional WMLs visualisation by the the brain magnetic resonance may greatly help to diagnose dementia in the elderly with a higher risk of falls. Regional white matter burden, independent of cognitive decline, correlates with balance/gait disturbance and predicts falls in elderly with aMCI and AD [59].

In dementia, many risk factors were studied. The most common risk factors for falls in patients with AD that are related to cognitive impairment and dementia are: gait and balance disturbances, behavioral disorders, visual problems, malnutrition, adverse effects of drugs, fear of falling, neurocardiovascular instability (particularly orthostatic hypotension), and environmental hazards.

Based on data from studies, a multifaceted intervention, including a physical exercise programme, and a modification of the risk factors may prevent falls in older people with cognitive impairment and dementia. Lorbach ER et al., considered [60] that age, history of falls, motor impairment, visual disturbance, cognitive disfunction, behavioral disturbance, side effects of prescription drugs, and the presence of risky behaviors are risk factors of falls. NutriAlz' study declared that the risk of falls are related with the history of falls, nutritional status and arthritis [61]. Walking is an automatic process until it is necessary to deviate from the learned program. Most of the locomotion involves intention and therefore, there are cognitive inputs of various degrees.

In AD and the other dementia diseases, cognitive impairment will have a negative effect on all aspects of gait performance and progressive decline in cognition. This may cause a concomitant disorganization of the network that controls locomotion, leading to an impaired gait timing and postural control.

A disintegration of a higher cortical sensory function and a particularly involving perceptual-motor integration may represent in AD patients. Because of this disintegration of the various components, previously learned routine motor functions "breaks down" due to visuo-spatial integration and other functions of higher cortical perception, an unconscious component in the network of motor control. In AD patients, both constructional and ideomotor apraxia at all stages of the disease occur. Alternatively, as a result of trying to compensate for an impaired higher cortical sensory integration and competition for attentional resources, the control of timing in the cerebellum executes programs with variable output, leading to the variability of stepping during the stride with subsequent gait unsteadiness and ultimately leads to falling [62].

Dementia and AD with frontal cognitive impairment is reported to cause deterioration of walking in patients [63]. In the study Coelho et al., [64] AD's mild/moderate stages indicate that the difference between the kinematic parameters is walking. Moderate stages of AD patients had shorter stride lengths and walked more slowly than patients who were in the mild stage. In the study of Maggio et al., [65] the caregivers are the risk factor of AD because of caregiver stress.

## 7. Other risk factors of falls in Alzheimer disease

Physiological and cognitive changes and other functional disabilities occur in patients with AD. The experimental or epidemiological studies show that there is more than one etiologic factor that may be responsible for the risk of falls.

**Age:** Age is seen as the most important etiologic factor. Both AD prevalence and falls increase with ageing. In Nutrialz study, the prevalence increase by 10% with ageing and is increases every 5 years [61]. It is known that, with ageing, dementia, AD, and falls increase. The loss of abilities is related to ageing.

**Education level:** In the study of Ott et al., [66] high education level is stated to be related to AD. It was especially noted that increased levels of education delay the onset of AD. With a higher education level, neural reserve and neural network capacities are higher, and this delayed the neurodegeneration [67,68]. The effects of education, job and entertainment experiences lead to the efficiency of neural reserves.

**Functional Ability and Falls:** Normal ageing involves vision, hearing, vestibular, and somatosensory changes in the primary sensory areas. Thus, a more cognitive effort may be required to accommodate these systemic changes. The progressive decline in cognitive functions may lead to the disorganization of the network that controls locomotion, leading to impaired gait speed, timing, and poor postural control [70].

**Recent Falling History**: The risk of falls is increasing with AD patients that have a previous falling history. This is influenced by, because of recent experiences, fear of falling. Fear of falling are influenced by spatial and temporal parameters [71-72]. In this subject, there are many evidences. Especially, the history of falling is the main risk factor in elderly people and in patients with AD.

**Gait:** In AD patients, stride length variability at all walking speeds may contribute to the increased incidence of falls [73].

**Global Brain Atrophy:** White matter lesions in older adults are also associated with gait and balance impairment, cognitive impairment, and frequent falling. Yamaha et al., [74]. stated that patients with cognitive disorders, global brain atrophy is an independent factor for falling in AD patients.

**Medication:** In AD patients, one of the risk factors for falls is the medication. In the study of Epstein et al., [75] the medication increases the falls. Even after the medication has been changed, medication side effects are still thought to be the cause of the vast majority of falls.

### 7.1. Preventing falls

Older adults can keep on their independence for their daily life activities and reduce their experience of falling through exercising regularly, asking their doctor to revise their medicine use due to dizziness, having their eyes checked, and making their homes safer [50,77,78].

Because half of all falls occur at home, below are some suggested steps that may be considered to make the home safer (Table 4) [51,79].

| |
|---|
| *Remove things you can trip over, such as papers, books, clothes, and shoes, from stairs and places where you walk.* |
| *Remove small throw rugs or use double-sided tape to keep the rugs from slipping.* |
| *Keep the items you use often in cabinets you can reach easily without using a step stool.* |
| *Have grab bars put next to your toilet and in the tub or shower.* |
| *Use non-slip mats in the bathtub and on shower floors.* |
| *Improve the lighting in your home. As you get older, you need brighter lights to see well. Lamp shades or frosted bulbs can reduce glare.* |
| *Put handrails and lights in all staircases.* |
| *Wear shoes that give good support and have thin non-slip soles. Avoid wearing slippers and athletic shoes with deep treads.* |

**Table 4.** Safety tips for preventing falls at home

Fall prevention for people with Alzheimer's Disease and other types of dementia is vital. The key point for reducing falls in people with dementia is to understand why they fall and what causes the falls (Figure 3) [78]. Restlessness, discomfort or pain, hunger or thirst, a need to use the bathroom, boredom, and loneliness were other contributors to falls [78-81].

Some studies indicate that cognitive impairment is associated with Alzheimer disease and increase fall risk among older adults. Strategies including multifactorial assessment should be considered to prevent the risk of falling [24,25,82]. Falls are a prevalent health problem in the geriatric population and can result in severe somatic and psychological consequences. Fall risk assessment can provide knowledge to make and develop suitable interventions for identifing persons at risk [21,83].

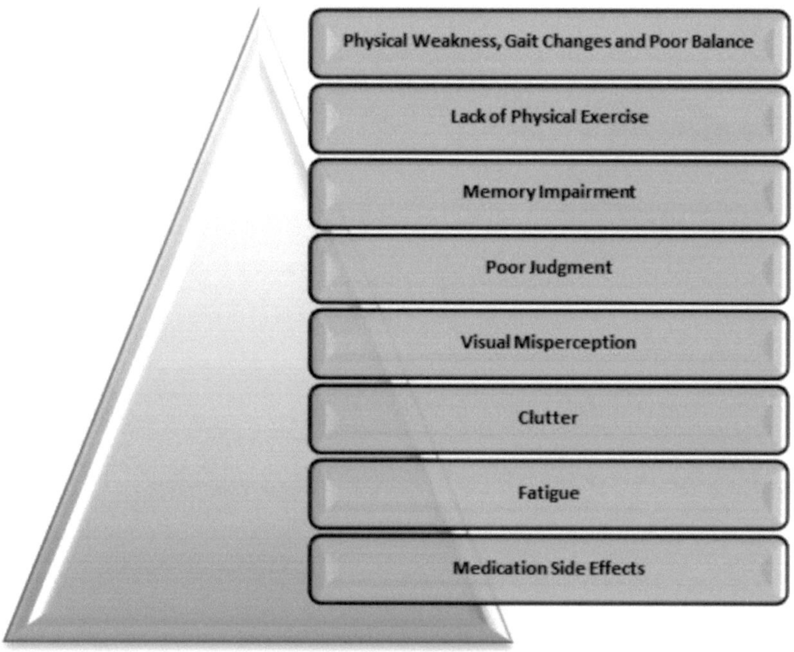


**Figure 3.** Causes of Falls among People with Alzheimer's Disease

## 8. How can we avoid accidents and reduce the risk of falls?

Aged people with dementia want to carry on their everyday life at home for as long as possible. However, it can be difficult managing everyday situations if you have dementia, particularly as the dementia progresses and as you get older. In conclusion, some people may not be as safe at home as they used to be. Some risk factors and suggested ways to manage them were mentioned below [84].

Occupational therapy provides practical support to help people do their day-to-day tasks, hobbies, interests, and activities (Figure 4 and 5). People who want to take an occupational therapy assessment can consult their local social services or their psychology experts related to occupational therapy [84].

Other preventions to reduce the risk of falls are: store dangerous substances safely, improve home environment, manage daily activities such as cooking or bathing through adaptations, avoid fire including fitting smoke alarms and carbon monoxide detectors, stay safe outdoors, use support networks, arrange access especially for family member or care worker, and record contact names and numbers belong to carers, friends, or family members [84].

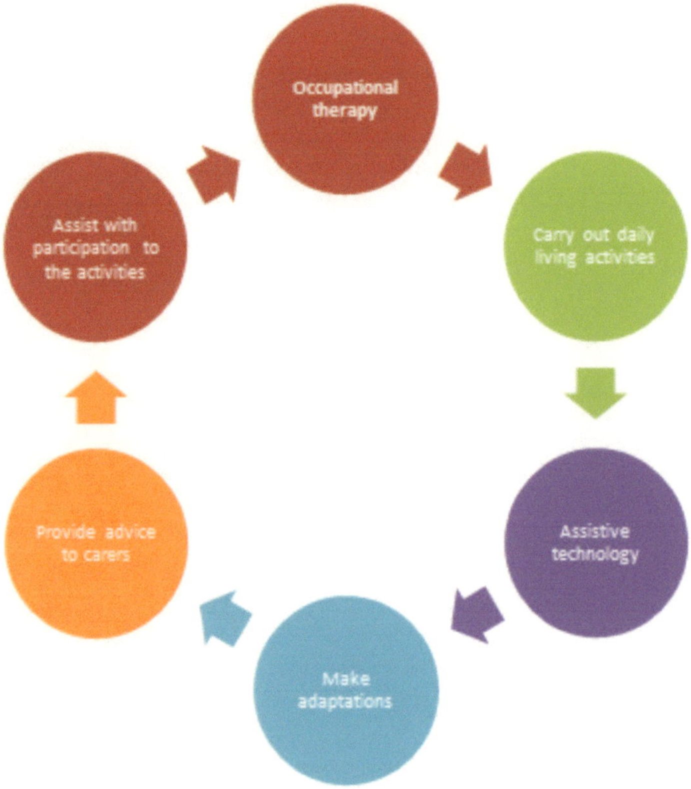
Occupational therapy
Carry out daily living activities
Assistive technology
Make adaptations
Provide advice to carers
Assist with participation to the activities

**Figure 4.** Seek advice from an occupational therapist.

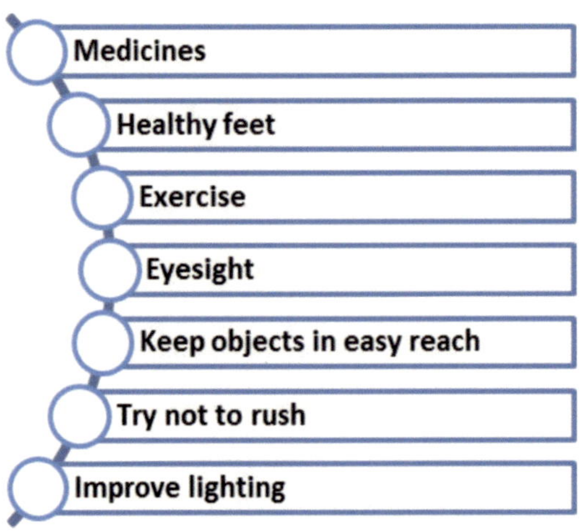


**Figure 5.** Steps to reduce the risk of falling at home.

## 9. Conclusion

With ageing, the risk of dementia and falls prevalence increases. Falls are one of the important risks for comorbidity and mortality in the aged population. Preventing strategies must be performed and must be related with the individual as well as the health services and the politics area. Only the implementation of prevention services may be solve this problem because the dementia and AD have a progressive decline process and there is currently no known alternative treatment for these pathologic conditions.

## Author details

Aysegul Uludag*, Sibel Cevizci and Ahmet Uludag

*Address all correspondence to: drayseguluudag@gmail.com

Canakkale Onsekiz Mart University, Faculty of Medicine, Department of Family Medicine, Canakkale, Turkey

## References

[1] Birren JE. The Psycology of Aging, Prentice Hall, Inc. New Jersey; 1982.

[2] Freedman VA, Martin LG, Schoeni RF. Recent trends in disability and functioning among older adults in the United States: a systematic review. JAMA 2002;288(24) 3137-46.

[3] Ferri CP, Prince M, Brayne C, Brodaty H, Fratiglioni L, Ganguli M, Hall K, Hasegawa K, Hendrie H, Huang Y et al. Alzheimer's Disease International. Global prevalence of dementia: a Delphi consensus study. Lancet 2005 17;366(9503) 2112-7.

[4] Thies W, Bleiler L. Alzheimer's disease facts and figures. Alzheimer's Dementia 2013;9(2) 208–45.

[5] Serrano-Pozo A, Frosch MP, Masliah E, Hyman BT. Neuropathological alterations in Alzheimer disease. Cold Spring Harb Perspect Med. 2011;1(1) 24-30.

[6] Morris JC, Rubin EH, Morris EJ, Mandel SA. Senile dementia of the Alzheimer's type: An important risk factor for serious falls. J Gerontol 1987;42 412–17.

[7] Tchalla AE, Lachal F, Cardinaud N, Saulnier I, Rialle V, Preux PM, Dantoine T. Preventing and managing indoor falls with home-based technologies in mild and moderate Alzheimer's disease patients: pilot study in a community dwelling. Dement Geriatr Cogn Disord. 2013;36(3-4) 251-61.

[8] http://www.mayoclinic.org/diseases-conditions/alzheimers-disease/basics/complications/con-20023871 (Accesed date August, 23,2014)

[9] De Groot JC, De Leeuw FE, Oudkerk M, et al. Cerebral white matter lesions and cognitive function: The Rotterdam scan study. Ann Neurol 2000;47 145–51.

[10] Maruyama M, Matsui T, Tanji H, et al. Cerebrospinal fluid tau protein and periventricular white matter lesions in patients with mild cognitive impairment: Implications for two major pathways. Arch Neurol 2004; 61 716–20.

[11] Turcotte M, Schellenberg G. A portrait of seniors in Canada [Internet]. Ottawa: Statistics Canada; 2006. http://www.statcan.gc.ca/pub/89-519-x/89-519-x2006001-eng.pdf (Accesed date August, 23,2014)

[12] Park CR. Cognitive effects of insulin in the central nervous system. Neurosci Biobehav Rev 2001;25(4) 311–23.

[13] Masud T, Morris RO. Epidemiology of falls. Age Ageing 2001;30(suppl 4) 3-7.

[14] Tinetti ME. Factors associated with serious injury during falls by ambulatory nursing home residents. Journal of the American Geriatrics Society 1987;35 644-48.

[15] WHO Global Report on Falls Prevention in Older Age. WHO 2007.

[16] Liang W, Liu Y, Weng X. An epidemiological study on injury of the community-dwelling elderly in Beijing. Chinese Journal of Disease Control and Prevention 2004; 8(6) 489-92.

[17] Yoshida H, Kim H. Frequency of falls and their prevention (in Japanese). Clinical Calcium 2006; 16(9) 1444-50.

[18] Rubenstein LZ. Falls in older people:epidemiology, risk factors and strategies for prevention. Age Ageing 2006;35 32-40.

[19] Stevens JA et al. Fatalities and Injuries From Falls Among Older Adults, United States, 1993-2003 and 2001-2005. Journal of the American Medical Association 2007; 297(1) 32-3.

[20] Division of Aging and Seniors, PHAC. Canada Report on senior's fall in Canada. Ontario, Division of Aging and Seniors. Public Health Agency of Canada 2005.

[21] Kannus P et al. Fall-induced deaths among elderly people. American Public Health Association 2005;95(3) 422-24.

[22] National Council on Ageing. Falls among older adults: risk factors and prevention strategies. In Fall free: promoting a national falls prevention action plan. J.A. Stevens Eds, 2005.

[23] Hernandez JL et al. Trend in hip fracture epidemiology over a 14-year period in a Spanish population. Osteoporosis International, 2006;17 464-70.

[24] World Health Organization. Active Ageing: A Policy Framework. Geneva 2002.

[25] United Nations (UN). World Population Prospects: The 2004 Revision. New York, USA.

[26] Tromp AM, Pluijm SMF, Smit JH, et al. Fall-risk screening test: a prospective study on predictors for falls in community-dwelling elderly. J Clin Epidemiol 2001;54(8) 837–44.

[27] Prevention of Falls and Fall-Related Injuries – Ontario Health Technology Assessment Series 2008;8 (2).

[28] Tinetti ME, Speechley M, Ginter SF. Risk factors for falls among elderly persons living in the community. N Engl J Med 1988;319 1701-7.

[29] Rubenstein LZ, Josephson KR. The epidemiology of falls and syncope. Clin Geriatr Med 2002;18 141-58.

[30] Centers for Disease Control and Prevention. Falls among older adults: summary of research findings. Accessed online January 26, 2005, at: http://www.cdc.gov/ncipc/pub-res/toolkit/SummaryOfFalls.htm

[31] Tinetti ME. Clinical practice. Preventing falls in elderly persons. N Engl J Med 2003;348:42-9.

[32] Nevitt MC, Cummings SR, Kidd S, Black D. Risk factors for recurrent nonsyncopal falls. A prospective study. JAMA 1989;261 2663-8.

[33] American Geriatrics Society, British Geriatrics Society, and American Academy of Orthopaedic Surgeons Panel on Falls Prevention. Guideline for the prevention of falls in older persons. J Am Geriatr Soc 2001;49 664-72.

[34] Leipzig RM, Cumming RG, Tinetti ME. Drugs and falls in older people: a systematic review and meta-analysis: II. Cardiac and analgesic drugs. J Am Geriatr Soc 1999;47 40-50.

[35] Leipzig RM, Cumming RG, Tinetti ME. Drugs and falls in older people: a systematic review and meta-analysis: I. Psychotropic drugs. J Am Geriatr Soc 1999;47:30-9.

[36] Rao SS. Prevention of Falls in Older Patients Am Fam Physician 2005;72 (81) 93-4.

[37] Papadimitropoulos EA, Coyte PC, Josse RG, et al. Current and projected rates of hip fracture in Canada. CMAJ. 1997;157(10) 1357–63.

[38] Canadian Community Health Survey. Detailed information for 2003.

[39] Peel NM, Kassulke DJ, McClure RJ. Population based study of hospi talised fall related injuries in older people. Inj Prev. 2002;8(4) 280–3.

[40] Maravic M, Le Bihan C, Landais P, et al. Incidence and cost of osteoporotic fractures in France during 2001. A methodological approach by the national hospital database. Osteoporos Int. 2005;16(12) 1475–80.

[41] U.S. Preventive Services Task Force. Guide to clinical preventive services: report of the U.S. Preventive Services Task Force. 2d ed. Baltimore: Williams & Wilkins, 1996.

[42] Robert P, Wilcock FKG. Dementia. J. Grimely Evans, T. Franklin Williams (Ed). Oxford Medical Publications, 2nd Edition. Oxford University Press, 2002.

[43] Takizawa C, Thompson PL, Van Walsem A, Faure C, Maier WC. Epidemiological and Economic Burden of Alzheimer's Disease: A Systematic Literature Review of Data across Europe and the United States of America J Alzheimer's Dis. 2014 26. [Epub ahead of print].

[44] Plassman BL, Havlik RJ, Steffens DC, Helms MJ, Newman TN, Drosdick D, et al. Documented head injury in early adulthood and risk of Alzheimer's disease and other dementias. Neurology 2000;55(8) 1158–66.

[45] Horikawa E, Matsui T, Arai H, et al. Risk of falls in Alzheimer's disease: a prospective study. Int Med. 2005;44:717–21.

[46] Webster KE, Merory JR, Wittwer JE. Gait variability in community dwelling adults with Alzheimer disease. Alzheimer Dis Assoc Disord. 2006;20 37-40.

[47] Glickstein J, Tideiksaar R. Risk of falls and injury in Alzheimer's disease. Focus Geriatr Care Rehabil. 1998;12 2-12.

[48] Chong RK, Horak FB, Frank J, Kaye J. Sensory organization for balance: specific deficits in Alzheimer's but not in Parkinson's disease. J Gerontol A Biol Sci Med Sci. 1999;54:122-28.

[49] CDC. Falls Among Older Adults: An Overview. http://www.cdc.gov/homeandrecreationalsafety/falls/adultfalls.html (Accessed August 15, 2013).

[50] Centers for Disease Control and Prevention, National Center for Injury Prevention and Control. Web–based Injury Statistics Query and Reporting System (WISQARS) [online]. Accessed August 15, 2013.

[51] Gang L, Sufang JYS. The incidence status on injury of the community-dwelling elderly in Beijing (in Chinese). Chinese Journal of Preventive Medicine, 2006;40(1) 3713.

[52] Gillespie, LD, Robertson, MC, Gillespie, WH, Sherrington C, Gates S, Clemson LM, Lamb SE. Interventions for preventing falls in older people living in the community. Cochrane Database of Systematic Reviews 2012;9.

[53] Olsson RH, Jr, Wambold S, Brock B, Waugh D, Sprague H. Visual spatial abilities and fall risk: an assessment tool for individuals with dementia. J Gerontol Nurs. 2005;31 45-51.

[54] Shaw FE. Falls in cognitive impairment and dementia. Clin Geriatr Med. 2002; 18 159-73.

[55] Sheridan PL, Hausdorff JM. The role of higher-level cognitive function in gait: executive dysfunction contributes to fall risk in Alzheimer's disease. Dement Geriatr Cogn Disord. 2007;24 125-37.

[56] Alexander NB, Hausdorff JM. Guest editorial: linking thinking, walking, and falling. J Gerontol A Biol Sci Med Sci 2008;63 1325–28.

[57] Liu-Ambrose TY, Ashe MC, Graf P, Beattie BL, Khan KM. Increased risk of falling in older community-dwelling women with mild cognitive impairment. Phys Ther 2008; 88 1482–91.

[58] Stark SL, Roe CM, Grant EA, Hollingsworth H, Benzinger TL, Fagan AM, et al. Preclinical Alzheimer disease and risk of Falls Neurology, 2013;82(5) 437-43.

[59] Ogama N, Sakurai T, Shimizu A, Toba K.J. Regional white matter lesions predict falls in patients with amnestic mild cognitive impairment and Alzheimer's disease. Am Med Dir Assoc. 2014;15(1) 36-41.

[60] Lorbach ER, Webster KE, Menz HB, Wittwer JE, Merory JR. Physiological falls risk assessment in older people with Alzheimer's disease. Dement Geriatr Cogn Disord. 2007;24 260-265.

[61] Salva A, Roque´ M, Rojano X, Inzitari M, Andrieu S, Schiffrin EC, Guigoz Y et al. Falls and Risk Factors for Falls in Community-Dwelling Adults With Dementia (NutriAlz Trial) Alzheimer Disease Ass. Disorder. 2012;26(1) 74-80.

[62] Sheridan PL, Hausdorff JM. The role of higher-level cognitive function in gait: executive dysfunction contributes to fall risk in Alzheimer's disease Dement Geriatr Cogn Disord. 2007; 24(2) 125–37.

[63] Holtzer R, Verghese J, Xue X, Lipton RB. Cognitive processes related to gait velocity: Results from the Einstein Aging Study. Neuropsychology 2006; 20 215–23.

[64] De Melo Coelho FG, Stella F, de Andrade LP, Barbieri FA, Galduróz RFS, et al. Gait and risk of falls associated with frontal cognitive functions at different stages of Alzheimer's disease Neuropsychology, Development, and Cognition. Section B, Aging, Neuropsychology and Cognition 2012;19(5) 644-56.

[65] Maggio D, Ercolani S, Andreani S, Ruggiero C, Mariani E, Mangialasche F, et al. Emotional and psychological distress of persons involved in the care of patients with Alzheimer disease predicts falls and fractures in their care recipients. Dement Geriatr Cogn Disord. 2010;30(1) 33-8.

[66] Ott A, Breteler MM, van Harskamp F, et al. Prevalence of Alzheimer's disease and vascular dementia: association with education. The Rotterdam study. BMJ 1995;310 970-3.

[67] Roe CM, Xiong C, Miller JP, Morris JC. Education and Alzheimer disease without dementia: support for the cognitive reserve hypothesis. Neurology 2007;68 223-8.

[68] Bennett DA, Wilson RS, Schneider JA, et al. Education modifies the relation of AD pathology to level of cognitive function in older persons. Neurology. 2003;60 1909-15.

[69] Sheridan PL, Hausdorff JM. The role of higher-level cognitive function in gait: executive dysfunction contributes to fall risk in Alzheimer's disease. Dement Geriatr Cogn Disord. 2007;24 125-37.

[70] Franssen EH, Souren LE, Torossian CL, Reisberg B. Equilibrium and limb coordination in mild cognitive impairment and mild Alzheimer's disease. J Am Geriatr Soc. 1999;47:463-9.

[71] Chamberlin ME, Fulwider BD, Sanders SL, Medeiros JM. Does fear of falling influence spatial and temporal gait parameters in elderly persons beyond changes associated with normal aging? J Gerontol A Biol Sci Med Sci. 2005;60 1163-7.

[72] Nakamura T, Meguro K, Sasaki H. Relationship between falls and stride length variability in senile dementia of the Alzheimer type. Gerontology 1996;42 108-13.

[73] Webster KE, Merory JR, Wittwer JE. Gait Variability in Community Dwelling Adults With Alzheimer Disease Alzheimer Dis Assoc Disord 2006;20 37–40

[74] Yamada M, Takechi H, Mori S, Aoyama T, Arai H. Global brain atrophy is associated with physical performance and the risk of falls in older adults with cognitive impairment Geriatr Gerontol Int 2013; 13 437–42.

[75] Epstein NU, Guo R, Farlow MR, Singh JP, Fisher M. Medication for Alzheimer's disease and associated fall hazard: a retrospective cohort study from the Alzheimer's Disease Neuroimaging Initiative. Drugs Aging. 2014;31(2) 125-9.

[76] Moyer VA. Prevention of Falls in Community-Dwelling Older Adults: U.S. Preventive Services Task Force Recommendation Statement. Annals of Internal Medicine 2012;157(3) 197–204.

[77] Nicole L. Baker, Michael N. Cook, H. Michael Arrighi and Roger Bullock: Hip fracture risk and subsequent mortality among Alzheimer's disease patients in the United Kingdom, 1988–2007 Oxford Textbook of Geriatric Medicine 2010;18.

[78] Heerema E. Causes of Falls in People with Dementia. Understanding Why People Fall Can Help Reduce and Prevent Falls. http://alzheimers.about.com/od/symptomsofalzheimers/a/Causes-of-Falls-in-People-With-Dementia.html (accessed August 13. 2014).

[79] Age and Ageing. Hip fracture risk and subsequent mortality among Alzheimer's disease patients in the United Kingdom, 1988–2007. Accessed September 25, 2012. http://ageing.oxfordjournals.org/content/40/1/49.abstract?sid=02dbc022-d8eb-4fb3-a547-3f781daf1540

[80] Fischer Center for Alzheimer's Research Foundation. People With Alzheimer's at High Risk of Falls and Injury. Accessed September 25, 2012. http://www.alzinfo.org/04/articles/people-alzheimers-high-risk-falls-injury

[81] The Royal Melbourne Hospital. Falls and Dementia. Accessed September 25, 2012. www.mednwh.unimelb.edu.au/vic_falls/pdf_docs/Eric_Seal.

[82] Mignardot JB, Beauchet O, Annweiler C, Cornu C, Deschamps T. Postural sway, falls, and cognitive status: a cross-sectional study among older adults. J Alzheimers Dis. 2014;41(2):431-9.

[83] Kalache A, Keller I (2000). The greying world: a challenge for the 21st century. Science Progress, 83(1):33-54.

[84] Falls. Safety in the home. http://alzheimers.org.uk/site/scripts/documents_info.php?documentID=145 (Accessed September 25, 2012)

Chapter 2

# The Cascade of Oxidative Stress and Tau Protein Autophagic Dysfunction in Alzheimer's Disease

Zhenzhen Liu, Peifu Li, Jiannan Wu, Yi Wang, Ping Li, Xinxin Hou, Qingling Zhang, Nannan Wei, Zhiquan Zhao, Huimin Liang and Jianshe Wei

Additional information is available at the end of the chapter

http://dx.doi.org/10.5772/59980

## 1. Introduction

Alzheimer's disease (AD) is the most common form of dementia in the elderly and a chronic neurodegenerative disease characterized by widespread degeneration of neurons. An estimated 37 million people worldwide currently have AD, which is estimated to increase to 65.7 million by 2030 and 115.4 million by 2050 [1]. It is a growing health concern in society because patients suffer from progressive functional impairments, emotional distress, loss of independence, and behavioral deficits. AD is characterized by the presence of two types of neuropathological hallmarks: senile plaques (SPs) and intracellular neurofibrillary tangles (NFTs). SPs predominantly consist of extracellular amyloid β-peptide (Aβ) deposits. NFTs are formed by intraneuronal aggregation of hyperphosphorylated tau. The amyloid cascade hypothesis theory proposes a dysregulation of amyloid precursor protein processing. This event leads to AD pathogenesis, which involves the aggregation of Aβ (particularly Aβ42), neuritic plaque formation, and consequently the formation of NFTs followed by the disruption of synaptic connections, neuronal death, and cognitive deficits (dementia) [2]. Increasing evidence suggests that Aβ oligomers may be the primary cause of AD because they have a greater correlation with dementia than insoluble Aβ42. Aβ also plays a crucial role in inducing neuronal oxidative stress [3]. Aβ-mediated mitochondrial oxidative stress causes hyperphosphorylation of tau in AD brains [4, 5]. Mounting evidence clearly links tau to neurodegeneration, indicating that tau hyperphosphorylation may be the necessary link in neural dysfunction and death. However, whether autophagic dysfunction is involved in neuronal death during this event still remains unknown. Recent studies have indicated the importance of defective autophagy in the pathogenesis of aging and neurodegenerative diseases, especially in AD. Autophagy may increase the formation of autophagosome in AD, and autophagic dysfunction may induce the pathogenesis of AD, particularly at the late stage of AD [6]. However, the relationship between oxidative stress, tau protein hyperphosphorylation, autophagic dysfunction and neuronal cells death in AD remains elusive. In this review, we summarize the latest progress in research focused on oxidative stress, tau hyperphosphorylation, and autophagic dysfunction, and their relationship with AD.

## 2. Oxidative stress in AD

Oxidative stress appears to be one of the earliest events and a major determinant of the pathogenesis and progression in AD. In experimental models and human brain studies of AD, oxidative stress has also been shown to play an important role in neuronal degeneration [7]. Several risk factors for AD may cause or promote oxidative damage, such as advanced age, apolipoprotein E (APOE) ε4 alleles [8], medical risk factors, environmental and lifestyle-related risk factors and so on. Generally, oxidative stress is caused by the imbalance between reactive oxygen species (ROS) ($O^{2-}$, $H_2O_2$ and OH), which associated with both the chronic formation of ROS derived from the mitochondrial electron transport chain and the acute and high output formation of ROS derived from nicotinamide adenine dinucleotide phosphate (NADPH) oxidase, and the breakdown of chemically reactive species, by reducing agents and antioxidant enzymes, such as superoxide dismutase (SOD). This disequilibrium may result from disease, stressors, or environmental factors. High ROS levels lead to the accumulation of oxidized proteins, lipids, and nucleic acids due to mitochondrial dysfunction, increased metal levels, inflammation, and Aβ peptides, thereby directly impairing cellular function if not be removed or neutralized [9]. Oxidative damage to cellular components is likely to result in the alteration of membrane properties, such as fluidity, ion transport, enzyme activities, protein cross-linking, and eventually cell death.

Structurally and functionally damaged mitochondria are more proficient at producing ROS [10]. Mitochondrial dysfunction may be an initial trigger for enhanced Aβ production during the aging process [11].Oxidative stress can promote Aβ deposition, tau hyperphosphorylation, and the subsequent loss of synapses and neurons in the development of AD. Several studies suggest that ROS are involved in Aβ fibrillization and NFT formation in AD and increases with Aβ and NFT pathology in AD. Both soluble and fibrillar Aβ may further accelerate oxidative stress, as well as mitochondrial dysfunction [12-14]. The transgenic (Tg) Thy1-APP751 (SL) mouse model of AD shows increased proteolytic cleavage of APP, increased production of Aβ, and impaired Cu/Zn-SOD activity [15]. Furthermore, oxidative stress is considered as a primary factor of NFT formation in AD. However, the relationship between oxidative stress and tau hyperphosphorylation remains unclear. Okadaic acid is used as a research model to induce tau phosphorylation and neuronal death in AD. Oxidative stress combined with Okadaic acid results in tau hyperphosphorylation [16], and mitochondrial $SOD_2$ deficiency also increases the levels of Ser396 phosphorylated tau in the Tg2576 mouse model of AD [4].

# 3. Tau protein in AD

## 3.1. Tau protein physiology and pathology

Tau protein (known as neuronal microtubule associated protein tau) plays a large role in the outgrowth of neuronal processes and the development of neuronal polarity. Tau protein in the central nervous system is predominantly expressed in neurons [17, 18], with its main function to promote microtubule assembly, stabilize microtubules, affect the dynamics of microtubules in neurons [19, 20], and inhibit apoptosis [21], particularly in axons [22, 23]. However, recent reports suggest that excess intracellular tau is released into the extracellular culture medium via membrane vesicles [24]. In the adult human brain, tau consists of six isoforms, and the tau gene contains 15 exons. The isoforms are generated by alternative splicing of exons 2, 3, and 10. Depending on the alternative splicing of exon 10, tau isoforms are termed 4R (with exon 10) or 3R (without exon 10). N-terminal exon (tau 1N), two N-terminal exons (tau 2N), or no N-terminal exons (tau 0N) at the N-terminal inserts mainly depend on the inclusion of exon 2, exon 2 and 3, or the exclusion of both. Biochemical analysis of postmortem AD brains indicate that 4R-tau is more abundant than 3R in isolated NFTs [25].

Tau protein normally stabilizes axonal microtubules in the cytoskeleton and plays a vital role in regulating the morphology of neurons. It has more than 30 phosphorylation sites. When tau is abnormally hyperphosphorylated, it destabilizes microtubules by decreasing the binding affinity of tau and resulting in its aggregation in NFTs. NFTs are composed of paired helical filaments (PHF) of abnormally hyperphosphorylated tau. The severity of dementia in AD was shown to correlate well with NFT load. In the transgenic mouse model, conditionally expressing the human tau P301L mutant, age-related NFTs develop, along with neuronal loss and behavioral impairment. After the suppression of transgenic tau, memory function recovered, and neuron numbers stabilized [26]. The pathogenesis of tau-mediated neurodegeneration is unclear but hyperphosphorylation, oligomerization, fibrillization, and propagation of tau pathology has been proposed as the likely pathological processes that induces the loss of function or gain of tau toxicity, which caused neurodegeneration [27]. Tau phosphorylation has been investigated at AD-related sites by using recombinant human tau phosphorylated by DNA damage-activated checkpoint kinase 1 (Chk1) and checkpoint kinase 2(Chk2) in vitro [28]. This study identified a total of 27 Ser/Thr residues as Chk1 or Chk2 target sites. Among these sites, 13 sites have been identified to be phosphorylated in AD brains [29]. The generation of a Tg mouse line overexpressing human tau 441 via V337M and R406W tau mutations has been shown to accelerate the phosphorylation of human tau, inducing tau pathology and cognitive deficits [30].

## 3.2. Tau protein kinases and phosphatase

Tau phosphorylation is mainly determined by a balance between the activation of various tau protein kinases and phosphatases, and its disruption results in the abnormal phosphorylation of tau, which is observed in AD. Each tau site is phosphorylated by one or more protein kinases. Tau kinases are grouped into three classes: (1) proline-directed protein kinases (PDPK) containing glycogen synthase kinase-3 (GSK3), cyclin-dependent protein kinase-5 (CDK5), and mitogen activated protein kinases (MAPK) (e.g. p38, Erk1/2 and JNK1/2/3); (2) non-PDPK, including tau-tubulin kinase 1/2 (e.g. casein kinase 1α/1δ/1ε/2), dual specificity tyrosine-phosphorylation-regulated kinase 1A/2, microtubule affinity regulating kinases, phosphorylase kinase, cAMP-dependent protein kinase A (PKA), PKB/Akt, protein kinase C, protein kinase N, and Ca2+/calmodulin-dependent protein kinase II (CaM kinase II); and (3) tyrosine protein kinases, including Src family kinase (SFK) members (e.g. Src, Lck, Syk, and Fyn), and c-Abelson kinase or Abl related gene kinase. Phosphatases are also usually classified into three classes according to their amino acids sequences, the structure of their catalytic site, and their sensitivity to inhibitors. These groups include: (1) phosphoprotein phosphatase (PPP), (2) metal-dependent protein phosphatase, and (3) protein tyrosine phosphatase (PTP).

GSK3 (particularly GSK3β) plays a key role in the pathogenesis of AD, contributing to Aβ production and Aβ-mediated neuronal death by phosphorylating tau in most serine and threonine residues and inducing hyperphosphorylation in paired helical filaments [31]. Inhibition of GSK3 prevents Aβ aggregation and tau hyperphosphorylation [32, 33].The involvement of CDK5 in tau phosphorylation is shown by the increase in its enzymatic activity and the absence of MT-2 cells neurite retraction in the presence of roscovitine or CDK5 siRNA [34]. Therefore, CDK5 may be a key candidate target for therapeutic gene silencing [35]. p38 MAPK has been identified as one of the kinases involved in the regulation of tau phosphorylation. Thus, under pathological conditions this kinase is likely to play a role in the hyperphosphorylation of tau [36]. CDKs and casein kinase 1 (CK1) are involved in the aggregation of Aβ peptides (forming extracellular plaques) and hyperphosphorylation of tau (forming intracellular NFTs). The expression pattern of CKIδ (an isoform of CK1) plays an important role in tau aggregation in AD [37]. Ser214, Ser262, and Ser409 are major phosphorylation sites of tau that are affected by PKA [38]. In P19 cells stably expressing human tau441, CaM kinase II has been shown to be involved in retinoic acid (RA)-induced tau phosphorylation- mediated apoptosis [39].

Tau protein phosphatase PPP group includes protein phosphatase [PP]1, PP2A, PP2B and proteinphophatase-5 [PP5]. In vitro, Overexpression of PP5 resulted in dephosphorylation of tau at multiple phosphorylation sites [40] and protected neurons against apoptosis induced by Aβ [41]. In vivo, PP5 interacts with the regulatory subunit A of PP2A [42], and the enzymatic activity level of PP5 has been reduced by 20% in AD brains [40]. PP2A contributes to abnormally hyperphosphorylated tau protein, and is the most efficient phosphatase. The inhibition of PP2A significantly plays a role in tau hyperphosphorylation [43-45]. PP2A is regulated by endogenous inhibitor-1 of PP2A (I1PP2A) and inhibitor-2 of PP2A (I2PP2A) in mammalian tissues [46].

Recently inactivation the nuclear translocation signal (179KRK181-AAA) along with 168KR169-AA mutations of I2PP2A (mNLS-I2PP2A), it was translocated from nucleus to the cytoplasm. Cytoplasmic retention of I2PP2A physically interacted with PP2A and inhibited its activity, induced Alzheimer-like abnormal tau protein hyperphosphorylation by the direct interaction of I2 PP2A with PP2A and GSK-3β [47]. In AD brain, I2PP2A is also translocated from neuronal nucleus to cytoplasm, leading to the inhibition of PP2A and abnormal phosphorylation of tau. I2PP2A directly inhibits the activity of PP2A activity without affecting its expression [48]. Over activation of GSK-3β inhibits PP2A through up regulation of I2PP2A. GSK-3 activation significantly contributes to tau hyperphosphorylation by inhibiting PP2A via the up-regulation of I2PP2A [49]. These data indicate that up-regulation or down-regulation of the phosphorylation system or dephosphorylation system, respectively of tau protein may be implicated in tau pathologies.

### 3.3. Tau protein and oxidative stress

#### *3.3.1. Tau protein hyperphosphorylation and oxidative stress*

Oxidative stress is believed to be a prominent early event in the pathogenesis of AD, contributing to tau phosphorylation and the formation of neurofibrillary tangles. However, the relationship and underlying mechanisms between oxidative stress and tau hyperphosphorylation remains elusive. Fatty acid oxidative products provide a direct link between the mechanism of how oxidative stress induces the formation of NFTs in AD [50]. Chronic oxidative stress increases the levels of tau phosphorylation at paired helical filaments (PHF-1) epitope (serine 399/404) via the inhibition of glutathione synthesis with buthionine sulfoximine (BSO) in an vitro model of chronic oxidative stress [5]. In primary rat cortical neuronal cultures stimulated by the combination of the copper chelator, cuprizone, and oxidative stress ($Fe^{2+}$/ $H_2O_2$), tau phosphorylation is significantly increased by the elevated activity of GSK-3 [51]. Furthermore, treatment of rat hippocampal cells and SHSY5Y human neuroblastoma cells with $H_2O_2$ at the early stages of oxidative stress exposure results in tau dephosphorylation at the Tau1 epitope by CDK5 via PP1 activation [52]. Several studies have suggested that oxidative stress is a causal factor in tau-induced neurodegeneration in Drosophila [53], and ROS generation is a key intracellular event that contributes to an induction of p38-MAPK activation and tau phosphorylation.

#### *3.3.2. GSK3β, PP2A, and oxidative stress*

Oxidative stress is likely to play a critical role in tau hyperphosphorylation, which is regulated by tau protein kinase activation and the suppression of phosphatase. Tau hyperphosphorylation may be induced by oxidative stress through the direct interaction with tau protein kinase and phosphatase, particularly GSK-3β and PP2A, respectively because they are predominant and play an important role.

The main site of ROS formation is mitochondrial complex I, inhibition of complex I induces a decrease in ATP levels and excessive production of ROS [54]. GSK-3β has been situated in the mitochondria and highly activated. Mitochondrial GSK3β activity controlled the mitochondrial complex I activity, promoted ROS production, and perturbed the mitochondrial morphology [55]. In contrast, GSK-3β activity is up-regulated under oxidative stress [56]. For example, in human embryonic kidney 293/Tau cells, $H_2O_2$ increases GSK-3β activity and tau is hyperphosphorylated at Ser396, Ser404, and Thr231. Mitochondrial superoxide activates the mitochondrial fraction of GSK-3α/β, resulting in the phosphorylation of the mitochondrial chaperone cyclophilin D [57]. This effect also provides a link between GSK-3β and oxidative stress.

Studies have also focused on the link between PP2A and oxidative stress. A recent report shows that rat cortical neurons treated with okadaic acid inhibits PP2A activity, resulting in an abnormal increase in mitochondrial ROS and mitochondrial fission [58]. Other findings reveal that ROS inhibits PP2A and PP5, leading to the activation of JNK and Erk1/2 pathways and subsequently caspase-dependent and -independent apoptosis of neuronal cells [59]. In vivo, after hypoxia exposure, the levels of activated form of GSK-3β was significantly increased in the hippocampus, while activated form of PP2A were significantly decreased [60]. Despite these studies, however, the relationship of GSK3 and PP2A with oxidative stress remains to be further investigated.

#### *3.3.3. Antioxidants and the tau protein*

In recent years, antioxidant therapy has received considerable attention as a promising approach for slowing the progression of AD. Research has focused on endogenous antioxidants (e.g. vitamins, coenzyme Q10, and melatonin) and the intake of dietary antioxidants, such as phenolic compounds that are flavonoids or non-flavonoids. This increased interest has thus strengthened the hypothesis that oxidative damage may be responsible for the cognitive and functional decline in AD patients. Melatonin is a free radical scavenger, clinical trial revealed that add-on prolonged-release melatonin had positive effects on cognitive functioning and sleep maintenance in AD patients compared with placebo [61]. The mechanism may be that melatonin can block tau hyperphosphorylation and microtubule disorganization under in vivo and vitro conditions [62-64] and also decreases the activity of GSK-3β [65]. Moreover, melatonin may be a potentially useful agent in the prevention and treatment of AD [66]. Demethoxycurcumin has been shown to inhibit the phosphorylation of both tau pS262 and pS396 in murine neuroblastoma N2A cells [67]. Curcumin reduced soluble tau and elevated heat shock proteins involved in tau clearance [68]. In addition, curcumin downregulated levels of phosphorylated tau, which may concerned with the upregulation in BAG2 levels in the neurons [69]. In addition, an association also exists between beta carotene and tau in AD patients [70]. Other experiments have shown that the active component of Ginkgo biloba, ginkgolide A, inhibits GSK3β and suppressed the phosphorylation level of tau [71]. Other antioxidants, such as Vitamins E and C [72, 73] and gossypin [74] are also reported to have a protective effect against neurotoxicity. These results have therefore led to further investigations of this compound as an antioxidant therapy strategy for AD.

## 4. Autophagy in AD

### 4.1. The Autophagic pathway

Autophagy is an essential lysosomal degradation pathway that turns over cytoplasmic constituents, including misfolded or aggregated proteins and damaged organelles, to facilitate the maintenance of cellular homeostasis. Autophagy is usually activated during nutrient deprivation and stress to enhance cellular survival, and its constitutive activity is recognized to control neuronal survival. Autophagic dysfunction has been reported to contribute to AD [75].

Autophagy includes macroautophagy, chaperone-mediated autophagy, and microautophagy. The most familiar of these types is macroautophagy, which is a process of cellular self-cannibalism in which portions of the cytoplasm are sequestered within double- or multimembraned vesicles (autophagosomes) and then delivered to lysosomes for bulk degradation. Autophagy is induced by two pathways in macroautophagy - mammalian target of rapamycin (mTOR)-dependent and -independent signaling pathways. mTOR is an important convergence point in the cell signaling pathway. mTOR kinase activity is modulated in response to various stimuli, such as trophic factors, mitogens, hormones, amino acids, cell energy status, and cellular stress. Rapamycin, as mTOR inhibitor, is a very important tool for autophagy [76, 77]. mTOR complex (mTORC) 1 is involved in autophagy and is the master regulator of cell growth enhancing the cellular biomass by up-regulating protein translation [78]. For cells to control cellular homoeostasis during growth, a close signaling interplay occurs between mTORC1 and two other protein kinases, AMP-activated protein kinase (AMPK) [79] and Unc51-like kinase (ULK1) [80]. Autophagy is inhibited by cytosolic p53 via the direct inhibition of AMPK [81]. mTORC1 controls autophagy by directly interacting with the ULK1, focal adhesion kinase family-interacting protein of 200 kDa (FIP200) and Atg13 complex [82]. Several mTOR-independent signals affect the autophagy pathway. When the level of free inositol and myoinositol-1,4,5- trisphosphate (IP3) decreases, autophagy is reduced [83]. Furthermore, lower levels of Bcl-2 lead to the release of more Beclin 1, thus forming the Beclin 1-PI3KCIII (class III phosphoinositide 3-kinase) complex to activate autophagy via the PI3K-AKT-mTOR pathway [84].

### 4.2. Autophagic dysfunction in AD pathology

A growing body of evidence suggests a link between AD and autophagy. Therefore, the pathological functions of autophagy may be a critical mediator of neurotoxicity [85]. Autophagy develops in AD brains because of the ineffective degradation of autophagosomes, which is controlled by many kinds of autophagy-related genes (Atg), including Atg1-Atg35. Atg8 (mammalian homolog is LC3) is an autophagosomal membrane protein and a marker of autophagosome formation [86]. Beclin-1 (the mammalian ortholog of yeast Atg6) plays a pivotal role in autophagy [87]. In an in vitro study of the pathogenesis of AD, Atg8/LC3 colocalizes with APP and LC3-positive autophagosomes are present [88]. Beclin-1 knockdown increases APP, APP-like proteins, APP-C-terminal fragments, and Aβ [89]. Atg5, Atg12, and LC3 are also associated with plaque, tangle pathologies, and neuronal death in AD [90]. Generally, autophagic vacuoles (AVs) are rare in the normal brain, but are increased in brains of AD patients. In the early stages of AD, the expression of lysosome-related component is significantly increased prior to the formation of plaques and NFTs, and autophagy is also induced at this stage, thus its activity is independent of extracellular Aβ deposition and NFT formation [91]. In the late stage of AD, AVs continue to accumulate in large numbers in dystrophic neurites. There are several causes for the dysfunction of autophagy in late-stage AD, including the enhanced processing of APP and Aβ degradation [92], and the toxic effect of high levels of intracellular Aβ on lysosomal function [93]. Inhibition of the AV-lysosome fusion is caused by impaired microtubule-associated retrograde transport, which in turn leads to increased accumulation of AV in dystrophic neurites. Lysosomal enzyme dysfunction may be associated with the accumulation of AVs [94, 95]. Autophagy plays an important role in the degradation of impaired mitochondria in AD. Dysfunction of the autophagy - lysosome system causes insufficient degradation of mitochondria [96]. Conversely, mitochondrial dysfunction may also impair this pathway [97].

### 4.3. Autophagy and the tau protein

#### *4.3.1. Tau protein degradation via autophagy*

A variety of forms of tau proteins have been shown to be degraded by the ubiquitin-proteasome system (UPS) and autophagy-lysosomal pathway (ALP). UPS may play an important role in the primary clearance of pathological tau. However, the importance of autophagy-mediated tau degradation, particularly at the late stage of NFT formation, is becoming more recognized. The autophagy-lysosomal pathway has the capacity to engulf protein aggregates and keep tau levels at a low level [98]. Autophagy is believed to be an evolutionarily conserved mechanism for intracellular degradation of proteins, such as Aβ and tau. mTOR in negatively regulating autophagy is an important convergence point in cell signaling. Increasing mTOR signaling facilitates tau pathology, and reducing this signaling ameliorates tau pathology [99]. Rapamycin has been reported to decrease tau phosphorylation at Ser214 in vitro, and reduce tau tangles and insoluble tau in vivo [100, 101]. In a tetracycline-inducible model [tau DeltaC (tauΔC)], tau is abnormally truncated at Asp $^{421}$, and is cleared predominantly by macroautophagy and degraded significantly faster than full-length tau [102]. Autophagy activation suppresses tau aggregation and eliminates cytotoxicity [99]. Moreover, trehalose (an enhancer of autophagy) directly inhibits tau aggregation in primary neurons [103]. Under in vitro conditions, the accumulation of tau species is increased with the autophagic inhibitor, 3-methyladenine, and decreased with trehalose [104]. Overall, these results suggest that tau degradation involves autophagy, and this activity is beneficial for neurons to prevent the accumulation of protein aggregates.

#### *4.3.2. Tau protein hyperphosphorylation leads to autophagic dysfunction*

The physiological function of tau protein is well known to be associated with microtubule binding and assembly. Autophagosome transport mainly depends on the movement along microtubules in the autophagic pathway. However, the link between tau hyperphosphorylation and autophagic dysfunction is still under debate. Frontotemporal dementia and parkinsonism linked to chromosome 17 (FTDP-17) - mediated tau mutations can disrupt lysosomal function in transgenic mice expressing human Tau with four tubulin-binding repeats (increased by FTDP-17 splice donor mutations) and three FTDP-17 missense mutations: G272V, P301L, and R406W [105]. In Tg mice expressing mutant human (P301L) tau, axonal spheroids have been shown to contain tau-immunoreactive filaments and AVs [106]. A recent study has revealed that PP2A upregulation stimulates neuronal autophagy, thus providing link between PP2A downregulation, autophagy disruption, and protein aggregation [107]. Furthermore, autophagosomes have been shown to be increased in rat neurons treated with okadaic acid [108]. Altogether, tau is known to regulate the stability of microtubules, and tau hyperphosphorylation may result in the destabilization of neuronal microtubules, thus affecting the placement and function of mitochondria and lysosomes. Therefore, tau hyperphosphorylation is likely to play a critical role in the process of autophagic dysfunction.

http://dx.doi.org/10.5772/59980

#### *4.3.3. Autophagic dysfunction induces tau protein aggregation*

The autophagy-lysosomal pathway is well recognized to play an important role in the clearance of abnormally modified proteins in cells. The hyperphosphorylation of tau and NFT formation results in the disruption of the neuronal skeleton, thereby contributing to neuronal dysfunction, cell death, and eventually the symptoms of AD. Abnormal lysosomal proteases are found in brains of AD patients. Several studies have shown that dysfunction of the autophagy-lysosomal pathway contributes to the formation of tau oligomers and insoluble aggregates [109, 110]. Both phosphorylated tau and GSK3β significantly accumulate in Atg7 conditional knockout brains, although NFTs are absent [111]. Therefore, the ALP system plays a crucial role in the clearance of tau, and its accumulation may be due to autophagic dysfunction in cells.

## 5. Conclusion

Oxidative stress, as the one of the earliest events in AD, induces tau phosphorylation with protein phosphatase and kinase imbance. Tau protein hyperphosphorylation destabilizes

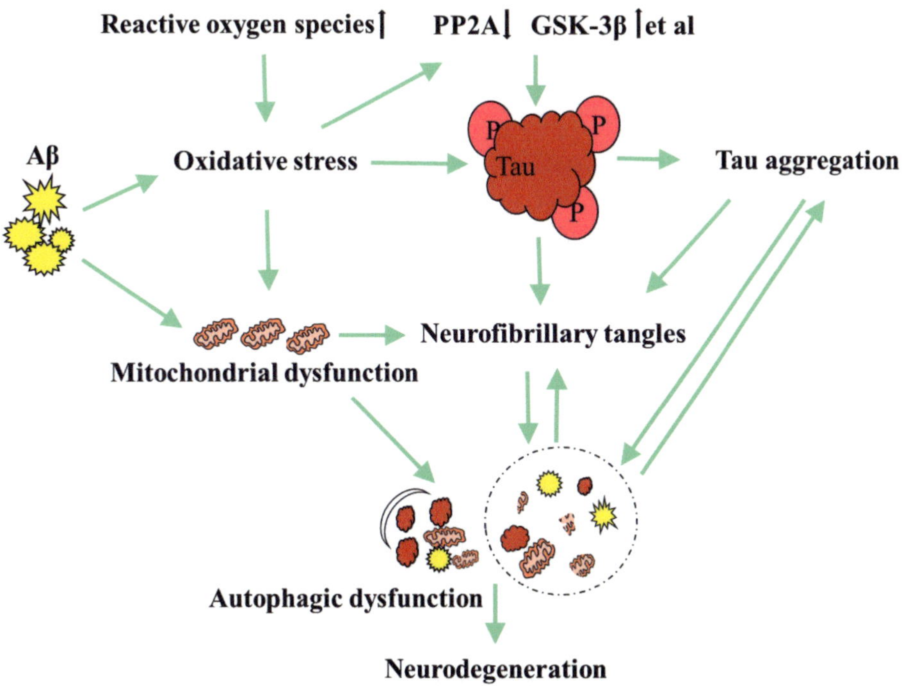


**Figure 1.** Tau protein NFTs formation and autophagic dysfunction in Alzheimer's disease. Aβ oligomers and ROS production intrigue oxidative stress and mitochondria dysfunction, which induce tau protein hyperphosphorylation and neurofibrillary tangles formation. These events converge to tau protein aggregation and autophagic dysfunction, then lead to neurodegeneration and cell death in AD.

microtubules by decreasing the binding affinity of tau, thereby resulting in the formation of NFTs in AD. Tau hyperphosphorylation may affect the autophagy- lysosomal pathway, and dysfunction of the ALP also promotes the accumulation of tau protein. These events initiate a series of cascades to induce neurodegeneration and cell death in AD (Figure 1). However, the relationships among oxidative stress, tau hyperphosphorylation and autophagic dysfunction and their accurate mechanisms on neurodegeneration in AD still require further research.

## Acknowledgements

The work has been generously supported by grant from the National Natural Science Foundation of China (81271410 to JW). The authors thank all other authors making contributions to the studies cited in this manuscript and apologize to those who made similar contributions in work not being cited due to space limitation. The authors have no competing financial interests.

## Author details

Zhenzhen Liu[1,2], Peifu Li[2], Jiannan Wu[1], Yi Wang[1], Ping Li[1], Xinxin Hou[2], Qingling Zhang[2], Nannan Wei[1], Zhiquan Zhao[1], Huimin Liang[1] and Jianshe Wei[1,2*]

*Address all correspondence to: jswei@henu.edu.cn

1 Laboratory of Brain Function and Molecular Neurodegeneration, Institute for Brain Science Research, School of Life Sciences, Henan University, Kaifeng, China

2 Institute of Neuroscience, Henan Polytechnic University, Jiaozuo, China

## References

[1] Cumming T, Brodtmann A. Dementia and stroke: The present and future epidemic. International Journal of Stroke 2010; 5(6): 453-454.

[2] Lee HG, Zhu X, Nunomura A, Perry G, Smith MA. Amyloid beta: the alternate hypothesis. Current Alzheimer Research 2006; 3(1): 75-80.

[3] De Felice FG, Velasco PT, Lambert MP, et al. Abeta oligomers induce neuronal oxidative stress through an N-methyl-D-aspartate receptor-dependent mechanism that is blocked by the Alzheimer drug memantine. Journal of Biological Chemistry 2007; 282(15): 11590-601.

[4] Melov S, Adlard PA, Morten K, Johnson F, et al. Mitochondrial oxidative stress causes hyperphosphorylation of tau. PLoS One 2007; 2(6): e536.

[5] Su B, Wang X, Lee HG, Tabaton M, Perry G, Smith MA, Zhu X. Chronic oxidative stress causes increased tau phosphorylation in M17 neuroblastoma cells. Neuroscience Letters 2010; 468(3): 267-71.

[6] Wolfe DM, Lee JH, Kumar A, Lee S, Orenstein SJ, Nixon RA. Autophagy failure in Alzheimer's disease and the role of defective lysosomal acidification. European Journal Neuroscience 2013; 37(12): 1949-61.

[7] Martínez E, Navarro A, Ordóñez C, et al. Oxidative stress induces apolipoprotein D overexpression in hippocampus during aging and Alzheimer's disease. Journal of Alzheimer's Disease 2013; 36(1): 129-44.

[8] Tayler H, Fraser T, Miners JS, Kehoe PG, Love S. Oxidative balance in Alzheimer's disease: relationship to APOE, Braak tangle stage, and the concentrations of soluble and insoluble amyloid-β. Journal of Alzheimer's Disease 2010; 22(4): 1363-73.

[9] Mattson MP, Magnus T. Ageing and neuronal vulnerability. Nature Reviews Neuroscience 2006; 7(4): 278-94.

[10] Wang X, Wang W, Li L, Perry G, Lee HG, Zhu X. Oxidative stress and mitochondrial dysfunction in Alzheimer's disease. Biochimica et Biophysica Acta 2014; 1842(8): 1240-7.

[11] Yao J, Irwin RW, Zhao L, Nilsen J, Hamilton RT, Brinton RD. Mitochondrial bioenergetic deficit precedes Alzheimer's pathology in female mouse model of Alzheimer's disease. Proceedings of the National Academy of Science of the United States of America 2009; 106(34): 14670-675.

[12] Yao J, Du H, Yan S, Fang F, et al. Inhibition of amyloid-beta (Abeta) peptide- binding alcohol dehydrogenase-Abeta interaction reduces Abeta accumulation and improves mitochondrial function in a mouse model of Alzheimer's disease. Journal of Neuroscience 2011; 31(6): 2313-20.

[13] Pensalfini A, Zampagni M, Liguri G, Becatti M, et al. Membrane cholesterol enrichment prevents Aβ-induced oxidative stress in Alzheimer's fibroblasts. Neurobiology of Aging 2011; 32(2): 210-22.

[14] Chen Z, Zhong C. Oxidative stress in Alzheimer's disease. Neuroscience Bulletin 2014; 30(2): 271-81.

[15] Schuessel K, Schafer S, Bayer TA, Czech C, et al. Impaired Cu/Zn-SOD activity contributes to increased oxidative damage in APP transgenic mice. Neurobiology of Disease 2005; 18(1): 89-99.

[16] Poppek D, Keck S, Ermak G, et al. Phosphorylation inhibits turnover of the tau protein by the proteasome: influence of RCAN1 and oxidative stress. Biochemical Journal 2006; 400(3): 511-20.

[17] Avila J, Lucas JJ, Perez M, Hernandez F. Role of tau protein in both physiological and pathological conditions. Physiological Reviews 2004; 84(2): 361-84.

[18] Gordon D, Kidd GJ, Smith R. Antisense suppression of tau in cultured rat oligodendrocytes inhibits process formation. Journal of Neuroscience Reseach 2008; 86(12): 2591-601.

[19] Kolarova M, García-Sierra F, Bartos A, Ricny J, Ripova D. Structure and pathology of tau protein in Alzheimer disease. International Journal of Alzheimer's Disease 2012; 2012: 731526.

[20] Fauquant C, Redeker V, Landrieu I, Wieruszeski JM, et al. Systematic identification of tubulin-interacting fragments of the microtubule-associated protein Tau leads to a highly efficient promoter of microtubule assembly. J Biological Chemistry 2011; 286(38): 33358-68.

[21] Li HL, Wang HH, Liu SJ, Deng YQ, Zhang YJ, Tian Q, et al. Phosphorylation of tau antagonizes apoptosis by stabilizing beta-catenin, a mechanism involved in Alzheimer's neurodegeneration. Proceedings of the National Academy of Sciences of the United States of America 2007; 104(9): 3591-96.

[22] Ballatore C, Brunden KR, Huryn DM, Trojanowski JQ, Lee VM, Smith AB 3rd. Microtubule stabilizing agents as potential treatment for Alzheimer's disease and related neurodegenerative tauopathies. Journal of Medicinal Chemistry 2012; 55(21): 8979-96.

[23] Rodríguez-Martín T, Cuchillo-Ibáñez I, Noble W, et al. Tau phosphorylation affects its axonal transport and degradation. Neurobiology of Aging 2013; 34(9): 2146-57.

[24] Simón D, García-García E, Royo F, Falcón-Pérez JM, Avila J. Proteostasis of tau. Tau overexpression results in its secretion via membrane Vesicles. FEBS Letters 2012; 586(1): 47-54.

[25] Iseki E, Yamamoto R, Murayama N, Minegishi M, et al. Immunohisto-chemical investigation of neurofibrillary tangles and their tau isoforms in brains of limbic neurofibrillary tangle dementia. Neuroscience Letters 2006; 405(1-2): 29-33.

[26] Santacruz K, Lewis J, Spires T, et al. Tau suppression in a neurodegenerative mouse model improves memory function. Science 2005; 309(5733): 476-81.

[27] Yoshiyama Y, Lee VM, Trojanowski JQ. Therapeutic strategies for tau mediated neurodegeneration. Journal of Neurology, Neurosurgery and Psychiatry 2013; 84(7): 784-95.

[28] Iijima-Ando K, Zhao L, Gatt A, Shenton C, Iijima K. A DNA damage-activated checkpoint kinase phosphorylates tau and enhances tau-induced neurodegeneration. Human Molecular Genetics 2010; 19(10): 1930-8.

[29] Mendoza J, Sekiya M, Taniguchi T, Iijima KM, Wang R, Ando K. Global Analysis of Phosphorylation of Tau by the Checkpoint Kinases Chk1 and Chk2 in vitro. Journal of Proteome Research 2013; 12(6): 2654-65.

[30] Flunkert S, Hierzer M, Löffler T, Rabl R, Neddens J, et al. Elevated levels of soluble total and hyperphosphorylated tau result in early behavioral deficits and distinct changes in brain pathology in a new tau transgenic mouse model. Neuro-degenerative Diseases 2013; 11(4): 194-205.

[31] Hernandez F, Lucas JJ, Avila J. GSK3 and tau: two convergence points in Alzheimer's disease. Journal of Alzheimer's Disease 2013; 33(Suppl 1): S141-4.

[32] Gao C, Hölscher C, Liu Y, Li L. GSK3: a key target for the development of novel treatments for type 2 diabetes mellitus and Alzheimer disease. Reviews in the Neurosciences 2011; 23(1): 1-11.

[33] Gandy JC, Melendez-Ferro M, Bijur GN, Van Leuven F, et al. Glycogen synthase kinase-3β (GSK3β) expression in a mouse model of Alzheimer's disease: a light and electron microscopy study. Synapse 2013; 67(6): 313-27.

[34] Maldonado H, Ramírez E, Utreras E, Pando ME, Kettlun AM, et al. Inhibition of cyclin-dependent kinase 5 but not of glycogen synthase kinase 3-β prevents neurite retraction andtau hyperphosphorylation caused by secretable products of human T-cell leukemia virus type I-infected lymphocytes. Journal of Neuroscience Research 2011; 89(9): 1489-98.

[35] López-Tobón A, Castro-Álvarez JF, Piedrahita D, Boudreau RL, et al. Silencing of CDK5 as potential therapy for Alzheimer's disease. Reviews in the Neurosciences 2011; 22(2): 143-52.

[36] Corrêa SA, Eales KL. The Role of p38 MAPK and Its Substrates in Neuronal Plasticity and Neurodegenerative Disease. Journal of Signal Transduction 2012; 2012: 649079.

[37] Li G, Yin H, Kuret J. Casein kinase 1 delta phosphorylates tau and disrupts its binding to microtubules. Journal of Biological Chemistry 2004; 279(16): 15938-45.

[38] Liu F, Liang Z, Shi J, Yin D, El-Akkad E, et al. PKA modulates GSK-3β- and cdk5-catalyzed phosphorylation of tau in site- and kinase-specific manners. FEBS Letters 2006; 580(26): 6269-74.

[39] Tsukane M, Yamauchi T. $Ca^{2+}$/calmodulin-dependent protein kinase II mediates apoptosis of P19 cells expressing human tau during neural differentiation with retinoic acid treatment. Journal of Enzyme Inhibition and Medicinal Chemistry 2009; 24(2): 365-71.

[40] Liu F, Grundke-Iqbal I, Iqbal K, Gong CX. Contributions of protein phosphatases PP1, PP2A, PP2B and PP5 to the regulation of tau phosphorylation. European Journal of Neuroscience 2005; 22(8): 1942-50.

[41] Sanchez-Ortiz E, Hahm BK, Armstrong DL, Rossie S. Protein phosphatase 5 protects neurons against amyloid-beta toxicity. Journal of Neurochemistry 2009; 111 (2): 391-402.

[42] Lubert EJ, Hong Y, Sarge KD. Interaction between protein phosphatase 5 and the A subunit of protein phosphatase 2A: evidence for a heterotrimeric form of protein phosphatase 5. Journal of Biological Chemistry 2001; 276(42): 38582-587.

[43] Landrieu I, Smet-Nocca C, Amniai L, Louis JV, et al. Molecular implication of PP2A and Pin1 in the Alzheimer's disease specific hyperphosphorylation of Tau. PLoS One 2011; 6(6): e21521.

[44] Rudrabhatla P, Pant HC. Role of protein phosphatase 2A in Alzheimer's disease. Current Alzheimer Research 2011; 8(6): 623-32.

[45] Park SS, Jung HJ, Kim YJ, Park TK, et al. Asp664 cleavage of amyloid precursor protein induces tau phosphorylation by decreasing protein phosphatase 2A activity. Journal of Neurochemistry 2012; 123(5): 856-65.

[46] Martin L, Latypova X, Wilson CM, Magnaudeix A, Perrin ML, Terro F. Tau protein phosphatases in Alzheimer's disease: the leading role of PP2A. Ageing Research Reviews 2013; 12(1): 39-49.

[47] Arif M, Wei J, Zhang Q, Liu F, Basurto-Islas G, Grundke-Iqbal I, Iqbal K. Cytoplasmic Retention of Protein Phosphatase 2A-Inhibitor 2 (I2PP2A) Induces Alzheimer-like Abnormal Hyperphosphorylation of Tau. Journal of Biological Chemistry 2014; 289(40): 27677-91.

[48] Arnaud L, Chen S, Liu F, Li B, Khatoon S, Grundke-Iqbal I, Iqbal K.. Mechanism of inhibition of PP2A activity and abnormal hyperphosphorylation of tau by I2(PP2A)/SET. FEBS Letters 2011; 585(17): 2653-59.

[49] Liu GP, Zhang Y, Yao XQ, Zhang CE, Fang J, Wang Q, Wang JZ. Activation of glycogen synthase kinase-3 inhibits protein phosphatase-2A and the underlying mechanisms. Neurobiology of Aging 2008; 29(9): 1348-58.

[50] Patil S, Chan C. Palmitic and stearic fatty acids induce Alzheimer-like hyperphosphorylation of tau in primary rat cortical neurons. Neuroscience Letters 2005; 384(3): 288-93.

[51] Lovell MA, Xiong S, Xie C, Davies P, Markesbery WR. Induction of hyperphosphorylated tau in primary rat cortical neuron cultures mediated by oxidative stress and glycogen synthase kinase-3. Journal of Alzheimer's Disease 2004 6(6): 659-671.

[52] Zambrano CA, Egaña JT, Núñez MT, et al. Oxidative stress promotes τ dephosphorylation in neuronal cells: the roles of cdk5 and PP1. Free Radical Biology and Medicine 2004; 36(11): 1393-402.

[53] Dias-Santagata D, Fulga TA, Duttaroy A, Feany MB. Oxidative stress mediates tau-induced neurodegeneration in Drosophila. Journal of Clinical Investigation 2007; 117(1): 236-45.

[54] Abou-Sleiman PM, Muqit MM, Wood NW. Expanding insights of mitochondrial dysfunction in Parkinson's disease. Nature Reviews Neuroscience 2006; 7(3): 207-19.

[55] King TD, Clodfelder-Miller B, Barksdale KA, Bijur GN. Unregulated mitochondrial GSK3beta activity results in NADH: ubiquinone oxidoreductase deficiency. Neurotoxicity Research 2008; 14(2): 367-82.

[56] Feng Y, Xia Y, Yu G, Shu X, Ge H, Zeng K, Wang J, Wang X. Cleavage of GSK-3β by calpain counteracts the inhibitory effect of Ser9 phosphorylation on GSK-3β activity induced by $H_2O_2$. Journal of Neurochemistry 2013; 126(2): 234-42.

[57] Chiara F, Gambalunga A, Sciacovelli M, et al. Chemotherapeutic induction of mitochondrial oxidative stress activates GSK-3α/β and Bax, leading to permeability transition pore opening and tumor cell death. Cell Death and Disease 2012; 3: e444.

[58] Cho MH, Kim DH, Choi JE, et al. Increased phosphorylation of dynamin-related protein 1 and mitochondrial fission in okadaic acid-treated neurons. Brain Research 2012; 1454: 100-110.

[59] Chen L, Liu L, Huang S. Cadmium activates the mitogen-activated protein kinase (MAPK) pathway via induction of reactive oxygen species and inhibition of protein phosphatases 2A and 5. Free Radical Biology and Medicine 2008; 45(7): 1035-44.

[60] Zhang CE, Yang X, Li L, Sui X, et al. Hypoxia-Induced Tau Phosphorylation and Memory Deficit in Rats. Neuro-degenerative Diseases 2014; 14(3): 107-16.

[61] Wade AG, Farmer M, Harari G, et al. Add-on prolonged-release melatonin for cognitive function and sleep in mild to moderate Alzheimer's disease: a 6-month, randomized, placebo-controlled, multicenter trial. Clinical Interventions in Aging 2004; 9: 947-61.

[62] Peng CX, Hu J, Liu D, Hong XP, Wu YY, Zhu LQ, Wang JZ. Disease- modified glycogen synthase kinase-3β intervention by melatonin arrests the pathology and memory deficits in an Alzheimer's animal model. Neurobiology of Aging 2013; 34(6): 1555-63.

[63] Benítez-King G, Ortíz-López L, Jiménez-Rubio G, Ramírez-Rodríguez G. Haloperidol causes cytoskeletal collapse in N1E-115 cells through tau hyperphosphorylation induced by oxidative stress: Implications for neurodevelopment. European Journal of Pharmacology 2010; 644(1-3): 24-31.

[64] Li XC, Wang ZF, Zhang JX, Wang Q, Wang JZ. Effect of melatonin on calyculin A-induced tau hyperphosphorylation. European Journal of Pharmacology 2005; 510(1-2): 25-30.

[65] Hoppe JB, Frozza RL, Horn AP, et al. Amyloid-beta neurotoxicity in organotypic culture is attenuated by melatonin: involvement of GSK-3beta, tau and neuroinflammation. Journal of Pineal Research 2010; 48(3): 230-38.

[66] Lin L, Huang QX, Yang SS, Chu J, Wang JZ, Tian Q. Melatonin in Alzheimer's disease. International Journal of Molecular Sciences 2013; 14(7): 14575-93.

[67] Villaflores OB, Chen YJ, Chen CP, Yeh JM, Wu TY. Effects of curcumin and demethoxy curcumin on amyloid-β precursor and tau proteins through the internal ribosome entry sites: a potential therapeutic for Alzheimer's disease. Taiwan Journal of Obstetrics and Gynecology 2012; 51(4): 554-64.

[68] Ma QL, Zuo X, Yang F, Ubeda OJ, et al. Curcumin suppresses soluble tau dimers and corrects molecular chaperone, synaptic, and behavioral deficits in aged human tau transgenic mice. Journal of Biological Chemistry 2013; 288(6): 4056-65.

[69] Patil SP, Tran N, Geekiyanage H, Liu L, Chan C. Curcumin-induced upregulation of the anti-tau cochaperone BAG2 in primary rat cortical neurons. Neuroscience Letters 2013; 554: 121-5.

[70] Stuerenburg HJ, Ganzer S, Müller-Thomsen T. Plasma beta carotene in Alzheimer's disease. Association with cerebrospinal fluid beta-amyloid 1-40, (Abeta40), beta-amyloid 1-42 (Abeta42) and total Tau. Neuro Endocrinology Letters 2005; 26(6): 696-8.

[71] Chen Y, Wang C, Hu M, et al. Effects of ginkgolide A on okadaic acid- induced tau hyperphosphorylation and the PI3K-Akt signaling pathway in N2a cells. Planta Medica 2012; 78(12): 1337-41.

[72] Galasko DR, Peskind E, Clark CM, et al. Antioxidants for Alzheimer disease: a randomized clinical trial with cerebrospinal fluid biomarker measures. Archives of Neurology 2012; 69(7): 836-41.

[73] Cente M, Filipcik P, Mandakova S, Zilka N, Krajciova G, Novak M. Expression of a truncated human tau protein induces aqueous-phase free radicals in a rat model of tauopathy: implications for targeted antioxidative therapy. Journal of Alzheimer's Disease 2009; 17(4): 913-920.

[74] Yoon I, Lee KH, Cho J. Gossypin protects primary cultured rat cortical cells from oxidative stress and beta-amyloid-induced toxicity. Archives of Pharmacal Research 2004; 27(4): 454-59.

[75] Funderburk SF, Marcellino BK, Yue Z. Cell "self-eating" (autophagy) mechanism in Alzheimer's disease. Mount Sinai Journal of Medicine 2010; 77(1): 59- 68.

[76] Bové J, Martínez-Vicente M, Vila M. Fighting neurodegeneration with rapamycin: mechanistic insights. Nature Reviews Neuroscience 2011; 12(8): 437-52.

[77] Cai Z, Yan LJ. Rapamycin, Autophagy and Alzheimer's Disease. Journal of Biochemical and Pharmacological Research 2013; 1(2): 84-90.

[78] Dunlop EA, Tee AR. The kinase triad, AMPK, mTORC1 and ULK1, maintains energy and nutrient homoeostasis. Biochemical Society Transactions 2013; 41(4): 939-43.

[79] Ishizuka Y, Kakiya N, Witters LA et al. AMP-activated protein kinase counteracts brain-derived neurotrophic factor-induced mammalian target of rapamycin complex 1 signaling in neurons. Journal of Neurochemistry 2013; 127(1): 66-77.

[80] Jung CH, Seo M, Otto NM, Kim DH. ULK1 inhibits the kinase activity of mTORC1 and cell proliferation. Autophagy 2011; 7(10): 1212-21.

[81] Maiuri MC, Malik SA, Morselli E, Kepp O, et al. Stimulation of autophagy by the p53 target gene Sestrin2. Cell Cycle 2009; 8(10): 1571-6.

[82] Chan EY, Longatti A, McKnight NC, Tooze SA. Kinase-inactivated ULK proteins inhibit autophagy via their conserved C-terminal domains using an Atg13-independent mechanism. Molecular and Cellular Biology 2009; 29(1): 157-71.

[83] Sarkar S, Floto RA, Berger Z, Imarisio S, Cordenier A, Pasco M, Cook LJ, Rubinsztein DC. Lithium induces autophagy by inhibiting inositol monophosphatase. Journal of Cell Biology 2005; 170(7): 1101-11.

[84] Zou J, Yue F, Jiang X, Li W, Yi J, Liu L. Mitochondrion-associated protein LRPPRC suppresses the initiation of basal levels of autophagy via enhancing Bcl-2 stability. Biochemical Journal 2013; 454(3): 447-57.

[85] Alirezaei M, Kiosses WB, Fox HS. Decreased neuronal autophagy in HIV dementia: a mechanism of indirect neurotoxicity. Autophagy 2008; 4(7): 963-6.

[86] Shpilka T, Weidberg H, Pietrokovski S, Elazar Z. Atg8: an autophagy-related ubiquitin-like protein family. Genome Biology 2011; 12(7): 226.

[87] Kang R, Zeh HJ, Lotze MT, Tang D. The Beclin 1 network regulates autophagy and apoptosis. Cell Death and Differentiation 2011; 18(4): 571-80.

[88] Lünemann JD, Schmidt J, Schmid D, Barthel K, et al. Beta-amyloid is a substrate of autophagy in sporadic inclusion body myositis. Annals of Neurology 2007; 61(5): 476-483.

[89] Jaeger PA, Pickford F, Sun CH, Lucin KM, Masliah E, Wyss-Coray T. Regulation of amyloid precursor protein processing by the Beclin 1 complex. PLoS One 2010; 5(6): e11102.

[90] Ma JF, Huang Y, Chen SD, Halliday G. Immunohistochemical evidence for macroautophagy in neurones and endothelial cells in Alzheimer's disease. Neuropathology and Applied Neurobiology 2010; 36(4): 312-19.

[91] Yu WH, Cuervo AM, Kumar A, Peterhoff CM, Schmidt SD, et al. Macroautophagy - a novel Beta-amyloid peptide-generating pathway activated in Alzheimer's disease. Journal of Cell Biology 2005; 171(1): 87-98.

[92] Perucho J, Casarejos MJ, Gomez A, Solano RM, et al. Trehalose protects from aggravation of amyloid pathology induced by isoflurane anesthesia in APP(swe) mutant mice. Current Alzheimer Research 2012; 9(3): 334-43.

[93] Lai AY, McLaurin J. Inhibition of amyloid-beta peptide aggregation rescues the autophagic deficits in the TgCRND8 mouse model of Alzheimer disease. Biochimica et Biophysica Acta 2012; 1822(10): 1629-37.

[94] Nixon RA, Yang DS, Lee JH. Neurodegenerative lysosomal disorders: a continuum from development to late age. Autophagy 2008; 4(5): 590-9.

[95] Wei J, Fujita M, Nakai M, Waragai M, Sekigawa A, et al. Protective role of endogenous gangliosides for lysosomal pathology in a cellular model of synucleinopathies. American Journal of Pathology 2009; 174(5): 1891-909.

[96] Cardoso SM, Pereira CF, Moreira PI, Arduino DM, Esteves AR, Oliveira CR. Mitochondrial control of autophagic lysosomal pathway in Alzheimer's disease. Experimental Neurology 2010; 223(2): 294-8.

[97] Silva DF, Esteves AR, Arduino DM, Oliveira CR, Cardoso SM. Amyloid-β- induced mitochondrial dysfunction impairs the autophagic lysosomal pathway in a tubulin dependent pathway. Journal of Alzheimer's Disease 2011; 26(3): 565-81.

[98] Wang Y, Mandelkow E. Degradation of tau protein by autophagy and proteasomal pathways. Biochemical Society Transactions 2012; 40(4): 644-52.

[99] Caccamo A, Magrì A, Medina DX, Wisely EV, et al. mTOR regulates tau phosphorylation and degradation: implications for Alzheimer's disease and other tauopathies. Aging Cell 2013; 12(3): 370-80.

[100] Liu Y, Su Y, Wang J, Sun S, Wang T, Qiao X, Run X, Li H, Liang Z. Rapamycin decreases tau phosphorylation at Ser214 through regulation of cAMP-dependent kinase. Neurochemistry International 2013; 62(4): 458-67.

[101] Ozcelik S, Fraser G, Castets P, Schaeffer V, Skachokova Z, et al. Rapamycin attenuates the progression of tau pathology in P301S tau transgenic mice. PLoS One 2013; 8(5): e62459.

[102] Dolan PJ, Johnson GV. A caspase cleaved form of tau is preferentially degraded through the autophagy pathway. Journal of Biological Chemistry 2010; 285(29): 21978-87.

[103] Krüger U, Wang Y, Kumar S, Mandelkow EM. Autophagic degradation of tau in primary neurons and its enhancement by trehalose. Neurobiology of Aging 2012; 33(10): 2291-305.

[104] Kim SI, Lee WK, Kang SS, Lee SY, et al. Suppression of autophagy and activation of glycogen synthase kinase 3beta facilitate the aggregate formation of tau. Korean Journal of Physiology and Pharmacology 2011; 15(2): 107-14.

[105] Lim F, Hernández F, Lucas JJ, Gómez-Ramos P, Morán MA, Avila J. FTDP-17 mutations in tau transgenic mice provoke lysosomal abnormalities and Tau filaments in forebrain. Molecular and Cellular Neurosciences 2001; 18(6): 702-14.

[106] Lin WL, Lewis J, Yen SH, Hutton M, Dickson DW. Ultrastructural neuronal pathology in transgenic mice expressing mutant (P301L) human tau. Journal of Neurocytology 2003; 32(9): 1091-105.

[107] Magnaudeix A, Wilson CM, Page G, Bauvy C, Codogno P, et al. PP2A blockade inhibits autophagy and causes intraneuronal accumulation of ubiquitinated proteins. Neurobiology of Aging 2013; 34(3): 770-90.

[108] Yoon SY, Choi JE, Kweon HS, Choe H, et al. Okadaic acid increases autophagosomes in rat neurons: implications for Alzheimer's disease. Journal of Neuroscience Research 2008; 86(14): 3230-9.

[109] Hamano T, Gendron TF, Causevic E, Yen SN, et al. Autophagic-lysosomal perturbation enhances tau aggregation in transfectants with induced wild-type tau expression. European Journal of Neuroscience 2008; 27(5): 1119-30.

[110] Wang Y, Martinez-Vicente M, Kruger U, Kaushik S, Wong E, Mandelkow EM, Cuervo AM, Mandelkow E. (2009). Tau fragmentation, aggregation and clearance: the dual role of lysosomal processing. Human Molecular Genetics 2009; 18(21): 4153-70.

[111] Inoue K, Rispoli J, Kaphzan H, Klann E, et al. Macroautophagy deficiency mediates age-dependent neurodegeneration through a phospho-tau pathway. Molecular Neurodegeneration 2012; 7: 48.

Chapter 3

# Neuroinflammation and Alteration of the Blood-Brain Barrier in Alzheimer´s Disease

Luis Oskar Soto-Rojas, Fidel de la Cruz-López,
Miguel Angel Ontiveros Torres,
Amparo Viramontes-Pintos,
María del Carmen Cárdenas-Aguayo,
Marco A. Meraz-Ríos, Citlaltepetl Salinas-Lara,
Benjamín Florán-Garduño and José Luna-Muñoz

Additional information is available at the end of the chapter

http://dx.doi.org/10.5772/60024

## 1. Introduction

Alzheimer's disease (AD) is a neurodegenerative disease, characterized by progressive memory loss, cognitive deterioration and personality changes. Neuropathologically AD brains are characterized by massive accumulation of neurofibrillary tangles (NFT). NFTs are composed by paired helical filaments (PHF), which main constituent is tau protein. Another hallmark lesions of AD are Neuritic plaques (NPs), constituted by extracellular amyloid peptide aggregates (Aβ), that are associated with distrophyc neurites (DNs). Amyloid precursor protein (APP) processing occurs via two pathways. A) The amyloidogenic and B) the non-amyloidogenic pathway. In the amyloidogenic pathway, the APP is proteolyzed by β-secretase. This truncation occurs at the N-terminus of APP. The cleavage produces a soluble N-terminal fragment of APP (sAPPβ) and a C-terminal transmembrane fragment (β-CTF). β-CTF is cut into the membrane by γ-secretase and generates the Amyloid beta (Aβ) peptide and the APP intracellular domain (AICD). Depending on the site of γ-secretase cleavage, two main species of Aβ are generated: Aβ 40 and Aβ 42 amino acids. Aβ 42 is more hydrophobic and more prone to aggregate, as compared to the Aβ 40 peptide. In the non-amyloidogenic pathway, APP is cleaved by the α-secretase. This cleavage occurs in the middle region of Aβ and produces an N-terminal fragment of soluble APPα (sAPPα) and a C-terminal transmembrane (α-CTF) fragment. The sAPPα have neurotrophic and neuroprotective functions.

Similarly to β-CTF, α-CTF after being cleaved by γ-secretase generates a 23-25 amino acid peptide designated as p3. Aβ aggregates promote an inflammatory response mediated by activated microglia and astrocytes, that may activate pathological signalling pathways, leading to neurodegeneration. Long-term activation of the innate immune system is able to trigger an inflammatory cascade that converges on alterations of the cytoskeleton (including aggregation of tau protein and formation of PHFs and microtube disassembling) promoting neuronal degeneration. One of the pathological signalling pathways that may lead to neurodegeneration is oxidative stress, defined by the generation of a large amount of reactive oxygen species (ROS), which are highly harmful since they lead to the alteration in the structure of proteins, lipids and nucleic acids and cellular death. High levels of copper and iron have been detected in the blood plasma of people with AD. These metals catalyse the production of ROS by the Fenton reaction resulting in the generation of highly reactive hydroxyl radical, so that the reactivity of these metals can give rise to cellular damage and neurodegeneration. In AD, it had been described oxidative stress caused by free radicals (FRs). The most important in human biology FRs are superoxide ($O_2$ -), hydroxyl (OH·), nitric oxide (NO·), and trichloromethyl ($CCl_3$·). In AD, there is an increase in iron concentration in the hippocampus. There is an accumulation of iron and aluminum in NPs and cerebrospinal fluid (CSF), which could contribute to this oxidative stress. In AD, neuroinflammation is involved in multiple pathological mechanisms. Clinicopathological and neuroimaging studies have shown that inflammation and microglial activation precede neuronal damage and that oxidative stress occurs prior to neurodegeneration. Aβ accumulation alters the normal neuronal function, cell death, even before the formation of NPs and NFTs. Aβ not only has been linked to the inflammatory response, but also in a lesser extent to tau pathology. The Aβ itself causes activation of microglia and astrocytes through toll-like receptors 2, 4, 9 (TLR); activated microglia produces neurotoxic molecules and is conveniently located to the vicinity of the NPs. The proinflammatory cascade generated by microglial activation, results in the release of cytotoxic molecules such cytokines, chemokines, matrix metalloproteinases, and complement factors. These cytotoxic molecules may enhance neuronal neurodegeneration increasing sensitivity to FRs. The neurotoxicity mediated by microglial cells depends on ROS and cytokines. The present chapter address the physiological and pathological role of proinflammatory cytokines and the induction of tau pathology including tau accumulation and the formation of NFTs, as well as the mechanisms involving extracellular deposits of beta amyloid species (Aβ1-42, Aβ1-40, Aβ3-42 and Aβ11-42), which generate neurotoxic microenvironment in AD. In relation with the mechanisms involved in AD neuroinflammation, we will discuss the participation of caspases in inflammation and its likely activation as a result of the accumulation of endothelial cells. We will also talk about how the accumulation of Aβ in blood vessels affects blood-brain barrier endothelial cells tight junctions, modifying its permeability and its implications in AD pathology.

## 2. Diagnosis of Alzheimer's disease

AD can be diagnosed with 70% of accuracy, with a battery of clinical analysis and cognition tests. However, the definitive diagnostic test for AD is done post-mortem through histological analysis of the brains of patients.

http://dx.doi.org/10.5772/60024

### 2.1. Gross microscopy pathology

Atrophy of the brain in a case of AD, is generally symmetrical and diffuse in the convolutions, which is evidenced by the decrease in thickness. An increase in the depth of the grooves, a dilatation of the ventricles (Fig 1A and B compared to Fig 1 C and D) and decreased brain weight and volume is noticeable. Atrophy, mainly affecting the hippocampus, and the adjacent area transenthorinal, entorhinal cortex and the temporal and frontal lobes (Fig 1 C,D).

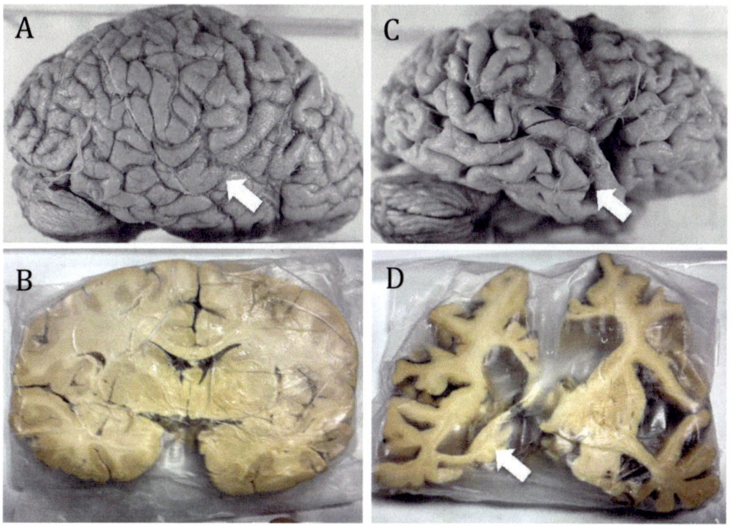


**Figure 1.** Neuroanatomical comparison of normal brain and Alzheimer´s disease brain. A,B) Normal Brain. C,D) Brain with pathology of AD. B) Prominent atrophy seen in fronto-temporal areas involved with association functions (arrows). B, D) Coronal sections of A) and C) respectively. Where observe an enlargement of the ventricles and selective hippocampal atrophy (arrow).

### 2.2. Histopathology of Alzheimer's disease

Microscopically, AD is characterized by the presence of lesions in the brain tissue known as neurofibrillary tangles (NFTs. Fig. 2 A, B. long arrows), dystrophic neurites (DNs. Fig. 1 C short arrows) and neuritic plaques (NPs, Fig. 1. C).

### 2.3. Neurofibrillary tangles

It has been shown that the severity of dementia in AD, correlates significantly with the density of NFTs in the neocortex and entorhinal cortex [1, 2]. At the stage of degeneration NFTs may be intracellular (iNFT, Fig. 2A) or extracellular (eNFT, Fig. 2B), [3] The formation of NFTs is associated with neuronal death [4-6] and found a strong correlation between neuronal degeneration and the transition between iNFT and eNFT [7]. The iNFT are characterized by a compact consistency and to be able to distinguish the cell membrane and the nucleus, although the nucleus may be displaced from its original position by the inclusion of fibrils. NFT is such a typical flame shape (Fig.2A). The eNFT show a fibrillar relax form and without nucleus (Fig 2B). These eNFT, are considered as the "skeleton" or "ghost" of the affected neuron (Fig 2B), are released into the extracellular space as a consequence of cell death, which remain stable due to its high insolubility and resistance to proteolysis.

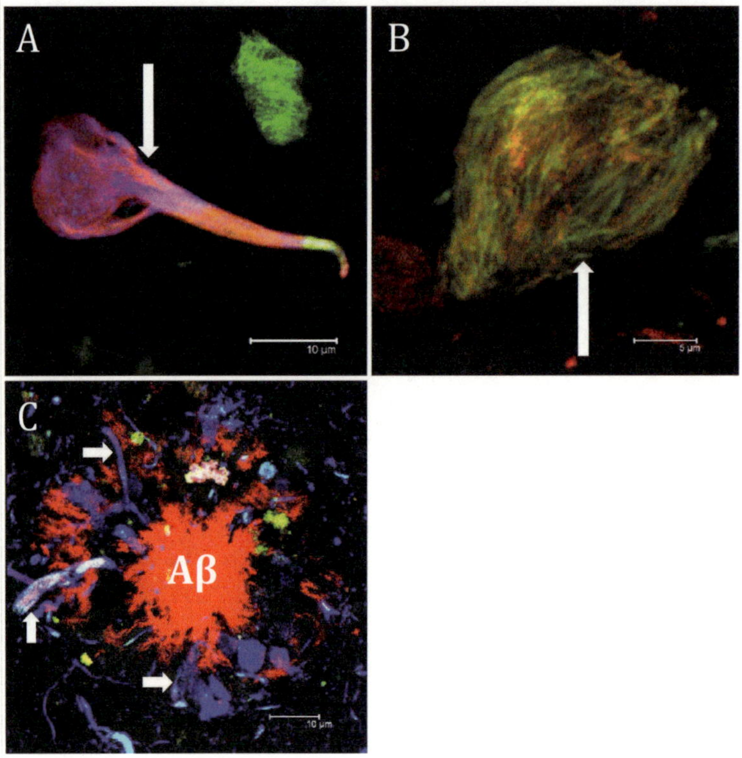


**Figure 2.** Hallmark characteristic of Alzheimer's disease brains. A) intracellular neurofibrillary tangle B) extracellular neurofibrillary tangle, are evidenced with antibodies against protein tau. C) Neuritic plaque. Evidenced by thiazine red dye (red channel) marker of beta-pleated sheet conformation and doble immunolabelling with two antibodies raised against tau protein to evidence dystrophic neurites (arrows), associated with these beta amyloid deposits (Aβ). Confocal microscope images (Leica SP8).

## 3. The tau protein and paired helical filaments

The NTFs and DNs (a component of NPs) are formed by the accumulation of abnormal polymers know as paired helical filaments (PHFs), due to their ultrastructural appearance [8]. The PHFs are characterized by its staining with thiazine red fluorescent dye, which has affinity for β-pleated structures [9], and have been used to differentiate between non-fibrillar (pre-assembled) amorphous and fibrillar states (assembled) of tau protein in AD [3, 10]. The main structural constituent of PHFs is tau protein, which is normally associated with microtubules.

### 3.1. Tau protein structure

Tau is the major component of the family of microtubule-associated proteins in the neuron. The tau gene was located on the long arm of chromosome 17 (17q21) and contains 16 exons[11]. Three of these exons (exon 4, 6 and 8), occurs only in the peripheral tissue RNA and these are not present in human brain mRNA, exons 1 and 14 are transcribed but not translated [12-15]. Exons 2, 3 and 10 have an alternative splicing and exon 3 never appears in the absence of exon 2 [15, 16]. Alternative splicing of three exons latter produces six isoforms of tau protein in the adult brain [12, 17]. Tau isoforms differ from each other by the presence or absence of one or two inserts (29 or 58 amino acids) in the amino terminal portion and by the presence of 3 to 4 repeated domains in the carboxyl terminal portion. The length of the various isoforms of tau varies from 352-441 aa's (Fig 3) [18].

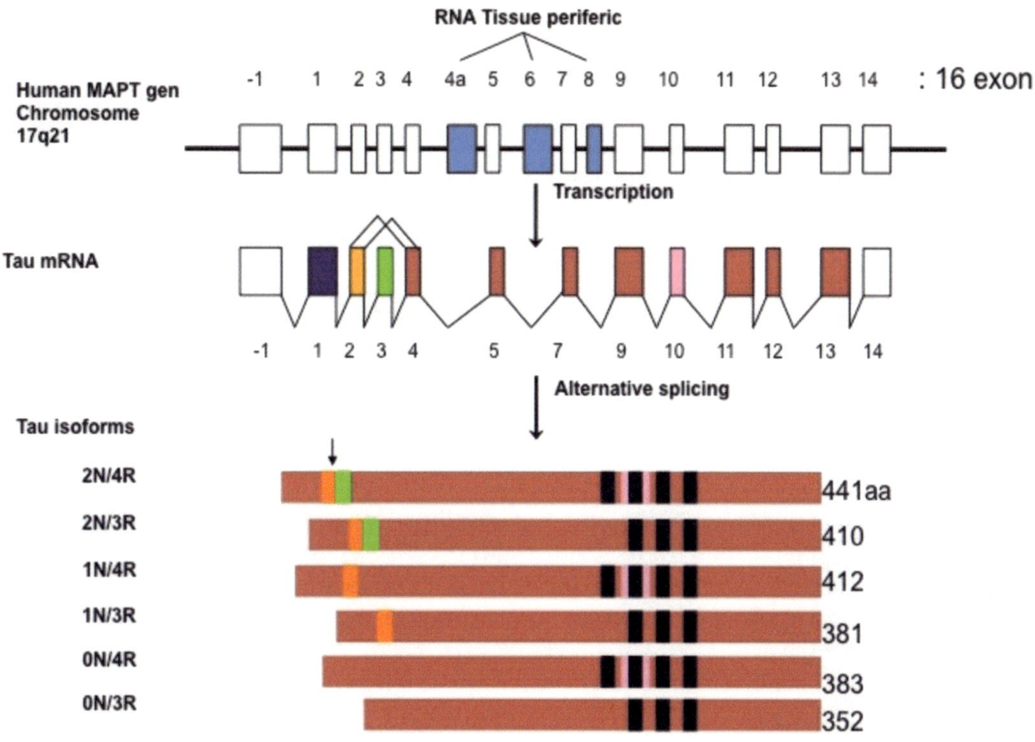


**Figure 3.** Schematic representation of tau protein gene. The MAPT gene encoding the tau protein is located on chromosome 17q21, which contains 16 exons. Isoforms of tau protein in human brain is encoded by 11 exons. Exons 2, 3 and 10 are alternatively spliced, favouring the synthesis of 6 isoforms. With a range of longitude between 352-441 amino acids. They differ by the presence or absence of one or two inserts of 29 amino acids at its amino terminal portion and by the presence of 3 or 4 microtubule binding domains in its C-terminal portion.

### 3.2. Post-translational modifications of tau protein in AD

It has not been reported for AD any change in the levels of RNAs messenger of any of the existing six isoforms of tau protein, which suggested, from the beginning, that abnormal forms of the protein found in PHFs originate from posttranslational modification rather than the novo synthesis [12]. There are two posttranslational modifications of tau protein, as the major molecular mechanisms involved in the pathophysiology of AD: the abnormal hyperphosphorylation and endogenous proteolysis [19, 20]. Both pathological processes are involved in the cascade of molecular events that lead to irreversible polymerization of tau protein into PHFs. Recently it has been described a series of tau conformational changes which appear to be associated, in fact, they appear to be the consequence of both the endogenous hyperphosphorylation and the truncation [21, 22].

## 4. Neuritic plaques

NPs are composed of extracellular deposits of insoluble amyloid fibrils that are made-up of Aβ peptide (Fig 2C), and these deposits are associated with neuritic component from dendritic and axonal origin (Fig. 2B arrows). There could also be AD brains with soluble non-fibrillar β-amyloid deposits without DNs associated, named senile plaques (SPs). SPs do not have a selective topographic distribution, however, their density is predominant in motor or sensory cortical areas than in primary hippocampal. The density of NPs in AD, in general, does not have a good correlation with the progression of dementia and the degree of neuronal loss [5, 23].

## 5. Amyloid precursor protein and amyloid-β peptide

Aβ originates from a large trans-membrane molecule, called APP. So far 8 isoforms of APP are known, were the predominats are the ones of 695, 751 and 770 aa's. The 695 isoform is the most abundant neuronal isoform. APP is a membrane glycoprotein with a single transmembrane domain, an intracytoplasmic portion and a extracellular long portion (Fig. 4). APP has an hydrophobic region of 23 aa's, by which it is anchored to cell membrane. The extracellular domain exposed to partial proteolysis by the action of three secretases (α, β and γ) (Fig 4). The proteolytic processing of APP, can occur via two types: the amyloidogenic and the non-amyloidogenic. By the action of both enzymes: γ (presenilin 1) [24] and β (transmembrane aspartyl protease called BACE) secretases, fragments of Aβ are generated, predominantly the fragments of 40 and 42 aa's. Alternatively to this proteolytic pathway amyloidogenic form, the action of α-secretase (metallo-protease and call disintegrin TACE) that cleaves the sequence of Aβ at aa's 16 and 17, represents a non-amyloidogenic processing. At first it was thought that the Aβ was produced only in pathological events, however, it was demonstrated that its production and secretion are physiological process, and Aβ is present in plasma and cerebrospinal fluid during the normal life of an individual [9, 25, 26]. In AD, APP metabolism is altered with a progressive increase in the production and abnormal deposition of Aβ. There are some Aβ deposits without neuritic component in elderly individuals without cognitive impairment

http://dx.doi.org/10.5772/60024

[27]. In general, it is thought that the abnormal accumulation of Aβ may be depend on certain alterations in the normal metabolic APP processes. Recent studies have emphasized a neurotoxic role of Aβ in *in vivo* animals models, which have led to reconsider the Aβ peptide, as one of the main factors related to the molecular pathogenesis of AD [28-30].

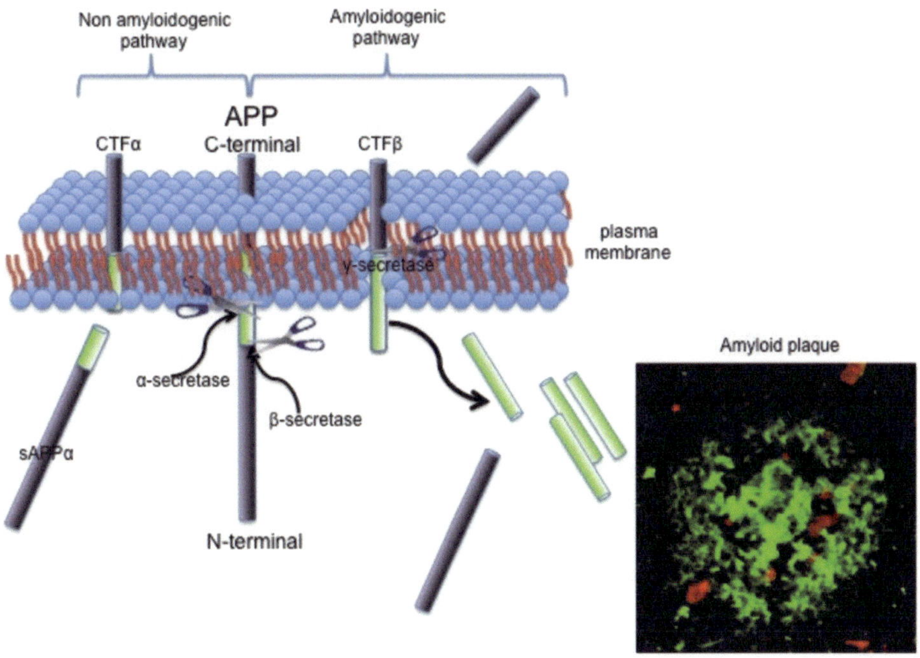


**Figure 4.** Amyloid precursor protein structure and metabolism. Schematic representation of APP processing by α-, β-, and γ-secretases. APP processing by secretase activities is divided into the non-amyloidogenic pathway on the left and the amyloidogenic pathway on the right. α- and β-secretase activities cleave APP in its extracellular domain to release respectively a soluble fragment sAPPα or sAPPβ in the extracellular space and generate carboxy-terminal fragments CTFα or CTFβ. These CTFs can subsequently be processed by γ-secretase complex to generate AICD and Aβ. The γ-secretase complex is composed of presenilin, nicastrin (NCT), γ-secretase activating protein (GSAP), pen-2, and aph-1.

## 6. Oxidative stress and Aβ

It is known that Aβ aggregates promote an inflammatory response, mediated mainly by microglia and astrocytes, which activate pathological signaling pathways, which may lead to neurodegeneration. A long-term activation of the innate immune system, is a mechanism capable of triggering an inflammatory cascade that culminates in cytoskeletal alterations (tau aggregation and formation of PHFs) with neurodegenerative consequences of this hypothesis, it has named "neuroimmunomodulation" [31].

One of these pathological signalling pathways that may lead to neurodegeneration, is oxidative stress, defined as the generation of a large amount of reactive oxygen species (ROS), which are highly harmful, leading to the alteration in the structure of proteins, lipids and nucleic acids and cell death [32]. AD described in the oxidative stress caused by free radicals (FRs). Major FRs in human biology are superoxide ($O_2$ -), the hydroxyl (OH ·), nitric oxide (NO ·), the thiyl (RS ·) and trichloromethyl ($CCl_3$ ·). There seem to be an accumulation of iron and aluminum in NPs and CSF [33], which could contribute to this oxidative stress [34].

Under physiological conditions, Aβ could regulate the release of NO, neurotransmitters, and hormones, long term potentiation and promotes cell survival. High levels of NO are generated under conditions of inflammation and may contribute to synaptic dysfunction, oxidation of proteins and lipids; culminating in neuronal death [35, 36] (Figure 5).

In AD, it has been shown that the A ▪ -peptide is able to promote the production of NO in microglia and activated astrocytes [37, 38] the release of proinflammatory cytokines such as IL-1β and TNF-$\alpha$ which contribute to the formation of NO and peroxynitrite [38, 39] and cause changes in proteins and lipids, mitochondrial damage, apoptosis and promotes the formation of Aβ, as well as increasing γ-secretase activity [40, 41] (Figure 3, 5). NO synthesis during development of AD could also contribute to the formation of NFTs (Fig 5), favouring the increase of tau phosphorylation [42].

## 7. Neuroinflammation as a trigger of neuronal death

Inflammation is involved in many pathological mechanisms in AD [43]. Clinicopathological and neuroimaging studies show that microglial activation and inflammation precede neuronal damage [44], and oxidative stress occurs before the histopathologycal lesion of AD appear [45]. But inflammation can be neuroprotective in its early stages [46] and the inability to resolve the activating stimulus can result in a chronic inflammatory response.

Under physiological conditions, glial cells and neurons express cytokines involved in modulating various functions including cellular homeostasis, metabolism, synaptic plasticity, and neural transmission. The Aβ plays a role in synaptic function and pathology [47], inducing degeneration, promoting the release of excitatory neurotransmitters by increasing intracellular calcium and ROS production (Figure 4) [48]. Aβ accumulation in the brain parenchyma and blood vessels promote microglial migration causing chronic and acute inflammatory response and induces production of FRs, proinflammatory cytokines and prostaglandins (PG), which may eventually promote neuronal death [49]. Aβ accumulation could disrupt the normal operation of the neurons, resulting in a significant cell dysfunction, which leads to apoptosis even before the formation of NPs and NFTs.

## 8. Glial cells key mediators of the inflammatory response in AD

Microglia cells are derived from monocytes during embryogenesis and are responsible for neuronal damage response [49]. Functions related to the immune response participate in a variety of neuroinflammatory processes [50].

The inflammatory response in AD includes morphological changes of microglia cells ranging from a branched cell "inactive" to the amoeboid appearance "active" [51, 52]. Activated microglia expresses several molecules on their surface, such as: Fc receptors required in phagocytosis of opsonized antigens by IgG, scavenger receptors *[53]*, cytokine and chemokine receptors, complement receptors as CD11b, CD11c, CD14, molecules of the major histocompatibility complex (MHC) [54], Toll-like receptors (TLR) family and Aβ receptors as the receptor for advanced glycation endproducts (RAGE). Cell surface microglial receptors are required for interaction with different types of immune cells, molecules involved in inflammatory responses in the brain and Aβ [55-57].

Aβ itself, causes activation of microglia and astrocytes through TLRs 2, 4 and 9 [54], when activated microglial cells produces neurotoxic molecules and strategically are located in the vicinity of the NPs. This proinflammatory cascade generated by microglial activation results in the release of cytotoxic molecules such as interleukins (IL-1 α, IL-1 β, IL-6, IL-10, IL-12, IL-16, IL-23), growth factors (transforming growth factor beta. TGF-β), chemokines, metalloproteinases (MMP-2, MMP-3, MMP-9), eicosanoids (PGD 2, leukotriene C4, cathepsins B and L) and complement factors (C1, C3, C4) also causing astrocytes chemotaxis around NPs [52]. Activated microglia also releases excessive amounts of glutamate and thereby inducing neurodegeneration These molecules can enhance cytotoxic neurodegeneration, increasing sensitivity to FRs [39]. Thus microglia-mediated neurotoxicity depends on ROS and cytokines [58, 59].

## 9. Astrocytic activation and their significance in the AD

Astrocytes represent the most abundant glial cell type in the CNS. They provide physical and metabolic support for neurons, and they are involved in the formation and maintenance of the BBB (Fig 5A), they produce neurotrophic and neuroprotective factors and are involved in repair processes within the CNS [60]. Attenuate the production of FRs and tumor necrosis factor α (TNF-α) [61], reduces microglial activation by Aβ [62] and alter their phagocytic activity [63]. They also decrease the cytotoxicity of A ▪ , both directly and indirectly through modulation of microglial cells [64].

In early stages of AD, activated astrocytes are located in two areas: in the molecular layer of the cerebral cortex and the amyloid deposits below the pyramidal cell layer. The activated astrocytes can phagocyte and degrade Aβ, suggesting that these cells are very important in the removal of parenchymal Aβ aggregates (Fig 5A and 6A. Arrowheads). As microglia, astrocytes are also activated by TLRs dependent pathways and RAGE receptors, therefore causing local inflammation and eventually favouring neuronal death [49]. Activated astrocytes produce numerous pro-inflammatory molecules as microglia, but unlike microglia, astrocytes produce S100β, which is highly expressed in the proximity of the Aβ deposits. Prolonged activation of astrocytes has a detrimental impact on neuronal survival and S100β could exacerbate this effect [65].

## 10. Monocytic cells derived from bone marrow function as a compensatory mechanism to remove amyloid deposits

There are 2 types of phagocytic cells within the CNS that are capable of initiating the innate immune response: microglia and peripheral macrophages [66]. These macrophages are recruited into the CNS by cytokines and chemokines, which are released during the microglial and astrocyte activation able to cross the blood brain barrier (BBB) [49]. Cells derived from bone marrow, can cross the BBB into the CNS and differentiate into microglia, which are located surrounding the amyloid deposits [67, 68]. This finding is very important, since if the resident activated microglia is incompetent to eliminate amyloid deposits, macrophages from the periphery could remove them by phagocytosis [69].

The presence of microvasculature in the brain promotes the release of chemokines such as IL-8, MPC-1, MIP-1, MIP-1$\alpha$ and MIP1-β and thereby promoting differentiation of monocytes into macrophages and migration through the BBB [70]. Analysis of the cerebrospinal fluid (CSF) of AD patients showed an increase in the levels of chemokines such as MCP-1 and IL-8 [71, 72]. In vitro models have demonstrated the ability of (CD4 and CD8) lymphocytes to cross the BBB [73] by increasing the level of MIP-1$\alpha$.

## 11. Effect of neuroinflammatory environment on BBB integrity

In AD brains, it has been observed a number of inflammatory reactions, surrounding brain microvasculature, together with A ▪ accumulation, which is associated with a dysfunction of the BBB. Morphological the BBB consists mainly of vascular endothelial cells, and other cellular components secondarily supporting the BBB that include pericytes found in the abluminal basal lamina, the perivascular astrocyte that form extensions towards capillaries around the basal lamina of the capillary wall and microglia.

The permeability and integrity of the BBB is regulated by the endothelial intercellular tight junctions (TJ), that consists of three integral membrane proteins: claudin, occludin and adhesion juntion molecules, as well as some accessory cytoplasmic proteins (ZO1, ZO2, ZO3 and cingulin). Cytoplasmic proteins are linked to actin cytoskeleton primary protein essential for the structural and functional maintenance of the endothelium [74]. While adherent junctions are formed by Vascular endothelium cadherin (VE-cadherin) which is a transmembrane glycoprotein catenin that its main function is to anchor the complex of cadherins and thereby the actin cytoskeleton, but also it is involved in the development of cellular signalling pathways (Figure 5) [75].

During neuroinflammation, leukocytes can infiltrate the brain microenvironment generating high levels of inflammatory mediators such as TNF-$\alpha$ and IFN-$\gamma$ [76]. Increased levels of TNF-$\alpha$ had been reported not only in endothelial and TJ modulating cytoskeletal rearrangement of brain endothelial cells (BEC) [77, 78], but also by causing an increase in the production of caspase-3 leading BEC to apoptosis [79]. However activation of this caspase 3, not always leads to apoptosis [80] and it has been shown that hypoxia can induce activation of caspases 3 and 9, without inducing neuronal apoptosis [81]. The caspase-3 has been involved in the disassembly of ZO-1 and claudin-5 in TJ regardless of fragmentation during cerebral ischemia (Fig. 5. blood Vessel) [82].

A recent study showed that TNF-$\alpha$ alone or in combination with IFN-$\gamma$ induces hypermeability, causing the leak of paracellular tracers and also induce degradation of ZO-1. Alterations in the function of brain endothelial cells (BEC) could lead to BBB breakdown, due to high concentrations of cytokines that correlates with expression of caspases 3 and 7 through activation of JNK signalling pathway and protein kinase C (PKC) and an increase in the number of apoptotic cells[83]. Treating peripheral microvascular endothelium with high concentrations of TNF-$\alpha$ and IFN-$\gamma$ results in a loss focal intercellular adhesion mediated by VE-cadherin generating endothelial rupture areas [76] whereas low concentrations of cytokines, also led to effector caspase activation, increased paracellular flux, and redistribution of zonula occludens-1 and VE-cadherin but failed to induce apoptosis. It was also suggested that cytokines have a dose dependent effect on the BEC. The BEC exposed to high levels of cytokines may be susceptible to caspase-mediated apoptosis and the BEC exposed to low concentrations of cytokine does not undergo apoptosis but results in alterations of the BBB [83].

## 12. Disruption of the blood-brain barrier as a marker of AD and other dementias

BBB dysfunction is a marker of neuroinflammatory diseases [84]. The BEC are the first physical barrier and expresses CNS binding complexes including TJ, and Adherent Junctions (AJ) [85]. In active inflammatory lesions, focal BEC show abnormalities in the distribution of occludin and ZO-1, including the absence or diffuse immunoreactivity at junctions and an increased immunoreactivity in the cytoplasm [86].

Occludin is vulnerable to the attack of matrix metalloproteinase (MMPs) [87]. MMPs can degrade the basal lamina proteins like fibronectin, laminin, and heparan sulfate after ischemic injury, which helps to break the BBB [88, 89]. It was demonstrated in a study the accumulation of occludin in neurons, astrocytes and microglia in AD, frontotemporal dementia (FTD) and vascular dementia (VaD) [90], suggesting a new function of occludin and proteins of the TJ in the pathogenesis of these dementias.

In this same study it was found that claudin 5 is degraded by MMP2 and MMP9 after ischemic damage, and therefore claudin and occludin were found surrounding astrocytes, but not in brain endothelium after an alteration in the BBB [91]. It is likely that the increase in occluding levels found in astrocytes and neurons in VaD, AD and FTD [90], may be a response to autophagy of TJ proteins by these cells after the rupture of the BBB caused by chronic hypoxia, aberrant angiogenesis or both [92].

## 13. Blood-brain barrier mechanisms of transport and regulation of brainAβ levels

According to the neural theory, Aβ is produced locally in the brain, in contrast to the vascular theory which suggests that the origin of Aβ comes from the circulation, and that the circulation of soluble Aβ (s- Aβ) may contribute to toxicity when it crosses BEC, which compromises the BBB (figure. 3) [93]. It has been proposed that specific receptors of Aβ are present in human brain capillaries and their distribution in the BEC transport could favour the peptide coupling to the BBB [94]. These receptors include RAGE and SR [95]. It is known that both RAGE and SR are receptors with multiple functions including cell endocytosis and transcytosis of macromolecules. RAGE and SR mediate binding of sA ▪ 1-40 at the apical side of human BBB, and RAGE is also involved in sA ▪ 1-40 transcytosis [94].

It has been shown that the interaction between Aβ/RAGE in the luminal membrane of the BBB participates in; 1). The diffusing of Aβ from the circulation to the brain through the BBB parenchyma, 2) Endothelial NF-KB mediated activation resulting in the secretion of pro-inflammatory cytokines (TNF-$\alpha$ and IL-6) and adhesion molecules expression (ICAM-1 and VCAM) and 3), generation of endothelin-1 decreases cerebral blood flow (CBF). The peptide Aβ / RAGE interaction contributes directly to neuronal death producing oxidative damage to neurons expressing RAGE and indirectly through activation of microglia [95]. Inhibition of RAGE/Aβ interaction in affected vasculature inhibits the production of cytokines, oxidative stress and Aβ peptide transport across the BBB [96]. Therefore it is suggested that RAGE could be an excellent therapeutic target in AD. It has been shown that RAGE inhibitors block its interaction to Aβ peptide and stabilizes the BBB functions, reducing neuroinflammation and improving the CBF.

## 14. Alterations of the neurovascular unit in AD

As previously described Aβ aggregates activate microglia and astrocytes, promoting the secretion of cytotoxic and pro-inflammatory factors culminating in neuronal and BBB dysfunction. Aβ can accumulate in the cerebral blood vessels, causing a morphofunctional alteration of neurovascular function.

Human brain receives 20% of the total cardiac output, if the cerebral blood flow (CBF) is stopped, so do brain functions in seconds and damage to neurons occurs in minutes [97]. The neuron-vessel relationship is critical for normal brain function. It has been estimated that each neuron in the human brain has its own capillary [98].

The length of brain capillaries is reduced in AD. These reductions can decrease vascular transport of substrates and nutrients through the BBB and reduce disposal of neurotoxins [99]. Vascular cells can directly affect the synaptic and neuronal functions through alterations in blood flow, the permeability of the BBB, nutrient supply, removal of toxic molecules, enzymatic functions, secretion of trophic factors and matrix molecules or through abnormal

http://dx.doi.org/10.5772/60024

expression of vascular receptors [100]. In response to vascular injury, astrocites and microglia are recruited, which when activated secrete several pro-inflammatory cytokines [101], that in turn, damage and exacerbates neuronal and synaptic dysfunction.

## 15. Stages of neurovascular dysfunction in AD

In early stages of AD, Aβ peptide removal through the BBB is impair, which could favour the accumulation of neurotoxic Aβ oligomers in the brain. Moreover, Aβ oligomers and focal reduction in capillary blood flow may affect synaptic transmission, causing neuronal damage and initiate the recruitment of microglial cells or blood within the brain [100].

In the early AD symptomatic stage, the BBB start missing Aβ removal properties, and activated endothelium and pro-inflammatory cytokines secreted to the CBF. This increases synaptic dysfunction, accumulation of intracellular tangles and activation of microglia. In late symptomatic AD stages, capillary unit is impair and contribute to the degeneration of the endothelial barrier. At this stage, there is a severe loss of the ability of the BBB to remove Aβ, resulting in amyloid deposits formation in the outer side of the capillary membrane, an increase in the number of NFT and activated microglia and astrocytes. At the final AD stages, the capillary unit is lost due to the amyloid deposits, therefore altering neuronal synapsis (Figure 6) [100].

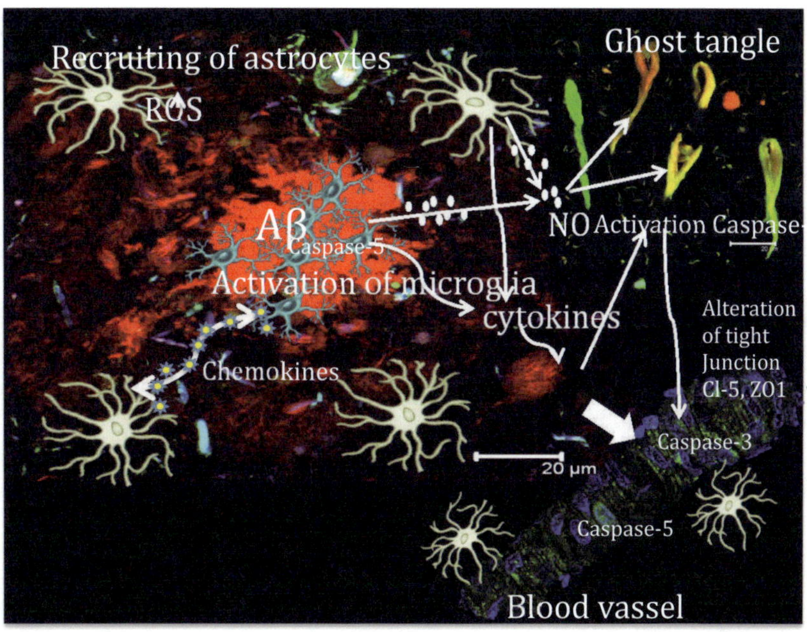


**Figure 5.** Schematic representation of neuroinflammatory environment and BBB alterations in AD. Aβ aggregates activate microglia and astrocytes, which will secrete pro-inflammatory cytokines and cytotoxic factors that will cause neuronal damage and disruption of the BBB (See more details in text).

## 16. Brain microvascular dysfunction as early event in AD

It is proposed that the breakdown of the BBB might be directly responsible for the pathogenesis of sporadic AD or at least could participate synergistically with other pathogenic mechanisms in the development of dementia [102]. Altering the BBB might occur as a result of hypoxia and complication of ischemic events, causing myocardial alterations commonly observed in AD. The breakdown of the BBB in AD is supported by the anatomical thickness and functional changes in the cerebral microvasculature [102] Deposits of A ▪ in the cerebral vasculature, leading to thickening of the basement membrane, stenosis of the vessel lumen and fragmentation of the internal elastic lamina, which can lead to stroke, brain haemorrhage or dementia [103, 104].

In AD there are ultrastructural changes [105] in the capillaries and changes in the its distribution and density [106]. It is believed that the accumulation of Aβ is one of the earliest events causing cerebrovascular alterations [107]. It has been detected changes in microvascular permeability and BBB dysfunction in AD brains [108]. BBB regulates the input of plasma derived Aβ and eliminates CNS Aβ through RAGE and the low-density lipoprotein receptor-related protein, (LRP1) respectively [95, 109].

The soluble peptide Aβ (s- Aβ) is normally produced by different cell types [110] and could be released into the circulation of the cerebrospinal fluid (CSF)[9] and brain parenchyma [111]. The Aβ 1-40 peptide represents about 90% of the total cerebrovascular amyloid [112]. High levels of Aβ and the presence of predisposing factors such as apoE4, genetic mutations in PS-1, PS-2 and APP [113], may favor the accumulation of Aβ as fibrillar amyloid in the wall vessel or in the brain parenchyma and could induce cytotoxic effects [95, 114] and contribute to neuronal loss and the development of the AD pathology [113].

Recent studies support the vascular theory to show that the brain distribution of Aβ receptors in the apical side of the BBB might be responsible for the interaction of Aβ circulating with the vascular wall and mediate its transit to the brain [115]. In AD many Aβ deposits are associated with microvessels [116] and with the presence of multiple inflammatory molecules that provide support for monocyte transmigration ability to neighbourhoods of Aβ deposit and in accordance with the clinical- pathological it has been suggested that neuroinflammation plays a role in patients with AD dementia [117]. In a study it was shown that Aβ peptide induced monocyte differentiation into macrophages and hypersecretion of inflammatory cytokines and chemokines [70]. In AD brains, a large number of core amyloid deposits in NPs are intimately associated with endothelial basal lamina and in many instances the lumen is lost [116]. It has also been found that calcium influx is induced by intracellular Aβ [118, 119], and that elevation of intracellular calcium leads to alteration of the TJ as the induction of MMPs [120].

Chronic transmigration of monocytes may result in subtle damage to the BBB. Disruption of the BBB would allow the passage of large amounts of circulating Aβ linked to other carrier proteins such as albumin [121], $\alpha$-2 macroglobulin [53] and Aβ components. Albumin levels in CSF of patients with early stages of AD, found to be significantly enhanced due to an increased permeability of the BBB [122]. Elevated levels of other proteins of high molecular weight as haptoglobin, had also been found in this conditions [123].

http://dx.doi.org/10.5772/60024

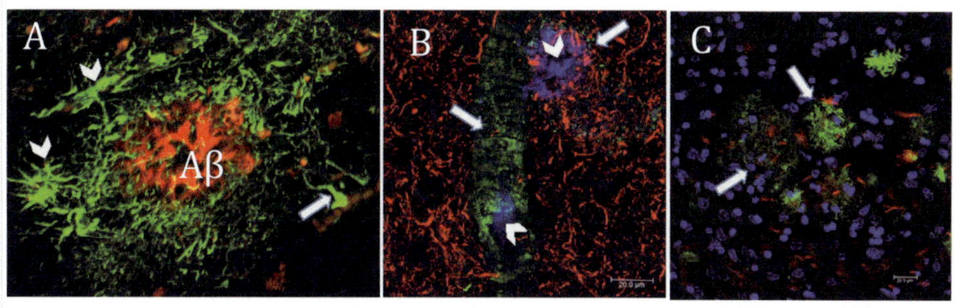


**Figure 6.** The extracellular deposits of amyloid-β peptide induces cronic inflammation in neuronal cell. A) Double immunostaining. Glial cell immunostaining evidenced by GFAP antibody (arrowheads), which is located in the perifery of the extracellular amyloid deposit evidenced by the thiazine red dye (Aβ). Microglial cell associated with a blood vessel. B) Triple immunostaining, where expression of caspase-5 (green channel) was detected in the cytoplasm of endothelial cells (the blood vessel, arrow). Adjacent to the blood vessel is possible to observed a extracellular Aβ deposit (amyloid plaque) evidenced by antibody BAM10 (arrowheads). In the red channel is the immunoreactivity of an antibody against tau protein. C) Double immunostaining with antibodies raised to Caspase-5 (green channel, arrows), which is strongly associated with amyloid plaques (as evidenced by the thiazine red staining, red channel), counterstained with Topro dye to show cell nuclei (blue channel). confocal microscopy, Leica SP8.

## 17. Amyloid beta peptide and intracellular caspase 5 in brain endothelial cells

Caspase-5 is expressed in a restricted manner in placenta, lung, liver, spleen, small intestine, colon and peripheral blood lymphocytes (1, 3) and it is located in the cell cytoplasm. It belongs to the family of proteins involved in apoptosis, inflammation, proliferation and differentiation. Caspase-5 operatively was associated with the caspases 1, 4 and 12.

Caspase-5 is regulated by lipopolysaccharide (LPS) and interferon-γ. Suggesting that caspase-5 may perform functions in inflammation and innate immune response. Likewise, it is associated with the complex of proteins that constitute the inflammasome. Caspase-5 also participates in IL-1β processing However the presence of caspase-5 and its role in neurodegenerative diseases is unknown.

In this review we have discuss the inflammatory role that is present in AD brains in response to Aβ accumulation and stress induced by this peptide, triggering a response in microglial and astroglial cells. Which are responsible for this inflammatory damage in AD. This proinflammatory cascade generated by microglial activation resulting from the release of cytotoxic molecules such as interleukins (IL-1 α, IL-1 β, IL-6, IL-10, IL-12, IL-16, IL-23), growth factors (transforming growth factor beta [TGF-β]), chemokines, matrix metalloproteinases (MMP-2, MMP-3, MMP-9), eicosanoids (PGD 2, leukotriene C4, cathepsins B and L) and complement factors (C1, C3, C4) also causing astrocytic chemotaxis around NPs (53). Activated microglia also releases excessive amounts of glutamate excitotoxicity, thereby inducing neurodegeneration. So far caspase-5 has been involved in Aβ induced neuroinflammation in AD brains. In our laboratory we have detect the presence of caspase-5 closely associated with Aβ deposits in blood vessels (Fig. 6 B arrows) and Aβ plaques (Fig. 6 B. arrowhead, Fig. 6. C arrows) in AD brains. NPs showed a high immunoreactivity to caspase-5. The presence of caspase-5 was observed in the area where active microglial cells are and poorly observed in the periphery of the NPs where the astroglial cells are (Fig. 6). This does suggest that microglial cells carry out active inflammatory activity and are responsible for the neurotoxic environment observed in AD.

A large numbers of studies have demonstrated an increase of endothelial cells activity in blood vessels. By double and triple immunostaining and confocal microscopy, we have demonstrated the presence of soluble Aβ and fibrillar Aβ (evidenced by the monoclonal antibody BAM10 and stained with thiazine red (TR), which is used to monitor the fibrillar state of tau and Aβ peptide, with a β pleated sheet conformation.) in endothelial cell soma. It is possible that the accumulation of extracellular Aβ peptide could be trigger by caspase-5 activity, causing an increase in the synthesis of IL, therefore modifying the permeability of cerebral blood vessels by altering tight junctions in AD brains. Consequently the presence and activity of caspase-5 could promote the prolonged and sustained inflammation described in AD brains.

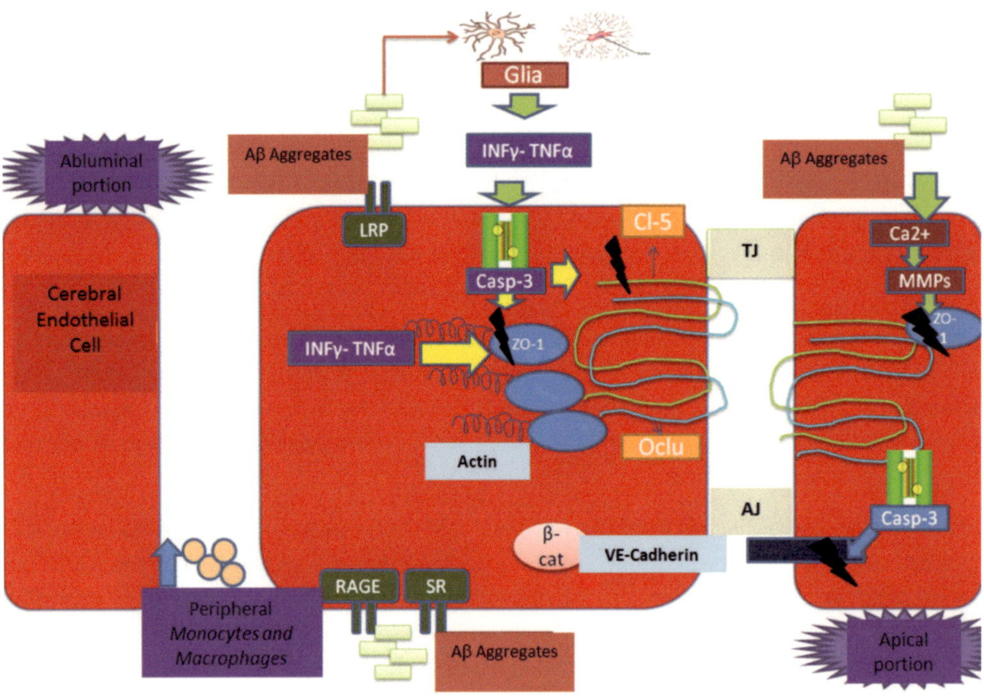


**Figure 7.** Disruption of the BBB in AD. Aβ aggregates activated glia, pro-inflammatory cytokines secretion, which in turn activate caspase 3, contributing to the disassembly of constitutive adherent junction proteins. The Aβ aggregates also contribute to activation of MMPs. BBB damage, allows monocytes, macrophages and peripheral Aβ aggregated to pass from outside the nervous system to the brain, increasing the neuroinflammatory environment.

http://dx.doi.org/10.5772/60024

## 18. Conclusions

Amyloid β peptide, which is aggregated extracellularly in the neuritic plaques, generates a constant inflammatory environment and prolonged, activation of microglial and astroglial cells that potentiate neuronal damage and have been involved in the alteration of the BBB, damaging the permeability of blood vessels. Maybe as a consequence of degradation of tight junctions proteins, favouring the loss of these junctions, altering the permeability of blood vessels. Understanding the mechanisms of action of different species of beta amyloid peptide could lead to new therapeutic interventions directed to inhibit Aβ aggregation at the level of oligomers, which are much more toxic than the fibrillary form. It is important to understand the mechanisms of action of caspase-5, in this pathological process of amyloid β peptide, emphasizing the clinical importance of casapasa-5 and its relation to the process of neuroinflammation.

## Acknowledgements

The authors wish to express their gratitude to the Mexican families who donate the brain of their loved ones affected with AD and made possible our research. We also want to thank Ms. Maricarmen De Lorenz for her outstanding technical and secretarial support and M en C Ivan J. Galván Mendoza, for hes support in confocal microscopy. This work was supported by the Grant from CONACYT, No. 142293.

## Author details

Luis Oskar Soto-Rojas[1,2,3], Fidel de la Cruz-López[2], Miguel Angel Ontiveros Torres[1], Amparo Viramontes-Pintos[1], María del Carmen Cárdenas-Aguayo[4], Marco A. Meraz-Ríos[4], Citlaltepetl Salinas-Lara[3,6], Benjamín Florán-Garduño[5] and José Luna-Muñoz[1*]

*Address all correspondence to: jluna@cinvestav.mx

1 Brain Bank-LaNSE CINVESTAV-IPN, Mexico

2 Departments of Physiology. ENCB IPN, México

3 FES Iztacala. UNAM, México

4 Molecular Biomedicine Department, CINVESTAV-IPN, Mexico

5 Physiology, Biophysics and Neurosciences Department, CINVESTAV-IPN, Mexico

6 INNN MVS, Mexico

## References

[1] Ball, M.J., et al., *Neuropathological definition of Alzheimer disease: multivariate analyses in the morphometric distinction between Alzheimer dementia and normal aging.* Alzheimer Dis Assoc Disord, 1988. 2(1): p. 29-37.

[2] Blessed, G., B.E. Tomlinson, and M. Roth, *The association between quantitative measures of dementia and of senile change in the cerebral grey matter of elderly subjects.* Br J Psychiatry, 1968. 114(512): p. 797-811.

[3] Mena, R., et al., *Monitoring pathological assembly of tau and beta-amyloid proteins in Alzheimer's disease.* Acta Neuropathol, 1995. 89(1): p. 50-6.

[4] Cras, P., et al., *Extracellular neurofibrillary tangles reflect neuronal loss and provide further evidence of extensive protein cross-linking in Alzheimer disease.* Acta Neuropathol, 1995. 89(4): p. 291-5.

[5] Gomez-Isla, T., et al., *Neuronal loss correlates with but exceeds neurofibrillary tangles in Alzheimer's disease.* Ann Neurol, 1997. 41(1): p. 17-24.

[6] Gomez-Isla, T., et al., *Profound loss of layer II entorhinal cortex neurons occurs in very mild Alzheimer's disease.* J Neurosci, 1996. 16(14): p. 4491-500.

[7] Bondareff, W., et al., *Evidence of subtypes of Alzheimer's disease and implications for etiology.* Arch Gen Psychiatry, 1993. 50(5): p. 350-6.

[8] Kidd, M., *Paired helical filaments in electron microscopy of Alzheimer's disease.* Nature, 1963. 197: p. 192-3.

[9] Seubert, P., et al., *Isolation and quantification of soluble Alzheimer's beta-peptide from biological fluids.* Nature, 1992. 359(6393): p. 325-7.

[10] Mena, R., et al., *Staging the pathological assembly of truncated tau protein into paired helical filaments in Alzheimer's disease.* Acta Neuropathol, 1996. 91(6): p. 633-41.

[11] Neve, R.L., et al., *A cDNA for a human microtubule associated protein 2 epitope in the Alzheimer neurofibrillary tangle.* Brain Res, 1986. 387(2): p. 193-6.

[12] Goedert, M., et al., *Multiple isoforms of human microtubule-associated protein tau: sequences and localization in neurofibrillary tangles of Alzheimer's disease.* Neuron, 1989. 3(4): p. 519-26.

[13] Goedert, M., et al., *Cloning and sequencing of the cDNA encoding an isoform of microtubule-associated protein tau containing four tandem repeats: differential expression of tau protein mRNAs in human brain.* Embo J, 1989. 8(2): p. 393-9.

[14] Sawa, A., et al., *Molecular diversity at the carboxyl terminus of human and rat tau.* Brain Res Mol Brain Res, 1994. 27(1): p. 111-7.

[15] Andreadis, A., W.M. Brown, and K.S. Kosik, *Structure and novel exons of the human tau gene.* Biochemistry, 1992. 31(43): p. 10626-33.

[16] Andreadis, A., J.A. Broderick, and K.S. Kosik, *Relative exon affinities and suboptimal splice site signals lead to non-equivalence of two cassette exons.* Nucleic Acids Res, 1995. 23(17): p. 3585-93.

[17] Kosik, K.S., et al., *Developmentally regulated expression of specific tau sequences.* Neuron, 1989. 2(4): p. 1389-97.

[18] Goedert, M., et al., *Tau proteins of Alzheimer paired helical filaments: abnormal phosphorylation of all six brain isoforms.* Neuron, 1992. 8(1): p. 159-68.

[19] Grundke-Iqbal, I., et al., *Abnormal phosphorylation of the microtubule-associated protein tau (tau) in Alzheimer cytoskeletal pathology.* Proc Natl Acad Sci U S A, 1986. 83(13): p. 4913-7.

[20] Novak, M., J. Kabat, and C.M. Wischik, *Molecular characterization of the minimal protease resistant tau unit of the Alzheimer's disease paired helical filament.* Embo J, 1993. 12(1): p. 365-70.

[21] Luna-Munoz, J., et al., *Earliest stages of tau conformational changes are related to the appearance of a sequence of specific phospho-dependent tau epitopes in Alzheimer's disease.* J Alzheimers Dis, 2007. 12(4): p. 365-75.

[22] Luna-Munoz, J., et al., *Regional conformational change involving phosphorylation of tau protein at the Thr231, precedes the structural change detected by Alz-50 antibody in Alzheimer's disease.* J Alzheimers Dis, 2005. 8(1): p. 29-41.

[23] Arriagada, P.V., et al., *Neurofibrillary tangles but not senile plaques parallel duration and severity of Alzheimer's disease.* Neurology, 1992. 42(3 Pt 1): p. 631-9.

[24] Saunders, A.M., *Apolipoprotein E and Alzheimer disease: an update on genetic and functional analyses.* J Neuropathol Exp Neurol, 2000. 59(9): p. 751-8.

[25] Haass, C., et al., *Amyloid beta-peptide is produced by cultured cells during normal metabolism.* Nature, 1992. 359(6393): p. 322-5.

[26] Shoji, M., et al., *Production of the Alzheimer amyloid beta protein by normal proteolytic processing.* Science, 1992. 258(5079): p. 126-9.

[27] Lemere, C.A., et al., *Sequence of deposition of heterogeneous amyloid beta-peptides and APO E in Down syndrome: implications for initial events in amyloid plaque formation.* Neurobiol Dis, 1996. 3(1): p. 16-32.

[28] Mattson, M.P., et al., *beta-Amyloid precursor protein metabolites and loss of neuronal Ca2+ homeostasis in Alzheimer's disease.* Trends Neurosci, 1993. 16(10): p. 409-14.

[29] Mattson, M.P., et al., *beta-Amyloid peptides destabilize calcium homeostasis and render human cortical neurons vulnerable to excitotoxicity.* J Neurosci, 1992. 12(2): p. 376-89.

[30] Shea, T.B., S. Prabhakar, and F.J. Ekinci, *Beta-amyloid and ionophore A23187 evoke tau hyperphosphorylation by distinct intracellular pathways: differential involvement of the calpain/protein kinase C system.* J Neurosci Res, 1997. 49(6): p. 759-68.

[31] Fernandez, J.A., et al., *The damage signals hypothesis of Alzheimer's disease pathogenesis.* J Alzheimers Dis, 2008. 14(3): p. 329-33.

[32] Lavados, M., et al., *Mild cognitive impairment and Alzheimer patients display different levels of redox-active CSF iron.* J Alzheimers Dis, 2008. 13(2): p. 225-32.

[33] Jellinger, K., et al., *Brain iron and ferritin in Parkinson's and Alzheimer's diseases.* J Neural Transm Park Dis Dement Sect, 1990. 2(4): p. 327-40.

[34] Pappolla, M.A., et al., *Immunohistochemical evidence of oxidative [corrected] stress in Alzheimer's disease.* Am J Pathol, 1992. 140(3): p. 621-8.

[35] Liu, B., et al., *Role of nitric oxide in inflammation-mediated neurodegeneration.* Ann N Y Acad Sci, 2002. 962: p. 318-31.

[36] Calabrese, V., et al., *Nitric oxide in the central nervous system: neuroprotection versus neurotoxicity.* Nat Rev Neurosci, 2007. 8(10): p. 766-75.

[37] Goodwin, J.L., M.E. Kehrli, Jr., and E. Uemura, *Integrin Mac-1 and beta-amyloid in microglial release of nitric oxide.* Brain Res, 1997. 768(1-2): p. 279-86.

[38] Rossi, F. and E. Bianchini, *Synergistic induction of nitric oxide by beta-amyloid and cytokines in astrocytes.* Biochem Biophys Res Commun, 1996. 225(2): p. 474-8.

[39] Combs, C.K., et al., *beta-Amyloid stimulation of microglia and monocytes results in TNFalpha-dependent expression of inducible nitric oxide synthase and neuronal apoptosis.* J Neurosci, 2001. 21(4): p. 1179-88.

[40] Keil, U., et al., *Amyloid beta-induced changes in nitric oxide production and mitochondrial activity lead to apoptosis.* J Biol Chem, 2004. 279(48): p. 50310-20.

[41] Guix, F.X., et al., *Modification of gamma-secretase by nitrosative stress links neuronal ageing to sporadic Alzheimer's disease.* EMBO Mol Med, 2012. 4(7): p. 660-73.

[42] Saez, T.E., et al., *Astrocytic nitric oxide triggers tau hyperphosphorylation in hippocampal neurons.* In Vivo, 2004. 18(3): p. 275-80.

[43] McGeer, P.L. and E.G. McGeer, *Inflammation, autotoxicity and Alzheimer disease.* Neurobiol Aging, 2001. 22(6): p. 799-809.

[44] Eikelenboom, P. and W.A. van Gool, *Neuroinflammatory perspectives on the two faces of Alzheimer's disease.* J Neural Transm, 2004. 111(3): p. 281-94.

[45] Zhu, X., et al., *Alzheimer's disease: the two-hit hypothesis.* Lancet Neurol, 2004. 3(4): p. 219-26.

[46] Wyss-Coray, T., et al., *Prominent neurodegeneration and increased plaque formation in complement-inhibited Alzheimer's mice.* Proc Natl Acad Sci U S A, 2002. 99(16): p. 10837-42.

[47] Kamenetz, F., et al., *APP processing and synaptic function.* Neuron, 2003. 37(6): p. 925-37.

[48] Gylys, K.H., et al., *Synaptic changes in Alzheimer's disease: increased amyloid-beta and gliosis in surviving terminals is accompanied by decreased PSD-95 fluorescence.* Am J Pathol, 2004. 165(5): p. 1809-17.

[49] Meraz-Rios, M.A., et al., *Inflammatory process in Alzheimer's Disease.* Front Integr Neurosci, 2013. 7: p. 59.

[50] Lund, S., et al., *The dynamics of the LPS triggered inflammatory response of murine microglia under different culture and in vivo conditions.* J Neuroimmunol, 2006. 180(1-2): p. 71-87.

[51] Suh, Y.H. and F. Checler, *Amyloid precursor protein, presenilins, and alpha-synuclein: molecular pathogenesis and pharmacological applications in Alzheimer's disease.* Pharmacol Rev, 2002. 54(3): p. 469-525.

[52] Glass, C.K., et al., *Mechanisms underlying inflammation in neurodegeneration.* Cell, 2010. 140(6): p. 918-34.

[53] Hughes, S.R., et al., *Alpha2-macroglobulin associates with beta-amyloid peptide and prevents fibril formation.* Proc Natl Acad Sci U S A, 1998. 95(6): p. 3275-80.

[54] Suzumura, A., *[Neurotoxicity by microglia: the mechanisms and potential therapeutic strategy].* Fukuoka Igaku Zasshi, 2009. 100(7): p. 243-7.

[55] El Khoury, J., et al., *Scavenger receptor-mediated adhesion of microglia to beta-amyloid fibrils.* Nature, 1996. 382(6593): p. 716-9.

[56] Lue, L.F., et al., *Involvement of microglial receptor for advanced glycation endproducts (RAGE) in Alzheimer's disease: identification of a cellular activation mechanism.* Exp Neurol, 2001. 171(1): p. 29-45.

[57] McGeer, P.L., et al., *Microglia in degenerative neurological disease.* Glia, 1993. 7(1): p. 84-92.

[58] Benzing, W.C., et al., *Evidence for glial-mediated inflammation in aged APP(SW) transgenic mice.* Neurobiol Aging, 1999. 20(6): p. 581-9.

[59] Mehlhorn, G., M. Hollborn, and R. Schliebs, *Induction of cytokines in glial cells surrounding cortical beta-amyloid plaques in transgenic Tg2576 mice with Alzheimer pathology.* Int J Dev Neurosci, 2000. 18(4-5): p. 423-31.

[60] Minagar, A., et al., *The role of macrophage/microglia and astrocytes in the pathogenesis of three neurologic disorders: HIV-associated dementia, Alzheimer disease, and multiple sclerosis.* J Neurol Sci, 2002. 202(1-2): p. 13-23.

[61] Smits, H.A., et al., *Activation of human macrophages by amyloid-beta is attenuated by astrocytes.* J Immunol, 2001. 166(11): p. 6869-76.

[62] von Bernhardi, R. and G. Ramirez, *Microglia-astrocyte interaction in Alzheimer's disease: friends or foes for the nervous system?* Biol Res, 2001. 34(2): p. 123-8.

[63] DeWitt, D.A., et al., *Astrocytes regulate microglial phagocytosis of senile plaque cores of Alzheimer's disease.* Exp Neurol, 1998. 149(2): p. 329-40.

[64] Ramirez, G., et al., *Protection of rat primary hippocampal cultures from A beta cytotoxicity by pro-inflammatory molecules is mediated by astrocytes.* Neurobiol Dis, 2005. 19(1-2): p. 243-54.

[65] Mori, T., et al., *Overexpression of human S100B exacerbates cerebral amyloidosis and gliosis in the Tg2576 mouse model of Alzheimer's disease.* Glia, 2010. 58(3): p. 300-14.

[66] Rezai-Zadeh, K., D. Gate, and T. Town, *CNS infiltration of peripheral immune cells: D-Day for neurodegenerative disease?* J Neuroimmune Pharmacol, 2009. 4(4): p. 462-75.

[67] Malm, T.M., et al., *Bone-marrow-derived cells contribute to the recruitment of microglial cells in response to beta-amyloid deposition in APP/PS1 double transgenic Alzheimer mice.* Neurobiol Dis, 2005. 18(1): p. 134-42.

[68] Simard, A.R., et al., *Bone marrow-derived microglia play a critical role in restricting senile plaque formation in Alzheimer's disease.* Neuron, 2006. 49(4): p. 489-502.

[69] Gate, D., et al., *Macrophages in Alzheimer's disease: the blood-borne identity.* J Neural Transm, 2010. 117(8): p. 961-70.

[70] Fiala, M., et al., *Amyloid-beta induces chemokine secretion and monocyte migration across a human blood--brain barrier model.* Mol Med, 1998. 4(7): p. 480-9.

[71] Galimberti, D., et al., *Chemokines in serum and cerebrospinal fluid of Alzheimer's disease patients.* Ann Neurol, 2003. 53(4): p. 547-8.

[72] Correa, J.D., et al., *Chemokines in CSF of Alzheimer's disease patients.* Arq Neuropsiquiatr, 2011. 69(3): p. 455-9.

[73] Man, S.M., et al., *Peripheral T cells overexpress MIP-1alpha to enhance its transendothelial migration in Alzheimer's disease.* Neurobiol Aging, 2007. 28(4): p. 485-96.

[74] Tsukita, S. and M. Furuse, *Occludin and claudins in tight-junction strands: leading or supporting players?* Trends Cell Biol, 1999. 9(7): p. 268-73.

[75] Stamatovic, S.M., R.F. Keep, and A.V. Andjelkovic, *Brain endothelial cell-cell junctions: how to "open" the blood brain barrier.* Curr Neuropharmacol, 2008. 6(3): p. 179-92.

[76] Wong, R.K., A.L. Baldwin, and R.L. Heimark, *Cadherin-5 redistribution at sites of TNF-alpha and IFN-gamma-induced permeability in mesenteric venules.* Am J Physiol, 1999. 276(2 Pt 2): p. H736-48.

[77] Forster, C., et al., *Differential effects of hydrocortisone and TNFalpha on tight junction proteins in an in vitro model of the human blood-brain barrier.* J Physiol, 2008. 586(7): p. 1937-49.

[78] de Vries, H.E., et al., *The influence of cytokines on the integrity of the blood-brain barrier in vitro.* J Neuroimmunol, 1996. 64(1): p. 37-43.

[79] Kimura, H., et al., *Cytotoxicity of cytokines in cerebral microvascular endothelial cell.* Brain Res, 2003. 990(1-2): p. 148-56.

[80] Kroemer, G. and S.J. Martin, *Caspase-independent cell death.* Nat Med, 2005. 11(7): p. 725-30.

[81] Garnier, P., et al., *Hypoxia induces caspase-9 and caspase-3 activation without neuronal death in gerbil brains.* Eur J Neurosci, 2004. 20(4): p. 937-46.

[82] Zehendner, C.M., et al., *Caspase-3 contributes to ZO-1 and Cl-5 tight-junction disruption in rapid anoxic neurovascular unit damage.* PLoS One, 2011. 6(2): p. e16760.

[83] Lopez-Ramirez, M.A., et al., *Role of caspases in cytokine-induced barrier breakdown in human brain endothelial cells.* J Immunol, 2012. 189(6): p. 3130-9.

[84] McQuaid, S., et al., *The effects of blood-brain barrier disruption on glial cell function in multiple sclerosis.* Biochem Soc Trans, 2009. 37(Pt 1): p. 329-31.

[85] Ballabh, P., A. Braun, and M. Nedergaard, *The blood-brain barrier: an overview: structure, regulation, and clinical implications.* Neurobiol Dis, 2004. 16(1): p. 1-13.

[86] Plumb, J., et al., *Abnormal endothelial tight junctions in active lesions and normal-appearing white matter in multiple sclerosis.* Brain Pathol, 2002. 12(2): p. 154-69.

[87] Rosenberg, G.A. and Y. Yang, *Vasogenic edema due to tight junction disruption by matrix metalloproteinases in cerebral ischemia.* Neurosurg Focus, 2007. 22(5): p. E4.

[88] Cheng, T., et al., *Activated protein C inhibits tissue plasminogen activator-induced brain hemorrhage.* Nat Med, 2006. 12(11): p. 1278-85.

[89] Zlokovic, B.V., *Remodeling after stroke.* Nat Med, 2006. 12(4): p. 390-1.

[90] Romanitan, M.O., et al., *Occludin is overexpressed in Alzheimer's disease and vascular dementia.* J Cell Mol Med, 2007. 11(3): p. 569-79.

[91] Yang, Y., et al., *Matrix metalloproteinase-mediated disruption of tight junction proteins in cerebral vessels is reversed by synthetic matrix metalloproteinase inhibitor in focal ischemia in rat.* J Cereb Blood Flow Metab, 2007. 27(4): p. 697-709.

[92] Wu, Z., et al., *Role of the MEOX2 homeobox gene in neurovascular dysfunction in Alzheimer disease.* Nat Med, 2005. 11(9): p. 959-65.

[93] Zlokovic, B., *Can blood-brain barrier play a role in the development of cerebral amyloidosis and Alzheimer's disease pathology.* Neurobiol Dis, 1997. 4(1): p. 23-6.

[94] Mackic, J.B., et al., *Human blood-brain barrier receptors for Alzheimer's amyloid-beta 1- 40. Asymmetrical binding, endocytosis, and transcytosis at the apical side of brain microvascular endothelial cell monolayer.* J Clin Invest, 1998. 102(4): p. 734-43.

[95] Yan, S.D., et al., *RAGE and amyloid-beta peptide neurotoxicity in Alzheimer's disease.* Nature, 1996. 382(6593): p. 685-91.

[96] Deane, R., et al., *RAGE mediates amyloid-beta peptide transport across the blood-brain barrier and accumulation in brain.* Nat Med, 2003. 9(7): p. 907-13.

[97] Girouard, H. and C. Iadecola, *Neurovascular coupling in the normal brain and in hypertension, stroke, and Alzheimer disease.* J Appl Physiol (1985), 2006. 100(1): p. 328-35.

[98] Zlokovic, B.V., *Neurovascular mechanisms of Alzheimer's neurodegeneration.* Trends Neurosci, 2005. 28(4): p. 202-8.

[99] Bailey, T.L., et al., *The nature and effects of cortical microvascular pathology in aging and Alzheimer's disease.* Neurol Res, 2004. 26(5): p. 573-8.

[100] Zlokovic, B.V., *The blood-brain barrier in health and chronic neurodegenerative disorders.* Neuron, 2008. 57(2): p. 178-201.

[101] Man, S., E.E. Ubogu, and R.M. Ransohoff, *Inflammatory cell migration into the central nervous system: a few new twists on an old tale.* Brain Pathol, 2007. 17(2): p. 243-50.

[102] Buee, L., P.R. Hof, and A. Delacourte, *Brain microvascular changes in Alzheimer's disease and other dementias.* Ann N Y Acad Sci, 1997. 826: p. 7-24.

[103] Weller, R.O. and J.A. Nicoll, *Cerebral amyloid angiopathy: both viper and maggot in the brain.* Ann Neurol, 2005. 58(3): p. 348-50.

[104] Rensink, A.A., et al., *Pathogenesis of cerebral amyloid angiopathy.* Brain Res Brain Res Rev, 2003. 43(2): p. 207-23.

[105] Vinters, H.V., et al., *Microvasculature in brain biopsy specimens from patients with Alzheimer's disease: an immunohistochemical and ultrastructural study.* Ultrastruct Pathol, 1994. 18(3): p. 333-48.

[106] Kalaria, R.N. and P. Hedera, *Differential degeneration of the cerebral microvasculature in Alzheimer's disease.* Neuroreport, 1995. 6(3): p. 477-80.

[107] Selkoe, D.J., *Alzheimer's disease: genes, proteins, and therapy.* Physiol Rev, 2001. 81(2): p. 741-66.

[108] Claudio, L., *Ultrastructural features of the blood-brain barrier in biopsy tissue from Alzheimer's disease patients.* Acta Neuropathol, 1996. 91(1): p. 6-14.

[109] Shibata, M., et al., *Clearance of Alzheimer's amyloid-ss(1-40) peptide from brain by LDL receptor-related protein-1 at the blood-brain barrier.* J Clin Invest, 2000. 106(12): p. 1489-99.

[110] Citron, M., et al., *Evidence that the 42- and 40-amino acid forms of amyloid beta protein are generated from the beta-amyloid precursor protein by different protease activities.* Proc Natl Acad Sci U S A, 1996. 93(23): p. 13170-5.

[111] Tabaton, M., et al., *Soluble amyloid beta-protein is a marker of Alzheimer amyloid in brain but not in cerebrospinal fluid.* Biochem Biophys Res Commun, 1994. 200(3): p. 1598-603.

[112] Masters, C.L., et al., *Amyloid plaque core protein in Alzheimer disease and Down syndrome.* Proc Natl Acad Sci U S A, 1985. 82(12): p. 4245-9.

[113] Wisniewski, T., J. Ghiso, and B. Frangione, *Biology of A beta amyloid in Alzheimer's disease.* Neurobiol Dis, 1997. 4(5): p. 313-28.

[114] Mattson, M.P. and R.E. Rydel, *Alzheimer's disease. Amyloid ox-tox transducers.* Nature, 1996. 382(6593): p. 674-5.

[115] Thomas, T., et al., *beta-Amyloid-mediated vasoactivity and vascular endothelial damage.* Nature, 1996. 380(6570): p. 168-71.

[116] Roher, A.E., et al., *beta-Amyloid-(1-42) is a major component of cerebrovascular amyloid deposits: implications for the pathology of Alzheimer disease.* Proc Natl Acad Sci U S A, 1993. 90(22): p. 10836-40.

[117] Mirra, S.S., M.N. Hart, and R.D. Terry, *Making the diagnosis of Alzheimer's disease. A primer for practicing pathologists.* Arch Pathol Lab Med, 1993. 117(2): p. 132-44.

[118] Griffin, W.S., et al., *Interleukin-1 expression in different plaque types in Alzheimer's disease: significance in plaque evolution.* J Neuropathol Exp Neurol, 1995. 54(2): p. 276-81.

[119] Hull, M., et al., *Occurrence of interleukin-6 in cortical plaques of Alzheimer's disease patients may precede transformation of diffuse into neuritic plaques.* Ann N Y Acad Sci, 1996. 777: p. 205-12.

[120] Quintanilla, R.A., et al., *Interleukin-6 induces Alzheimer-type phosphorylation of tau protein by deregulating the cdk5/p35 pathway.* Exp Cell Res, 2004. 295(1): p. 245-57.

[121] Biere, A.L., et al., *Amyloid beta-peptide is transported on lipoproteins and albumin in human plasma.* J Biol Chem, 1996. 271(51): p. 32916-22.

[122] Mecocci, P., et al., *Blood-brain-barrier in a geriatric* population: barrier function in degenerative and vascular dementias. Acta Neurol Scand, 1991. 84(3): p. 210-3.

[123] Mattila, K.M., et al., Altered blood-brain-barrier function in Alzheimer's disease? Acta Neurol Scand, 1994. 89(3): p. 192-8.

Chapter 4

# Metals Involvement in Alzheimer's Disease — A Patho-Genetic View

Carlo Salustri, Mariacristina Siotto,
Serena Bucossi and Rosanna Squitti

Additional information is available at the end of the chapter

http://dx.doi.org/10.5772/60447

## 1. Introduction

As Alois Alzheimer himself first observed, the brain of an individual affected by Alzheimer's disease (AD) shows aggregations of the peptide beta-amyloid (Aβ) and tau proteins, which form characteristic plaques and neurofibrillary tangles respectively [1].

Since Aβ is known to participate in many normal body functions, its precipitation into plaques, often referred to as 'amyloid cascade', has been for a long time the only recognized, yet unexplained mechanism of AD pathogenesis [2]. In time, however, diverse phenomena, such as oxidative stress, aberrant inflammations, impaired energy metabolism and more have been gradually discovered to contribute to the cascade [3].

The observation that Aβ aggregation in plaques is an age-dependent phenomenon, whereas Aβ production is not, suggested that some other age-dependent mechanism must play a role in transforming Aβ into a neurotoxic element. The fact that some metals, such as copper and zinc, are known to modulate glutamatergic neurotransmission [4] led researchers to hypothesize that late-age abnormalities in the homeostasis of one or more transition metals may play a role in the amyloid cascade.

Moreover, much evidence gathered on AD depicts an improperly functioning ceruloplasmin, an enzyme synthesized by the liver, which controls iron oxidization state. There is also evidence that a functional failure of systemic ceruloplasmin may be behind the iron-related redox processes that produce oxidative stress in the AD brain [5, 6]. Ceruloplasmin is the 'crosstalk' factor linking copper to iron metabolism, thus its failure is very likely to be a major actor in the dysfunctional metal metabolism affecting AD individuals. Aβ may gain toxicity upon some interaction with copper, in a process involving ceruloplasmin, even though the molecular mechanism still remains elusive.

This notion was further supported by the fact that the Amyloid precursor protein (APP) was discovered to possess selective copper binding sites, which mediate redox activities causing precipitation of Aβ even at low concentrations [7]. Aβ itself has been reported to possess selective high- and low-affinity metal-binding sites which, in normal conditions, bind equimolar amounts of either copper or zinc but, in conditions of acidosis, see zinc completely displaced by copper [8]. Thus, hyper-metallation was suggested to be the mechanism that gives Aβ its redox properties, triggering redox cycles through production of $H_2O_2$ that lead to self-oxidation of Aβ, formation of oligomers with diverse grades of complexity and finally to Aβ precipitation into plaques (Figure 1) [4, 9].

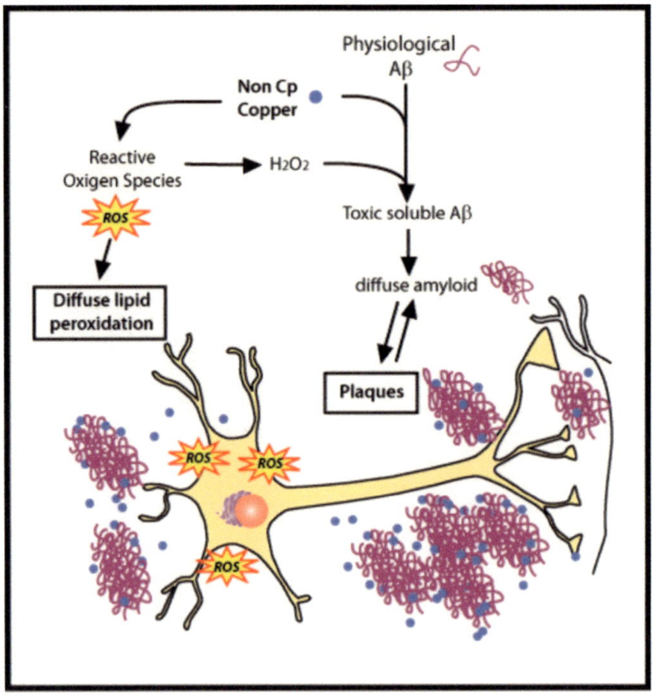


**Figure 1.** Systemic Non-Cp-copper in AD passes through the Blood Brain Barrier and causes an imbalance of copper in the brain. Here Non-Cp-copper can interact with physiological amyloid-β (Aβ), forming clusters of metal-toxic soluble Aβ that evolve in diffuse amyloid and, finally, in toxic plaques. Non-Cp-Copper can also interact with reactive oxygen species (ROS), which are responsible for lipid peroxidation in neuron membranes, protein oxidation, and cleavage of DNA and RNA molecules.

Diverse animal studies support the toxic role of copper in AD pathogenesis.

White et al. [10] showed that the copper contents of both liver and cerebral cortex in $APP^{-/-}$ and amyloid precursor-like protein ($APLP2^{-/-}$) knockout mice were significantly increased, supporting the authors' hypothesis that the *APP* gene modulates hepatic and cortical copper levels. However, the mechanism leading to increased brain copper content (due to *APP* gene knockout) remains known. Serum copper levels were not significantly more altered in *APP*$^{-/-}$ and *APLP2*$^{-/-}$ mice than in wild-type mice. It appears that a failure of copper excretion from the brain to the blood or, more likely, an imbalance of copper distribution between the Cp-bound and unbound fractions could be associated with the deposition of excessive copper levels in the brain in this knockout model. Besides demonstrating that the AβPP is an important regulator of brain copper homeostasis, White et al. also demonstrated that it potentiates the Aβ-mediated neurotoxicity by increasing oxidative stress.

Sparks and Schreurs [11] demonstrated that adding 0.12 ppm (0.12 mg/L) of copper to water given to a cholesterol-fed rabbit AD-model resulted in significantly enhanced cognitive waning and also exacerbated amyloid plaque deposition. This finding led to serious concerns in some Government Environmental Agencies about the content of copper in drinking water delivered to households via copper pipes. It must be kept in mind that cholesterol, though vital for neuronal transmission, synaptic plasticity and cell function, is also a well-established risk factor for atherosclerosis and AD [12]. Cholesterol to 7-hydroxy cholesterol oxidation, caused by Aβ, is extremely toxic for neurons [13]. Cp levels measured using o-dianisidine dihydrochloride as a substrate in the plasma of cholesterol-fed rabbit model after adding copper to drinking water, suggest an increase, although the change did not reach statistical significance. This suggests that a Non-Cp copper increase is a vehicle of copper within the brain.

In a different investigation [14], Sparks reconfirmed this earlier finding, reporting that other animal models, like spontaneously hyper-cholesterolemic Watanabe rabbits, cholesterol-fed beagles and rabbits, and *PS1* and *APP* transgenic mice showed considerably increased brain levels of Aβ when given copper-rich (0.12 ppm) drinking water. Notably, non-cholesterol fed *PS1* and *APP* transgenic mice models of AD demonstrated significantly enhanced levels of Aβ due to copper exposure via drinking water, demonstrating that the mouse model of AD exhibits vulnerability to copper even in the absence of cholesterol in the diet. This observation highlights the fact that both cholesterol and copper are separate causative factors whose interaction further enhances the formation of Aβ plaques.

In another study [15], Lu at al. confirmed the findings of Sparks and colleagues'. The authors demonstrated that Kunming strain mice fed with a high-cholesterol diet and distilled water containing 0.21 ppm copper exhibited significantly increased level of *APP* mRNA, coupled with the activation of caspase-3 in the brain, suggesting apoptosis mediated neurotoxicity. Strikingly, copper also increased cholesterol-induced learning and memory impairment in mice.

Moreover, it has been reported [16] that, in Sprague-Dawley rats, which underwent bilateral common carotid artery occlusion (2VO) and were administered with 250 ppm copper containing water for 3 months, chronic copper toxicity exacerbated memory impairment induced by 2VO coupled with an augmented expression of brain AβPP and β-site AβPP-cleaving enzyme 1 (BACE1) at both mRNA and protein levels. However, these copper-aggravated changes were ameliorated after copper was withdrawn from the drinking water.

As a whole, these experimental animal models demonstrated the toxicity mediated by copper in the AD cascade, showing that increased level of copper ingested with drinking water, or more generally through the diet, affects AD neuropathology.

All this evidence has eventually led to the proposal of the so called Metal Hypothesis of AD (Bush et al. 2008), which is based on the concept that it is the interaction of Aβ with specific metals, especially copper, that actually drives the amyloid cascade and AD pathogenesis.

One question remained: how does copper actually reach the brain? In fact, we normally ingest copper through the diet - via food, drinking water, beverage, supplements - and copper status in the body is regulated by the balance between duodenal absorption (intestine) and biliary excretion (liver). After crossing the intestinal lumen, copper is transported via portal circulation to the liver, where it is partly stored and partly redistributed to other organs. In the hepatocyte, copper is incorporated into ceruloplasmin, whose dimensions don't allow an easy crossing of the blood-brain-barrier (BBB).

An answer to the question came with the discovery that, although the vast majority of human copper circulates tightly bound to ceruloplasmin [17, 18], a faulty copper metabolism leads to the creation of a small pool of copper that goes into circulation loosely bound to and constantly exchanged among albumin, $\alpha 2$ macroglobulin, peptides, amino acids and other low-molecular-weight compounds. Due to the loose character of the bindings, this portion is normally referred to as Non Ceruloplasmin copper (Non–Cp copper). The key difference between bound (to ceruloplasmin) and Non-Cp copper lies in the fact that the low-molecular-weight compounds can easily cross the BBB [18], thus carrying Non-Cp copper into the brain. There, copper can enter cycles of Haber-Weiss or Fenton reactions producing ·OH, against which our body has no defenses [19], and generate pleiotropic effects on the amyloid cascade [3].

The metal hypothesis has also gained support from consistent reports of enhanced concentrations of labile copper in areas of the brain that are considered critical for AD [20].

There is by now a solid body of literature reporting *in vitro* [8, 21, 22], experimental (reviewed in [23, 24]) and clinical evidence gathered over the last years which have shown that some systemic abnormalities in copper metabolism are shared between the AD and the Wilson's disease (WD). Wilson's disease is the paradigmatic disease of copper toxicosis or accumulation [18]. Although much less severe than in WD, it has been shown that the increases in Non-Cp copper correlate with some typical AD deficits, with the 'core' markers of AD in the cerebrospinal fluid [25], a poor prognosis of the disease [26], and the conversion from Mild Cognitive Impairment (MCI) to full dementia [27]. Meta-analyses have confirmed increased levels of total copper and Non-Cp copper in general circulation of AD patients compared with healthy control subjects [28-30]. A higher intake of copper in the diet was also associated with cognitive decline or with an increase in overall mortality. Specifically, in the 'Chicago Health and Aging Project' (3718 subjects followed from 1993 to 2002), a diet with a content of 2.75 mg / day of copper on average, along with a high saturated and trans fat intake, has been proved to be associated with cognitive decline, which was estimated to be equivalent to an extra nineteen years of aging [31]. In the 'Iowa Women's Health Study' (38772 older women followed from

1986 to 2008), the use of dietary supplements of copper has been shown to be associated with a 18% increase in total mortality [32]. Recently, it was shown that the increase of copper in the soil in 26 provinces and 3 municipal districts in China, between 1991 and 2000, is associated with an increased AD-related mortality. In geographic areas with higher concentrations of copper, the relative risk of AD-related death is 2.6 times higher than that in geographical areas with a lower content copper in the soil [33].

Also results of a recently completed Phase II clinical trial, based on using metal attenuating complexing compounds or Zinc therapy [34-37], appear to support the notion of a copper dysfunction in AD. The available evidence has now reached such a quantitative and qualitative level that the notion of a copper-related phenotype in AD has now started to be accepted [23]. This is a very important step, since many translational hypotheses may develop from this notion, in terms of both diagnostic and prognostic tools, with important repercussions in terms of preventive and therapeutic approaches. However, most of the literature dealing with the relationship between copper and AD focuses on local copper abnormal distribution, especially in those specific areas of the brain that are considered critical for the disease. Recently, this vision has started to appear limited. There is now a bulk of evidence suggesting that all modifications should be viewed in a wider framework of systemic, rather than local, metal dishomeostasis. This concept can be better understood looking at recent studies of the link between the status of serum ceruloplasmin and AD clinical signs and/or Aβ markers in the CSF [23]. Torsdottir et al. [38] reported a decrease in ceruloplasmin activity in AD patients. Lower levels of circulating ceruloplasmin in AD patients with different CSF markers of AD were reported by Brewer's [39], Arnal's [40] and Kessler's [41] groups. In 2008, our laboratory demonstrated a consistent and measurable increase of apo-ceruloplasmin (a defective form of ceruloplasmin, lacking copper and its ferroxidase activity) in the serum and CSF of AD patients [42, 43].

Since both WD and the early-onset form of AD are known to have a genetic origin determining the hereditability of the disease, researchers have embarked in a wide range of studies in the attempt to find genes that cause the late-onset AD or at least contribute to it via damaging phenomena, such as oxidative stress, inflammation, apoptosis or an increased expression of Aβ. In order to encompass as much as possible of the huge genome world, researchers have also embarked in so-called large-scale genome-wide association studies (GWAS). These studies search for DNA sequence variations that appear more common in individuals with a certain disease than in individuals without that disease. GWAS typically analyze a multitude of single gene variations, generally called single-nucleotide polymorphisms (SNPs), and verify their association, if any, with the traits of a disease.

## 2. AD and *APOE*

So far, no specific gene has been found that can be reliably considered a cause of AD. Even genes, whose mutations have been found responsible for early-onset AD, appear to have a minor, or at least not a pivotal role in the late-onset form. However, numerous risk factors have been identified in the last few years. Historically, the first one to be established is the inheritance of the ε4 allele of the apolipoprotein E (*APOE*), found on chromosome 19. *APOE* is the gene encoding the protein that carries cholesterol and other fats into circulation and manifests itself in a number of alleles, of which ε2, ε3 and ε4 are the most common. The allele ε3, the most common of the three, appears totally unrelated to the risk of developing AD. The slightly less common ε4, instead, has been definitely established to increase the risk of developing AD. The rare variant ε2 seems instead to provide some form of protection by delaying the onset age of the disease.

Individuals inherit two copies of the *APOE* gene, one from each parent, which can be different alleles. If one of the inherited alleles is ε4, the carrier has about a 3-fold increased risk of developing AD. Two copies of ε4 make this risk is much higher, reaching a 15-fold increase of the risk. In other words, it can be stated that *APOE*ε4 carriers have a 90% statistical risk of contracting AD if they are heterozygote and close to 100% if homozygote [44].

It must be emphasized, though, that we are dealing here with statistical risk: in fact, not all individuals who have one or two ε4 develop AD and AD occurs also in people who have no ε4. Thus, *APOE*ε4 is a 'susceptibility' gene, i.e., a gene that affects risk but is not the cause.

## 3. Other genes

The fact that *APOE*ε4 is neither necessary nor sufficient for the development of the disease has supported the quest for more genetic risk factors and GWAS have led to the identification of numerous genes now widely accepted as risk factors for AD. Major examples include:

*CLU* – The *CLU* gene on chromosome 8 encodes the protein clusterin, or apolipoprotein J, which is implicated in multiple biological processes, such as lipid transport, membrane recycling, cell adhesion and apoptosis. Two GWAS have independently found a statistical association between a SNP within *CLU* and the risk of having AD [45, 46]. Despite the fact that people who already have AD have more clusterin in their blood, and that clusterin blood levels correlate with faster cognitive decline in individuals with AD, there is no indication that levels of this protein can predict the onset of AD.

*SORL1* – an *APOE* receptor in the neural system. Some variants on chromosome 11 have been related to AD [47], since a significant decrease in their expression has been found in AD patients and some authors have described a link between *SORL1* and APP regulation.

*CR1* – encodes the protein C3b/C4b receptor, whose deficiency may contribute to chronic inflammation in the brain. Some specific variant of this gene have been identified as contributors to AD [46, 47].

*PICALM* - located on chromosome 11, encodes phosphatidylinositol-binding clathrin assembly protein, which is linked to the process by which brain nerve cells (neurons) communicate with each other. GWAS have identified several functional SNPs in the *PICALM* gene [45-50]

In AD, GWAS have consistently shown that the effect size and the strength of association of *APOE* variants are greater than the best of *APOE*-unrelated associations. This stresses the relevance of *APOE* as risk factor for AD, although also other explanations should be considered: firstly, most GWAS do not study the variants' true susceptibility but are rather based on the identification of their tagging markers. The latter generally show much greater heterogeneity than the former in terms of both alleles and extent of linkage. Consequently, it is possible that some variants have in reality bigger effect sizes than the ones seen by GWAS. Secondly, current GWAS platforms are often insufficient to detect rare variants. Thus, the existence of some variants that have a big effect size but happen to be rare can remain undetected. Moreover, the linear modeling framework often used in GWASs considers only one SNP at a time, thus ignoring the genomic and environmental context of each SNP [51]. This is an important limitation since the genotype-phenotype relationship is most likely characterized by significant genetic heterogeneity and complex gene-gene and gene-environment interactions [52]. Recently, there has been a shift away from the 'one SNP at a time' method toward a more holistic approach that includes the gene's environmental context.

Another approach is selecting a candidate gene on the basis of hypotheses regarding the disease and then analyze all sequence changes of that gene. Direct sequencing has proven an effective way to discover rare variants with large effect sizes. Recently, studies using next-generation sequencing have led to the identification of rare frequency coding variants in *PLD3* [53] and *TREM2* genes [54, 55] associated with the risk of AD.

### 3.1. *ATP7A* and *ATP7B*

Two serious disorders are today recognized to be due to a dyshomeostasis in copper metabolism: Menkes disease (MD) and Wilson's disease (WD). Both are caused by a mutation of one gene: *ATP7A* in MD and *ATP7B* in WD, which generate a dysfunction of the proteins they encode: ATP7A and ATP7B, respectively [56]. These two proteins are copper pump proteins or transporting ATPase and, although they have somewhat different distributions in diverse cell types, both are key in regulating copper levels in the body.

The *ATP7A* gene is located on the long (q) arm of the X chromosome. The protein it encodes, ATP7A, is found virtually everywhere in the body except in the liver and delivers copper wherever it is needed within tissue cells. In the small intestine, it contributes to control the absorption of copper from food. Mutations of the *ATP7A* gene lead to synthesis of dysfunctional proteins, of which some engage in disorderly copper transport while others are even unable to bind the metal. More than 100 mutations the have been identified as causes of MD.

*ATP7B* is a gene of chromosome 13, expressed mainly in the liver, although it has also been detected in the brain, heart, kidney, lung, mammary gland and placenta [57]. The protein it encodes, ATP7B, maintains the body copper homeostasis. In the hepatocyte, ATP7B receives copper from ATOX1 and it moves across the trans Golgi network where it incorporates this metal into apo-ceruloplasmin generating a holo-active form. When intracellular copper levels exceed cell needs, ATP7B moves toward the bile canaliculi and carries out the excretion of copper [58].

Technically, mutations of the two genes have somewhat opposite effects: in MD, the dysfunctional *ATP7A* results in an unbalanced distribution of copper throughout the body. Copper accumulates in some tissues while it remains insufficient in others, where the decreased supply reduces the activity of enzymes that are necessary for the health of numerous body parts, such as bone, skin, blood vessels, and the nervous system. In WD, instead, the dysfunctional ATP7B causes: (i) a failure in the incorporation of copper into the holo-ceruloplasmin, resulting in increased levels of Non-Cp copper being released into the blood stream and in low circulating levels of that protein; (ii) decreased levels of copper released into the bile canaliculi, causing cell over-feeding and intracellular copper deposits, which accelerate apoptotic cell death [59].

We know that in WD huge amounts of Non-Cp copper enter the brain through the BBB, where labile copper accumulates and leads to neurodegeneration. WD is considered the hallmark of copper toxicosis.

Since increased copper levels characterizing WD are shared in a smaller scale by AD patients, the *ATP7B* gene and its variations have of course become the focus of much of our research focusing on copper. Some authors have expressed doubts about this research direction by pointing out that neurodegeneration in WD leads to movement disorders with little or no effect on cognition, while AD neurodegeneration affects chiefly cognition. Moreover, onset ages are very different in the two pathologies as WD appears typically in childhood, whereas late-onset AD by definition after 60-65y. In other words, even accepting the fact that the two pathologies share copper toxicity, manifestations are so different that it seems unreasonable to claim that the same gene causes both of them. In reply to this valid concern, other authors have argued that *ATP7B* has a high variability. Thus, the possibility that this gene is a causative gene for WD when in homozygosis and a susceptibility gene for AD (interacting with environmental factors and other risk genes) cannot be ruled out. Other genes have shown unexpected diverse effects. *ATP7A*, for example, which is causative of MD, has been recently recognized to be associated with a mild form of occipital horn syndrome [60]. Moreover, recent evidence has demonstrated that certain missense mutations of this gene can cause a syndrome restricted to progressive distal motor neuropathy even without signs of copper deficiency [61].

Our laboratory has pursued the link between copper and AD pathogenesis on the assumption that the excessive Non-Cp copper production in the body is actually due to a faulty ATP7B causing a flaw in the incorporation of copper into nascent ceruloplasmin in the liver [56]. On this basis, we have embarked in an extensive study of the *ATP7B* gene and of the protein ATP7B, which is the only one known to catalyze that incorporation.

Unfortunately, analysis of the *ATP7B* gene is not an easy task, due to its huge variability. The 1000 Genomes project has identified 1,358 variations of *ATP7B* in human populations. At least 500 of them have been recognized as disease-causing [62]. Worldwide detection of *ATP7B* mutations is actually difficult [63] since most mutations are rare, reported only within single families and often prevalent in specific ethnic groups [32]. As a result, the database regarding both the gene's properties and the possible dysfunctions of the proteins they encode is still largely insufficient [64].

The first significant information on the structure of the ATP7B protein was gained from a homology modeling study [65]. Some more light was later shed by nuclear magnetic resonance (NMR) spectroscopy studies [66-70]. Recently, significant progress in the comprehension of

ATP7B structural organization has come from the solution of the crystal structure of the bacterial copper ATPase LCopA [71]. The LCopA protein model has been employed as a template to analyze ATP7B core domain on the basis of its sequence homology to build interpretations of WD mutations [64].

We know that mutations leading to a complete abolition of ATP7B function, chiefly early stop mutations and mutations in regions of the gene that have a high functional importance, lead to an early and predominantly hepatic dysfunction. Conversely, point mutations in regions that are functionally less important are associated with a later onset and predominantly neurological or psychiatric dysfunctions [17].

An effective strategy to characterize genetic compositions, which has become popular in recent years, is the so-called *in-silico* analysis, i.e., performed via computer simulations. Several computational procedures have been developed to analyze the effects of genetic variants on the protein function. The advantage of this type of analysis is that it allows analysis of huge amounts of data, delivered by high-throughput sequencing technologies, in relatively short time. These procedures take into account different factors associated with the protein properties, such as chemistry constraints, three dimensional structure, and amino acid sequences of homologous and orthologous proteins [72].

Our laboratory has used a new in-silico approach based on amino acid sequence, utilizing four among the most used bioinformatics tools (i.e. Polyphen- 2, SIFT, Panther, and PhD-SNPs). We have applied this approach to non-synonymous SNP (nsSNPs) detected in the *ATP7B* gene to profile WD-causing and WD-non-causing mutations, while obtaining at the same time useful information about the gene's domains that could potentially harbor loci of susceptibility for other disorders related to copper metabolism [73].

### 3.2. rs7323774 and rs2147363

In pursuit of the identification of regions in the *ATP7B* gene linked to copper dishomeostasis, our laboratory has embarked in an investigation of the association between copper-related biochemical markers in serum (bound copper, Non-Cp copper and ceruloplasmin) and variants of the *ATP7B* gene.

In one study of 399 AD patients and 303 healthy elderly controls, we focused our attention on a set of four SNPs that had been reported to be informative of the *ATP7B* gene structure [74]: rs1801243 (missense substitution: Ser406Ala), rs2147363 (intronic variant: c.1544-53A>C), rs1061472 (missense substitution: Lys832Arg) and rs732774 (missense substitution: Arg952Lys). We had already found in a previous study that those SNPs among the four that lay in the transmembrane domains appear to have an association with AD [75].

We first stratified the AD and control groups into three 'classes' according to their Non-Cp copper levels: 'low Non-Cp copper' (<1 μmol/L), 'medium Non-Cp copper' (≥1, <1.6 μmol/L) and 'high Non-Cp copper' (≥1.6 μmol/L) (Figure 2). Results showed antithetic distributions for patients and controls: the 'low Non-Cp copper' class accounted for 27% of AD cases vs. 61% of controls; the 'medium Non-Cp copper' for 11% of AD vs. 10% of controls and the 'high Non-Cp copper' for 62% of AD versus 29% of controls. The serum copper profile was then analyzed in relation to the selected gene variants in the sole 'high Non-Cp copper' class (patients with AD, n = 109; controls, n = 53).

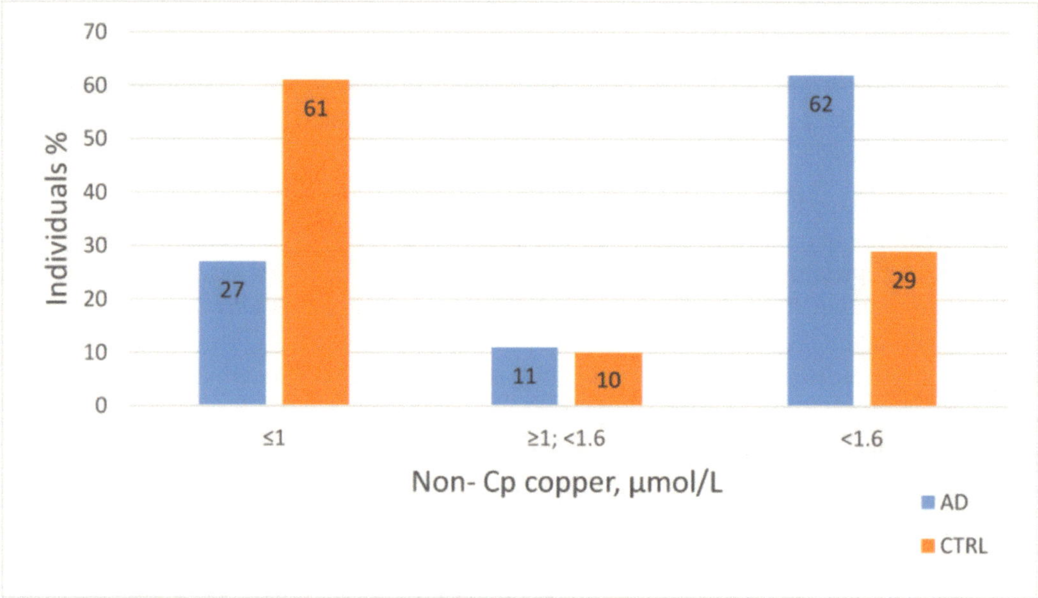


**Figure 2.** Stratification of the AD and control groups (CTRL) into three 'classes' according to their Non-Cp copper levels: 'low Non-Cp copper' (<1 µmol/L), 'medium Non-Cp copper' (≥1, <1.6 µmol/L) and 'high Non-Cp copper' (≥1.6 µmol/L). The bar graph reports the percentage of AD (first bar from left) and CTRL (second bar from left) for each class.

The main result of this study was that individuals who are GG homozygous for *ATP7B* rs7323774 SNP have higher levels of Non-Cp copper in their serum. This was true for the entire sample of patients and controls but was definitely more pronounced in AD individuals. Non-Cp copper distributions of AD patients turned out antithetic to those of controls and results showed that this is due to those *ATP7B* variants that are located in regions encoding ATP7B transmembrane domains, i.e., variants that we know to be associated with copper dyshomeostasis in AD. It must be noted, however, that we selected the variants on the basis of the information they could deliver on the *ATP7B* gene structure, not for their impact on gene function. Consequently, it is obvious that rs1801243, rs2147363, rs1061472 and rs732774, even though significantly associated with AD [74], could not be the loci responsible for the effects of the *ATP7B* gene on AD, either in terms of Non-Cp copper derangement or in terms of an increased risk of the AD [76].

In another study of 286 AD patients and 283 controls we focused on the rs2147363 and rs7334118 variants of the *ATP7B* gene. All genotype frequencies in our controls were within the ranges reported previously in the European origin populations of the HapMap project (available on http://hapmap.ncbi.nlm.nih.gov).

http://dx.doi.org/10.5772/60447

We analyzed the genetic association between SNPs and AD risk. Our study revealed a significant association between rs2147363 and AD. When data were adjusted for confounding variables (i.e., age, gender, and *APOE* genotype), significant results were obtained for the recessive model (OR: 1.63, 95% CI: 1.03–2.57; p = 0.035) and Log-additive model (OR: 1.51, 95% CI: 1.05–2.16; p = 0.025).

In order to verify whether rs2147363 has any functional variants in LD, we also analyzed the SNPs that showed a complete LD (D' = 1) with this *ATP7B* variant in Tuscans in Italy (TSI), which is the HapMap population most genetically related to our sample. We identified ten SNPs in complete LD with the rs2147363. We prioritized these variants using FastSNP. This analysis highlighted that one variant is a non-synonymous SNP (medium-high risk), four are intronic enhancers (very low-low risk), four are intronic with no known function (no effect), and one is a downstream variant with no known function (no effect) (Table 1).

| SNP ID (rs) | Possible Functional Effects | Region | SIFT | PolyPhen2 |
|---|---|---|---|---|
| *rs7334118* | *Missense (non-conservative); Splicing regulation* | *coding* | *Damaging* | *Possibly Damaging* |
| **rs4943053** | Intronic enhancer | intronic | - | - |
| **rs9535803** | Intronic enhancer | intronic | - | - |
| **rs9535809** | Intronic enhancer | intronic | - | - |
| **rs2147362** | Intronic enhancer | intronic | - | - |
| **rs11839458** | Intronic with unknown function | intronic | - | - |
| **rs9526820** | Intronic with unknown function | intronic | - | - |
| **rs9535827** | Intronic with unknown function | intronic | - | - |
| **rs9535794** | Downstream with unknown function | 3-UTR | - | - |
| **rs9535806** | Intronic with unknown function | intronic | - | - |

**Table 1.** Prioritization and functional analysis of *ATP7B* SNPs in LD with **rs2147363**.

To predict the functional impact of the non-synonymous SNP (rs7334118), we used two different bioinformatics tools: SIFT and Polyphen2. The application of both the SIFT algorithm using orthologous sequences and the Polyphen2 tool highlighted that this coding variant may have an adverse effect on the ATP7B protein.

To verify the hypothesis that genetic association of rs2147363 is due to LD with the rs7334118 SNP, 176 AD subjects and 169 healthy controls among the study population were genotyped for the SNP rs7334118. Two AD patients were carriers of the rs7334118G allele, whereas no healthy individual with this *ATP7B* mutation was identified. Even though this coding variant was identified only in AD patients, its allele frequency in the AD group is in line with the minor allele frequency observed in a general population of European origin (information available at dbSNP). Thus, this result has to be confirmed in a bigger healthy control sample.

To test whether the intronic region, in which rs2147363 is located, plays a role in the regulation of the *ATP7B* gene function, the GERP++ and is-rSNP algorithms were used. rs2147363 nucleotide position resulted non-conserved, whereas, in the intronic region around this SNP, 7 nucleotide positions on the 16 analyzed (43%) achieve the GERP threshold [77]. Table 2 describes the findings of the is-rSNP algorithm. This analysis predicted the presence of binding sites of 8 transcription factors (TF) binding sites, and, in two cases (i.e., Zfp423 and PLAG1), the prediction results were significant (adjusted $p < 0.05$). The main result of this detailed genetic analysis is that the significant association between rs2147363 SNP and AD can be explained on the basis of the presence of TFs binding sites in the region in which this variant is located. Thereby, rs2147363 may be associated with a cis-regulatory function. Specifically, we observed two of the genetic models of rs2147363 SNP associated with AD: a recessive model that suggested a 1.63-fold increased, and a log-additive model that suggested a 1.51-fold increase in the risk of having AD. The Akaike Information Criterion (AIC) and Bayesian Information Criterion (BIC) analyses highlighted that log-additive model achieved the most reliable outcome. This suggests that C allele of rs2147363 SNP is additive: its presence in one gene copy will lead to an increase in AD risk; its presence in both gene copies will lead to a further increase. Additionally, we tested the reliability of our coding or noncoding hypotheses to explain this intronic association. When we considered the coding hypothesis, we analyzed the SNPs in complete LD (D' = 1) with rs2147363 in TSI. The functional prediction analysis showed that the SNP rs7334118 has a complete LD (D' = 1) with rs2147363. Moreover, rs7334118 has been recorded in the Wilson's Disease Mutation database (available at http://www.wilson-disease.med. ualberta.ca) and in Human Genome Mutation Database (available at http://www.hgmd.cf.ac.uk/) as a Wilson's disease-causing variant, it corresponds to H1207R, located into the P-domain, the domain in which phosphorylation of ATP7B occurs; in particular the residue lies in the ATP-hinge which connects the nucleotide-binding domain (N-domain) and the P-domain (Figure 3). Even though the genotype analysis in our case-control population revealed the presence of two carriers of the rs7334118G allele in AD patients and none in healthy controls, this *ATP7B* mutation could not alone explain the genetic association observed for rs2147363. Specifically, two AD patients heterozygous for the rs7334118G mutation were also carriers of the C allele in rs2147363 (1%). On the contrary, the other 166 AD patients, carriers of the C allele in rs2147363, were negative for the rs7334118 WD mutation (99%). However, this result does not exclude additional rare variants with large functional effects may explain this intronic association.

We used the HapMap database to identify functional coding variants, in which only few rare variants are present. Using other genomic databases, such as the database of 1,000 Genomes Project, may deliver new candidate variants that could be tested to explain our intronic association. Conversely, in-silico analyses on rs2147363 revealed that this intronic SNP can have a regulatory role on ATP7B function. In particular, the GERP analysis highlighted that the intronic region around rs2147363 resulted significantly conserved, and the is-rSNP algorithm significantly predicted the presence of two TF-binding sites in the rs2147363 region. These independent findings suggested that this genomic region has a regulatory function, and consequently rs2147363 can be associated with clinical phenotypes related to ATP7B dysfunction.

| Position | Nucleotide | GERP++ score |
|---|---|---|
| **chr13: 52542783** | **C** | **2.17** |
| **chr13: 52542784** | **A** | **2.37** |
| **chr13**: 52542785 | G | -7.84 |
| **chr13: 52542786** | **G** | **4.09** |
| **chr13**: 52542787 | G | 0.889 |
| **chr13**: 52542788 | C | -1.02 |
| **chr13**: 52542789 | C | 1.93 |
| **chr13**: 52542790 | T | -0.596 |
| **chr13: 52542791** | **C** | **4.11** |
| **chr13**: 52542792 | T | -3.02 |
| **chr13: 52542793** | **A** | **2.98** |
| **chr13**: 52542794 | G | -3.44 |
| **chr13: 52542795** | **G** | **2.55** |
| **chr13**: 52542796 | T | -7.19 |
| **chr13: 52542797** | **T** | **3.25** |
| **chr13: 52542798** | **G** | **4.87** |

**Table 2.** GERP analysis of the genomic region around rs2147363. Conserved positions are highlighted in bold.

Specifically, Zfp423 and PLAG1 have been predicted to have a binding-site in the genetic region of rs2147363. Both these TFs are involved in complex metabolic processes. For example, Zfp423 has been reported to regulate neural and adipocyte development [78], whereas *PLAG1* is a proto-oncogene that activates genes involved in uncontrolled cell proliferation (e.g., *IGFII, CRLF1, CRABP2, CRIP2,* and *PIGF*) [79]. In this framework, our data on Zfp423 support the hypothesis that *ATP7B* can be involved in molecular pathways linked to brain activity regulation, suggesting new perspectives in the interpretation of neurologic signs of WD and AD. This conclusion fits well with our original hypothesis that *ATP7B* can harbor variants that may account for some of the missing hereditability of AD [80]. In particular, the present data furnished a new insight into the copper hypothesis: non-coding regions can play a role in the *ATP7B* function, and, thereby, genetic variation in *ATP7B* cis-regulatory elements within non-coding regions may be associated with AD risk. Furthermore, genetic data adjusted for age confounding effect confirmed the association between rs2147363 and AD risk. However, although in-silico analyses support our hypothesis, further functional studies are necessary to confirm the role of non-coding variants in the *ATP7B* gene function and in AD risk.

| SNPs | Exon | ATP7B sequence NM_000053.3:c | ATP7B sequence NP_000044.2:p | ATP7B domains |
|---|---|---|---|---|
| rs1801243 | 2 | 1216T>G | missense substitution: Ser406Ala | Metal Binding Unit 4 |
| rs2147363 | Intron 3 | 1544-53A>C | - | - |
| rs1061472 | 10 | 2495A>G | missense substitution: Lys832Arg | A-domain |
| rs732774 | 12 | 2855G>A | missense substitution: Arg952Lys | Luminal Loop between TM5-TM6 |
| rs7334118 | 17 | 3620A>G | missense substitution: His1207Arg | P-domain: ATP hinge |

Linkage Disequilibrium

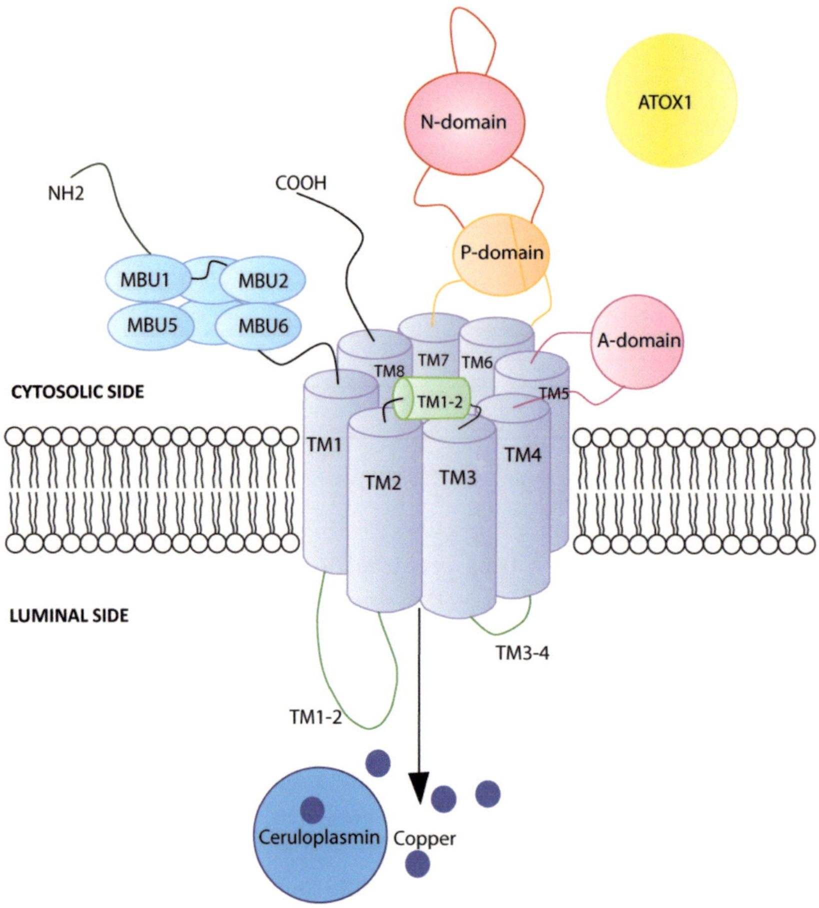


**Figure 3.** Schematic representation of human ATP7B on the basis of homology-modeled structure [71]. The table reports the *ATP7B* SNPs studied from our group and the specific nucleotide and amino acid substitutions, standing in a specific ATP7B domain.

### 3.3. K832R (rs1061472) and R952K (rs732774)

In a recent study, we focused our attention on two functional changes in the *ATP7B* gene in particular: K832R (rs1061472) and R952K (rs732774).

K832R corresponds to a non synonymous amino acid substitution and the corresponding AAG>AGG mutation in exon 10 specifies this amino acid change in the A-domain, within the ATP binding domain region of the protein. R952K (AGA>AAA) corresponds to a non-synonymous substitution in the loop between Tm 5-Tm6 of the protein (Figure 3). Our aim was to verify whether and in what way these amino acid changes have a disturbing effect on the function of the ATP7B protein in terms of metal binding properties or ATP hydrolysis, which can eventually result in copper dyshomeostasis.

We recruited 251 AD patients and 201 controls. As reported in the original article [76], for the K832R substitution, the minor allele frequency (MAF) resulted 40% in Italian Tuscans, 45% in Utah residents with Northern and Western European ancestry, while 42% in our controls. For the R952K substitution, MAF was 39% in Italian Tuscans, 44% in Utah residents and 43% in controls. The LD analysis revealed an association between K832R and R952K substitutions in both AD patients (D′ = 0.79) and controls (D′ = 0.81). A high LD between K832R and R952K was confirmed also in all HapMap populations.

Allele frequency distributions of both *ATP7B* SNPs differed between AD and controls: K832R substitution genotype frequencies were K832/K832 10%, K832/R832 47%, and R832/R832 43% ($\chi 2$ test, $p = 0.022$) in AD patients, while K832/K832 15%, K832/R832 54%, and R832/R832 31% in our controls. R832/R832 genotype was more frequent in AD and this frequency variation was maintained also when taking into account the Bonferroni correction ($\alpha = 0.025$) as well as in the logistic regression analysis, which took into account age and gender as confounding factors. Our analysis revealed that patients with the *ATP7B* homozygous R832 genotype had a 1.71-fold higher risk of developing AD than controls [adjusted OR= 1.71 (1.12–2.60); $p = 0.012$]. Genotype frequencies of the R952K substitution were R952/R952 15%, R952/K952 41%, and K952/K952 45% in AD patients, and R952/R952 16%, R952/K952 54%, and K952/K952 30% in our controls.

The $\chi 2$ test indicated that two distributions differed ($p = 0.006$) and the association between the risk allele K952 and AD was maintained after checking for age and gender as possible confounders in a logistic regression model. In summary, patients with the *ATP7B* homozygous K952 genotype had a 1.82-fold increased risk of AD compared with controls [adjusted OR= 1.82 (1.19–2.80); $p = 0.006$].

We also performed a haplotype association analysis for the two SNPs in order to investigate their combined effect on AD risk. The most common haplotype was R832/K952, which contained a risk allele at each SNP locus. It was distributed as follows: 60.2% in AD patients and 53.2% in controls ($X2 = 4.85$; $p = 0.028$).

The second more frequent haplotype was K832/R952, which contained no risk alleles and its frequencies differed between the two cohorts, being 28.8% in patients and 37.3% in controls ($X2 = 7.21$; $p = 0.007$).

A logistic regression model was used to check these associations when taking into account age as a possible confounder. The model confirmed the association ($p = 0.018$) and revealed that the haplotype K832/R952 confers some protection against AD [adjusted OR= 0.68 (0.49–0.93)]. Thus, the haplotype association analysis revealed that the presence of alleles with normal function, i.e., K832 and R952, is protective, even though the haplotype lies in a gene with significant disease-risk.

It is important to notice that the SNPs of *APOE*ε4 and *ATP7B* (both K832R and R952K) are independent AD risk factors, as there was no difference in the frequency of the *ATP7B* alleles between carriers and non-carriers of the *APOE*ε4 variant (consistently $p > 0.2$), even when the analysis was restricted to assessment of only the AD population (consistently $p > 0.2$). In summary, the RR genotype in K832R raises the relative risk of developing AD by 71%, while KK in R952K by 82%. The haplotype R832/K952, instead, appears to confer protection against the disease by reducing the relative risk by 32%.These results seem in conflict with the fact that GWASs carried out so far have never found an association between AD and the 13q14.3 chromosomal region where the *ATP7B* gene lies. However, we already described above how GWAS, which are not well equipped to detect rare variants and fail to take into account the genomic and environmental context of the investigated diseases, may underestimate *ATP7B* haplotypes that are instead significantly associated with high risk of AD in individuals exposed to inorganic copper [80].

## 4. Conclusions

The form of AD that has been the subject of this chapter accounts for about 95% of all AD cases and appears rather late in life, normally after 60. For this reason it is called late-onset Alzheimer's disease (LOAD), a term that well differentiates it from the inherited form, familial AD, which is called early-onset AD because it develops much before 60 and accounts for the remainder 5%. In opposition to familial AD, LOAD was initially called "sporadic" because early researchers saw no link between the disease and hereditary factors and assumed that the appearance of the disease was occasional and totally casual.

As we have seen above, this appeared untrue later, when researchers discovered the role of several polymorphisms of the *APOE* gene in the disease pathogenesis. The term sporadic continued to be widely used but we now know that LOAD is strongly influenced by both genetic and environmental factors and appears to have a complex pattern of inheritance. It remains true, however, that so far no gene has been found to be fully causative of LOAD, a fact that is often referred to as *missing heritability*.

Due to the lack of a secure culprit, the role of genetic mutations in LOAD is often understated. In an attempt to compensate, this chapter has described some of the most meaningful evidence constituting the genetic background believed to provide a combined contribution to susceptibility (to become sick), which remains a statistical entity. It must be kept in mind that not only genetic heterogeneity contributes to susceptibility but also other factors, such as *reduced penetration*, a term describing that a predisposing genotype might be present without the pathology necessarily appearing, or even *phenocopy*, in which there are no predisposing genotypes and yet the pathology develops due to environmental factors. The distinction between *genetic inheritance* and *genetic risk* is fundamental and has helped understand how the disease incidence can be decreased by changes in life style.

The chapter has also described GWAS, which have linked a substantial number of genes to the pathogenesis of AD. It is important to notice that each gene, when taken alone, accounts only for a small percentage of the disease incidence and often lacks clinical significance: the above mentioned *CLU* gene, for example, has a proven correlation with AD-related cognitive decline but its odds ratio tells us that it increases the risk of developing LOAD just 0.1-0.15 times. Moreover, this gene has no clinical relevance since it does not predict the disease onset.

However, all the genetic evidence presented here should be regarded as the framework in which systemic metal unbalances develop. For this reason, we have described in a consequential but also factual fashion the role of systemic copper in the toxic processes leading to AD, which we believe to be among the most important phenomena in AD pathogenesis.

We conclude with the introduction of an important, and somewhat innovative, notion concerning copper in AD. We have shown how multiple variants of the *APOE* gene have an actual effect on the statistical risk to develop AD and how they are also linked to level variations of the portion of copper that does not bind to ceruloplasmin. These variants are also in linkage disequilibrium with rare mutations, which can have a relevant effect on the risk of the disease. We are now starting to explore this field by searching for multiple rare variants in the *ATP7B* gene, which may account for portions of the odds of developing AD, defining a new gene for AD susceptibility. Looking at all these associations as a whole, genetics appears as the factor guiding the association between copper abnormalities and the clinical picture of the disease. In other words, the fact that *ATP7B* multiple rare variants in practice modify the copper homeostasis of an individual and have an effect on his/her risk of developing AD is an expression of the causative character of this gene on the susceptibility of the disease.

## Author details

Carlo Salustri[1], Mariacristina Siotto[2], Serena Bucossi[3] and Rosanna Squitti[3,4]

1 Institute of Cognitive Sciences and Technologies (CNR), Fatebenefratelli Hospital, Isola Tiberina, Rome, Italy

2 Don Carlo Gnocchi Foundation ONLUS, Milan, Italy

3 Laboratory of Neurodegeneration, IRCCS San Raffaele Pisana, Rome, Italy

4 Fatebenefratelli Foundation, AFaR Division; Fatebenefratelli Hospital, Isola Tiberina, Rome, Italy

## References


[1] Querfurth, H.W. and F.M. LaFerla. *Alzheimer's disease.* N Engl J Med 2010;362(4) 329-44.

[2] Hardy, J.A. and G.A. Higgins. *Alzheimer's disease: the amyloid cascade hypothesis.* Science 1992;256(5054) 184-5.

[3] Frautschy, S.A. and G.M. Cole. *Why pleiotropic interventions are needed for Alzheimer's disease.* Mol Neurobiol 2010;41(2-3) 392-409.

[4] Bush, A.I. and R.E. Tanzi. *Therapeutics for Alzheimer's disease based on the metal hypothesis.* Neurotherapeutics 2008;5(3) 421-32.

[5] Loeffler, D.A., et al. *Increased regional brain concentrations of ceruloplasmin in neurodegenerative disorders.* Brain Res 1996;738(2) 265-74.

[6] Squitti, R., et al. *Ceruloplasmin/Transferrin ratio changes in Alzheimer's disease.* Int J Alzheimers Dis 2010;2011 231595.

[7] Multhaup, G., et al. *The amyloid precursor protein of Alzheimer's disease in the reduction of copper(II) to copper(I).* Science 1996;271(5254) 1406-9.

[8] Atwood, C.S., et al. *Copper catalyzed oxidation of Alzheimer Abeta.* Cell Mol Biol (Noisy-le-grand) 2000;46(4) 777-83.

[9] Cherny, R.A., et al. *Aqueous dissolution of Alzheimer's disease Abeta amyloid deposits by biometal depletion.* J Biol Chem 1999;274(33) 23223-8.

[10] White, A.R., et al. *Copper levels are increased in the cerebral cortex and liver of APP and APLP2 knockout mice.* Brain Res 1999;842(2) 439-44.

[11] Sparks, D.L. and B.G. Schreurs. *Trace amounts of copper in water induce beta-amyloid plaques and learning deficits in a rabbit model of Alzheimer's disease.* Proc Natl Acad Sci U S A 2003;100(19) 11065-9.

[12] Atwood, C.S., et al. *Dramatic aggregation of Alzheimer abeta by Cu(II) is induced by conditions representing physiological acidosis.* J Biol Chem 1998;273(21) 12817-26.

[13] Nelson, T.J. and D.L. Alkon. *Oxidation of cholesterol by amyloid precursor protein and beta-amyloid peptide.* J Biol Chem 2005;280(8) 7377-87.

[14] Sparks, D.L., et al. *Trace copper levels in the drinking water, but not zinc or aluminum influence CNS Alzheimer-like pathology.* J Nutr Health Aging 2006;10(4) 247-54.

[15] Lu, J., et al. *Trace amounts of copper induce neurotoxicity in the cholesterol-fed mice through apoptosis.* FEBS Lett 2006;580(28-29) 6730-40.

[16] Mao, X., et al. *The effects of chronic copper exposure on the amyloid protein metabolisim associated genes' expression in chronic cerebral hypoperfused rats.* Neurosci Lett 2012;518(1) 14-8.

[17] Hoogenraad, T., *Wilson's disease.* 2001, Amsterdam/Rotterdam: Intermed Medical Publishers

[18] Scheinberg, I.H. and I. Sternlieb. *Wilson's Disease.* Annu Rev Med 1965;16 119-34.

[19] Gutteridge, J.M. and B. Halliwell. *The measurement and mechanism of lipid peroxidation in biological systems.* Trends Biochem Sci 1990;15(4) 129-35.

[20] James, S.A., et al. *Elevated labile Cu is associated with oxidative pathology in Alzheimer disease.* Free Radic Biol Med 2012;52(2) 298-302.

[21] Atwood, C.S., et al. *Copper mediates dityrosine cross-linking of Alzheimer's amyloid-beta.* Biochemistry 2004;43(2) 560-8.

[22] White, A.R., et al. *The Alzheimer's disease amyloid precursor protein modulates copper-induced toxicity and oxidative stress in primary neuronal cultures.* J Neurosci 1999;19(21) 9170-9.

[23] Pal, A., et al. *Towards a Unified Vision of Copper Involvement in Alzheimer's Disease: A Review Connecting Basic, Experimental, and Clinical Research.* J Alzheimers Dis 2014.

[24] Squitti, R., M. Siotto, and R. Polimanti. *Low-copper diet as a preventive strategy for Alzheimer's disease.* Neurobiol Aging 2014;35 Suppl 2 S40-50.

[25] Squitti, R., et al. *Excess of nonceruloplasmin serum copper in AD correlates with MMSE, CSF [beta]-amyloid, and h-tau.* Neurology 2006;67(1) 76-82.

[26] Squitti, R., et al. *Longitudinal prognostic value of serum "free" copper in patients with Alzheimer disease.* Neurology 2009;72(1) 50-5.

[27] Squitti, R., et al. *Value of serum nonceruloplasmin copper for prediction of mild cognitive impairment conversion to Alzheimer disease.* Ann Neurol 2014;75(4) 574-80.

[28] Bucossi, S., et al. *Copper in Alzheimer's disease: a meta-analysis of serum,plasma, and cerebrospinal fluid studies.* J Alzheimers Dis 2011;24(1) 175-85.

[29] Schrag, M., et al. *Oxidative stress in blood in Alzheimer's disease and mild cognitive impairment: a meta-analysis.* Neurobiol Dis 2013;59 100-10.

[30] Squitti, R., et al. *Meta-analysis of serum non-ceruloplasmin copper in Alzheimer's disease.* J Alzheimers Dis 2014;38(4) 809-22.

[31] Morris, M.C., et al. *Dietary copper and high saturated and trans fat intakes associated with cognitive decline.* Arch Neurol 2006;63(8) 1085-8.

[32] Mursu, J., et al. *Dietary supplements and mortality rate in older women: the Iowa Women's Health Study.* Arch Intern Med 2011;171(18) 1625-33.

[33] Shen, X.L., et al. *Positive Relationship between Mortality from Alzheimer's Disease and Soil Metal Concentration in Mainland China.* J Alzheimers Dis 2014;42(3) 893-900.

[34] Brewer, G.J. *Copper excess, zinc deficiency, and cognition loss in Alzheimer's disease.* Biofactors 2012;38(2) 107-13.

[35] Lannfelt, L., et al. *Safety, efficacy, and biomarker findings of PBT2 in targeting Abeta as a modifying therapy for Alzheimer's disease: a phase IIa, double-blind, randomised, placebo-controlled trial.* Lancet Neurol 2008;7(9) 779-86.

[36] Ritchie, C.W., et al. *Metal-protein attenuation with iodochlorhydroxyquin (clioquinol) targeting Abeta amyloid deposition and toxicity in Alzheimer disease: a pilot phase 2 clinical trial.* Arch Neurol 2003;60(12) 1685-91.

[37] Squitti, R., et al. *d-penicillamine reduces serum oxidative stress in Alzheimer's disease patients.* Eur J Clin Invest 2002;32(1) 51-9.

[38] Torsdottir, G., et al. *Ceruloplasmin and iron proteins in the serum of patients with Alzheimer's disease.* Dement Geriatr Cogn Dis Extra 2011;1(1) 366-71.

[39] Brewer, G.J., et al. *Copper and ceruloplasmin abnormalities in Alzheimer's disease.* Am J Alzheimers Dis Other Demen 2010;25(6) 490-7.

[40] Arnal, N., et al. *Clinical utility of copper, ceruloplasmin, and metallothionein plasma determinations in human neurodegenerative patients and their first-degree relatives.* Brain Res 2010;1319 118-30.

[41] Kessler, H., et al. *Cerebrospinal fluid diagnostic markers correlate with lower plasma copper and ceruloplasmin in patients with Alzheimer's disease.* J Neural Transm 2006;113(11) 1763-9.

[42] Capo, C.R., et al. *Features of ceruloplasmin in the cerebrospinal fluid of Alzheimer's disease patients.* Biometals 2008;21(3) 367-72.

[43] Squitti, R., et al. *Ceruloplasmin fragmentation is implicated in 'free' copper deregulation of Alzheimer's disease.* Prion 2008;2(1) 23-7.

[44] Corder, E.H., et al. *Gene dose of apolipoprotein E type 4 allele and the risk of Alzheimer's disease in late onset families.* Science 1993;261(5123) 921-3.

[45] Harold, D., et al. *Genome-wide association study identifies variants at CLU and PICALM associated with Alzheimer's disease.* Nat Genet 2009;41(10) 1088-93.

[46] Lambert, J.C., et al. *Genome-wide association study identifies variants at CLU and CR1 associated with Alzheimer's disease.* Nat Genet 2009;41(10) 1094-9.

[47] Lambert, J.C., et al. *Meta-analysis of 74,046 individuals identifies 11 new susceptibility loci for Alzheimer's disease.* Nat Genet 2013;45(12) 1452-8.

[48] Naj, A.C., et al. *Common variants at MS4A4/MS4A6E, CD2AP, CD33 and EPHA1 are associated with late-onset Alzheimer's disease.* Nat Genet 2011;43(5) 436-41.

[49] Seshadri, S., et al. *Genome-wide analysis of genetic loci associated with Alzheimer disease.* JAMA 2010;303(18) 1832-40.

[50] Corneveaux, J.J., et al. *Association of CR1, CLU and PICALM with Alzheimer's disease in a cohort of clinically characterized and neuropathologically verified individuals.* Hum Mol Genet 2010;19(16) 3295-301.

[51] Moore, J.H., F.W. Asselbergs, and S.M. Williams. *Bioinformatics challenges for genome-wide association studies.* Bioinformatics 2010;26(4) 445-55.

[52] Stranger, B.E., E.A. Stahl, and T. Raj. *Progress and promise of genome-wide association studies for human complex trait genetics.* Genetics 2011;187(2) 367-83.

[53] Cruchaga, C., et al. *Rare coding variants in the phospholipase D3 gene confer risk for Alzheimer's disease.* Nature 2014;505(7484) 550-4.

[54] Guerreiro, R., et al. *TREM2 variants in Alzheimer's disease.* N Engl J Med 2013;368(2) 117-27.

[55] Jonsson, T., et al. *Variant of TREM2 associated with the risk of Alzheimer's disease.* N Engl J Med 2013;368(2) 107-16.

[56] Gaggelli, E., et al. *Copper homeostasis and neurodegenerative disorders (Alzheimer's, prion, and Parkinson's diseases and amyotrophic lateral sclerosis).* Chem Rev 2006;106(6) 1995-2044.

[57] Michalczyk, A.A., et al. *Defective localization of the Wilson disease protein (ATP7B) in the mammary gland of the toxic milk mouse and the effects of copper supplementation.* Biochem J 2000;352 Pt 2 565-71.

[58] Lutsenko, S., et al. *Function and regulation of human copper-transporting ATPases.* Physiol Rev 2007;87(3) 1011-46.

[59] Behari, M. and V. Pardasani. *Genetics of Wilsons disease.* Parkinsonism Relat Disord 2010;16(10) 639-44.

[60] Moller, L.B., et al. *Similar splice-site mutations of the ATP7A gene lead to different phenotypes: classical Menkes disease or occipital horn syndrome.* Am J Hum Genet 2000;66(4) 1211-20.

[61] Kennerson, M.L., et al. *Missense mutations in the copper transporter gene ATP7A cause X-linked distal hereditary motor neuropathy.* Am J Hum Genet 2010;86(3) 343-52.

[62] Lepori, M.B., et al. *Mutation analysis of the ATP7B gene in a new group of Wilson's disease patients: contribution to diagnosis.* Mol Cell Probes 2012;26(4) 147-50.

[63] Ferenci, P. *Regional distribution of mutations of the ATP7B gene in patients with Wilson disease: impact on genetic testing.* Hum Genet 2006;120(2) 151-9.

[64] Schushan, M., et al. *A structural model of the copper ATPase ATP7B to facilitate analysis of Wilson disease-causing mutations and studies of the transport mechanism.* Metallomics 2012;4(7) 669-78.

[65] Fatemi, N. and B. Sarkar. *Structural and functional insights of Wilson disease copper-transporting ATPase.* J Bioenerg Biomembr 2002;34(5) 339-49.

[66] Achila, D., et al. *Structure of human Wilson protein domains 5 and 6 and their interplay with domain 4 and the copper chaperone HAH1 in copper uptake.* Proc Natl Acad Sci U S A 2006;103(15) 5729-34.

[67] Banci, L., et al. *Solution structures of the actuator domain of ATP7A and ATP7B, the Menkes and Wilson disease proteins.* Biochemistry 2009;48(33) 7849-55.

[68] Banci, L., et al. *Metal binding domains 3 and 4 of the Wilson disease protein: solution structure and interaction with the copper(I) chaperone HAH1.* Biochemistry 2008;47(28) 7423-9.

[69] Dmitriev, O., et al. *Solution structure of the N-domain of Wilson disease protein: distinct nucleotide-binding environment and effects of disease mutations.* Proc Natl Acad Sci U S A 2006;103(14) 5302-7.

[70] Fatemi, N., et al. *NMR characterization of copper-binding domains 4-6 of ATP7B.* Biochemistry 2010;49(39) 8468-77.

[71] Gourdon, P., et al. *Crystal structure of a copper-transporting PIB-type ATPase.* Nature 2011;475(7354) 59-64.

[72] Gonzalez-Castejon, M., et al. *Functional non-synonymous polymorphisms prediction methods: current approaches and future developments.* Curr Med Chem 2011;18(33) 5095-103.

[73] Squitti, R., et al. *In silico investigation of the ATP7B gene: insights from functional prediction of non-synonymous substitution to protein structure.* Biometals 2014;27(1) 53-64.

[74] Squitti, R., et al. *Linkage disequilibrium and haplotype analysis of the ATP7B gene in Alzheimer's disease.* Rejuvenation Res 2013;16(1) 3-10.

[75] Squitti, R., et al. *ATP7B variants as modulators of copper dyshomeostasis in Alzheimer's disease.* Neuromolecular Med 2013;15(3) 515-22.

[76] Bucossi, S., et al. *Association of K832R and R952K SNPs of Wilson's Disease Gene with Alzheimer's Disease.* J Alzheimers Dis 2012;29(4) 913-9.

[77] Bucossi, S., et al. *Intronic rs2147363 variant in ATP7B transcription factor-binding site associated with Alzheimer's disease.* J Alzheimers Dis 2013;37(2) 453-9.

[78] Gupta, R.K., et al. *Transcriptional control of preadipocyte determination by Zfp423.* Nature 2010;464(7288) 619-23.

[79] Van Dyck, F., et al. *PLAG1, the prototype of the PLAG gene family: versatility in tumour development (review).* Int J Oncol 2007;30(4) 765-74.

http://dx.doi.org/10.5772/60447

[80] Squitti, R. and R. Polimanti. *Copper Hypot*hesis in the Missing Hereditability of Sporadic Alzheimer's Disease: ATP7B Gene as Potential Harbor of Rare Variants. J Alzheimers Dis 2012;29(3) 493-501.

Section 2

# The Role of Lipids and Cholesterol

Chapter 5

# Lipids and Lipoproteins in Alzheimer's Disease

Sophie Stukas, Iva Kulic, Shahab Zareyan and
Cheryl L. Wellington

Additional information is available at the end of the chapter

http://dx.doi.org/10.5772/59808

## 1. Introduction

Cholesterol is a key structural component of the brain, and cholesterol transport and distribution within the central nervous system (CNS) is mediated by a lipid metabolic cycle that includes generation of apolipoproteins as lipid carriers, lipidation by cholesterol and phospholipid transporters, enzyme remodeling of these particles and their receptor-mediated uptake and turnover in cells. It is becoming increasingly appreciated that Alzheimer's Disease (AD) patients often have comorbid conditions such as cardiovascular disease, type II diabetes mellitus, or hypertension, each of which can greatly affect lipoprotein metabolism, especially at the vessel wall and thereby possibly contribute to AD pathogenesis. Here we review the known biology of lipids and lipoproteins in the CNS and discuss how alterations in lipid metabolism may impact AD pathogenesis. Apolipoprotein E (*APOE*) is the best established genetic risk factor for AD and the major apolipoprotein expressed in the brain. In addition, genome-wide association studies (GWAS) have identified several other genes associated with AD risk that function in lipid or lipoprotein metabolism, including clusterin (*CLU*), ATP binding cassette (ABC) transporter A7 (*ABCA7*), and apoE receptors. Understanding how lipid/lipoprotein metabolism in the brain and body affect cognitive function may therefore offer new insights in developing more effective therapeutic approaches for dementia.

## 2. Lipid and lipoprotein metabolism in the CNS

### 2.1. General biology and function of lipids and lipoproteins in the CNS

The brain is the most cholesterol-rich organ in the body, with an average cholesterol content of 15-20 mg/g wet weight compared to 2 mg/g for peripheral tissues in the adult mouse [1].

The majority of the brain's sterol content is located in free cholesterol, 70-80% of which is in myelin. Cholesterol, sphingomyelin and phospholipids form the major structural components of cellular membranes, with cholesterol, phosphatidylcholine and phosphatidylethanolamine being the most abundant lipids in synaptic vesicles [2]. Many lipids also participate in important signaling pathways in the brain, with lipid-mediated second messengers derived from sphingomyelin and phosphatidylinositol, activation of G- protein coupled receptors and nuclear receptor activation being particularly important [1, 3].

| Name | Major Sites of Production in the Brain | Main Functions in Healthy Brain | Potential Role in AD |
|---|---|---|---|
| **ApoE** | • Astrocytes<br>• Microglia | • Lipid transport<br>• Aβ homeostasis<br>• BBB integrity<br>• Cerebrovascular health<br>• Innate immune response<br>• Reelin signaling | • Involved in Aβ metabolism: deposition, transport across the BBB, clearance through ISF and the CSF pathways, and enzymatic degradation<br>• Regulation of inflammation<br>• ApoE4, the most established AD genetic risk factor, is associated with:<br>1. Impaired Aβ degradation and clearance<br>2. Increased tau phosphorylation and formation of NFT<br>3. Ineffective lipid transport<br>4. Impaired synaptic integrity<br>5. Reduced ability to suppress inflammation |
| **Clusterin** | • Astrocytes<br>• Choroid plexus epithelial cells<br>• Neurons | • Golgi chaperone<br>• Inflammatory response<br>• Complement regulation<br>• Cell Cycle regulation<br>• Reelin signaling | • Third most highly associated susceptibility locus for AD.<br>• Potentially involved in Aβ sequestration, degradation and clearance |
| **ApoA-I** | • Not produced in the brain | • Reverse cholesterol transport<br>• Vascular endothelial health | • AD comorbidities such as type II diabetes and hypercholesterolemia lead to apoA-I dysfunction<br>• Reduction of CAA, neuroinflammation, and oxidative stress in mouse models of AD |

**Table 1.** Major Apolipoproteins in the Brain

As lipids are insoluble in aqueous environments, neutral lipids are transported through bodily fluids on lipoprotein particles consisting of amphipathic apolipoproteins that surround and stabilize their lipid cargo. The general structure of mature spherical lipoproteins consists of a core of neutral cholesterol ester and triglycerides surrounded by amphipathic free cholesterol and phospholipids at the exposed surface, all of which are encapsulated by apolipoproteins

[3]. Four major lipoprotein classes, defined by their buoyant density, are found in the circulation: high density lipoproteins (HDL), low density lipoproteins (LDL), very low density lipoproteins (VLDL) and chylomicrons. While LDL, VLDL and chylomicrons are triglyceride rich, HDL is triglyceride poor, and the HDL-like lipoprotein species found within the CNS contain even less triglyceride than plasma HDL. As apolipoprotein B (apoB), the major apolipoprotein of chylomicrons, VLDL, and LDL, is not found in the CNS, lipoprotein metabolism in the brain and cerebrospinal fluid (CSF) is based entirely on a lipoprotein class that most resembles plasma HDL with respect to size, shape, and density [4-11]. In rodents, astrocytes secrete apoE-containing lipoproteins that are primarily composed of phospholipids (~6 μg/ml) and cholesterol (~13 μg/ml), 0-18% of which is found in the esterified form. These nascent lipoprotein particles are discoidal, ranging from 9-17 nm in diameter with a density of 1.00-1.12 g/ml [7, 10]. Clusterin, also known as apolipoprotein J (apoJ), is also produced by astrocytes but is secreted virtually free of lipids [7, 10, 12]. Conversely, whereas lipoprotein particles found in CSF are of a similar diameter (11-20 nm) and density (1.063-1.12 g/ml) to those secreted by astrocytes, they are distinguished by their spherical shape and a greater proportion of phospholipids and cholesterol, with approximately 70% of cholesterol found as cholesterol esters [5, 7, 8, 10, 13]. ApoE and apolipoprotein A-I (apoA-I) are the major apolipoproteins present in CSF by mass, with apolipoproteins A-II, A-IV, D, CI, CIII, and clusterin also present to a lesser extent [5, 8-11]. In the healthy CNS, lipoproteins regulate the transport, delivery and distribution of lipids. In addition, lipoproteins are also thought to regulate many functions in the CNS including inflammation, oxidative stress, vascular tone, cerebral blood flow, and blood brain barrier (BBB) integrity (Table 1) [14].

### 2.2. Apolipoproteins present in the CNS

ApoE is present at 2-10 μg/ml in human and mouse CSF [8, 13, 15, 16] and at 10-50 ng/ml in interstitial fluid (ISF) from both wild-type mice as well as in targeted replacement mice that express human apoE [17]. ApoE is the most abundant apolipoprotein expressed within the brain, where it is synthesized and secreted by astrocytes and, to a lesser extent, microglia [5]. Secreted apoE particles are lipid-rich, containing equal amounts of apoE and lipid, and carry cholesterol secreted by astrocytes [10, 18]. Indeed, lipidation of apoE is essential for its stability and function [19-21]. Humans express three *APOE* isoforms that differ from one another by two amino acid residues; *APOE2* (cys112, cys158), *APOE3* (cys112, arg158) and *APOE4* (arg112, arg158), with the *APOE3* allele being the most common and the *APOE2* allele being the least frequent in the general population [19]. The resulting apoE2, apoE3 and apoE4 proteins therefore have both structural differences with respect to protein folding as well as functional interactions with respect to their ability to bind to lipids and apoE receptors [22]. In addition to mediating cholesterol transport to neurons, apoE has other functions in the brain such as regulating vascular health and the innate immune system (Table 1) [23].

Brain tissue has one of the highest concentrations of clusterin, which is expressed in astrocytes, epithelial cells of the choroid plexus, and selected neuronal subsets [24]. As a result, clusterin is present in CSF at concentrations of 4-6.5 μg/ml in healthy human adults [25]. In humans, due to the presence of three alternative mRNA start sites, the clusterin gene *CLU* is expressed as three transcriptional isoforms. At the protein level, clusterin exists in two major forms: a 50 kDa nuclear form and a 75-80 kDa glycosylated secreted form [26]. Although clusterin is best known for its role as a chaperone, it also appears to be involved in the inflammatory response and complement regulation, the cell cycle, and endocrine functions (Table 1) [27].

Unlike apoE and clusterin, apoA-I is not expressed in either murine or human brain [28-31], suggesting that its presence in the CNS reflects transport across the BBB and/or the blood-CSF-barrier (BCSFB) following its production from hepatocytes and enterocytes. Although *in vitro* experiments suggest that apoA-I can transcytose across cultured endothelial cells [32], an *in vivo* study shows that peripherally injected apoA-I rapidly localizes to choroid plexus epithelial cells with negligible association in cerebrovascular endothelial cells, suggesting that peripherally derived apoA-I may gain access to the CNS primarily by crossing the BCSFB [31]. The concentration of apoA-I in CSF is ~3-4 μg/mL, or 0.26% of plasma levels, in humans [8, 13, 15, 33] and 0.02 μg/mL, or 0.01% of plasma levels, in wild-type mice [31]. The physiological functions of apoA-I in the CNS are not well understood but are hypothesized to be similar to those of CNS apoE (Table 1) [14].

In addition to apoE, clusterin, and apoA-I, other apolipoproteins are also detected in the CNS, including apoD, apoC-I, apoC-III, apoA-II, and apoA-IV [8, 9, 11], each of which is detected in human CSF [5, 8-11]. It has been shown that apoD, an apolipoprotein with antioxidant and anti-inflammatory properties, is produced in neuroglial cells, pia mater cells, and perivascular cells in the human brain [34, 35].

### 2.3. Cholesterol and Phospholipid Transporters

Lipid-poor apolipoproteins receive cholesterol and phospholipids from membrane bound transporters that are part of the ABC transporter family. The ubiquitously expressed transporter ABCA1 mediates the transfer of cellular cholesterol and phospholipids from cellular membranes to lipid-poor apolipoprotein acceptors including apoA-I and apoE [36- 39], a process that is essential for the production of both plasma and CSF HDL. HDL plays a critical role in the regulation of lipid homeostasis, and is particularly important for cells such as macrophages and microglia that form part of the innate immune system. ABCA1 activity in these phagocytic cells is exquisitely sensitive to cholesterol accumulation, and by catalyzing efflux of excess cholesterol and phospholipids to apoA-I and apoE acceptors, ABCA1 activity helps to maintain intracellular cholesterol balance. In humans, mutations that block ABCA1 function cause Tangier Disease, which is characterized by a 95% loss of plasma HDL cholesterol and apoA-I levels due to rapid catabolism of lipid-poor apoA-I by the kidney. ABCA1-dependent lipidation of CNS apoE is also critical for its stability as both total body and brain-specific loss of ABCA1 in mice leads to a significant 60-80% reduction of brain and CSF apoE [20, 21, 30]. Whether ABCA1 also regulates apoE levels in the brain of Tangier Disease patients is not known. Notably, Wahrle et al. did not observe significant differences in CSF apoE levels between control subjects versus those with ten different *ABCA1* single nucleotide polymorphisms (SNPs), suggesting that these SNPs may not have a significant effect on human ABCA1 function in the CNS [16]. In mice, total body deletion of ABCA1 results in a significant and proportional reduction of apoA-I levels by 60-90% in plasma, brain tissue and CSF [40].

Intriguingly, brain-specific deletion of ABCA1 in mice leads to a significant increase of apoA-I protein levels in brain tissue and CSF [30]. The mechanisms that regulate the distribution of apoA-I between peripheral and CNS compartments remain to be fully determined.

Highly homologous to ABCA1, ABCA7 is also abundantly expressed in microglia, oligodendrocytes, neurons, and astrocytes in both humans [41] and mice [42, 43]. Although the potential for ABCA7 to act as a cholesterol and/or phospholipid transporter in the CNS is unknown, when overexpressed in human embryonic kidney cells, ABCA7 can mediate the transfer of phospholipids and sphingomyelin, but not cholesterol, to lipid-poor apoA-I and apoE [42]. The relative contribution of ABCA7 to the *in vivo* generation of plasma HDL cholesterol appears to be minimal and may be influenced by sex, as decreases in plasma total cholesterol and HDL cholesterol are only detected in female *Abca7-/-* mice [43]. Instead, ABCA7 may be more involved is modulating the phagocytic activity of macrophages, particularly following injury or infection; whether this is also true in brain microglia will be important to address in the future [44, 45]. One critical difference between ABCA1 and ABCA7 is the distinct manner in which they are regulated by cholesterol. Whereas ABCA1 expression is induced by activation of the Liver-X-Receptor (LXR) pathway in response to increased cellular cholesterol content, ABCA7 induction is unaffected [42, 43]. Instead, ABCA7 expression is primarily regulated by sterol regulatory element binding protein 2 (SREBP-2) and is thus repressed in cholesterol-laden cells [44].

Following initial lipidation, nascent HDL lipoproteins can receive additional lipids from the cholesterol transporters ABCG1 and ABCG4 [46], which are abundantly expressed in grey and white matter of the brain [47]. Unlike ABCG4, whose expression appears to be restricted to neurons, astrocytes, and the retina, ABCG1 is widely expressed throughout the body and is found in the liver, intestine, lungs, kidney and spleen in addition to neurons, astrocytes, microglia, and choroid plexus epithelial cells [47, 48]. In addition to lipid efflux activity, ABCG1 and ABCG4 are also believed to regulate intracellular transport of cholesterol and sterols and vesicle trafficking in the brain [47, 48].

### 2.4. Enzymes involved in lipoprotein metabolism

Many enzymes involved in lipoprotein metabolism are found in CSF, although for most, their CNS expression patterns and functional roles have not been explored to the same extent as in the periphery. For example, lecithin cholesterol acyltransferase (LCAT), phospholipid transfer protein (PLTP), and cholesteryl ester transfer protein (CETP) are all detectable in brain tissue and CSF [13, 49-53] and, as they have established roles in plasma lipoprotein metabolism, it is of interest to understand whether they function similarly in the brain.

In plasma, LCAT is the enzyme responsible for generating the cholesterol ester core characteristic of mature circulating lipoproteins, including HDL. As the more hydrophobic cholesterol esters migrate to the core of the lipoprotein particle, the discoidal nascent particle takes on its mature spherical shape. LCAT-mediated esterification of cholesterol serves not only to generate mature HDL particles, but also to maintain the downward cholesterol gradient between the cell and the lipoprotein particle, enabling further cholesterol efflux [54]. LCAT is present in human CSF at levels corresponding to 2.2-2.5% of that in serum and migrates with γ-like lipoproteins [13, 49]. In mice, LCAT is secreted mainly by astrocytes, can be activated by both apoA-I and apoE, and esterifies free cholesterol contained on glial-derived apoE-containing lipoproteins [55]. LCAT may therefore play a role in maturation of discoidal lipoprotein particles secreted from glia to the spherical particles that circulate in CSF by catalyzing the cholesterol esterification of immature CNS lipoprotein particles [5, 7, 56].

PLTP is another enzyme intimately involved in the maturation and turnover of lipoprotein particles within the circulation and CNS. PLTP's primary activity involves the transfer of phospholipids between HDL particles, thus modulating HDL size and composition, and transferring lipids between apoB-containing lipoproprotein particles and HDL [53]. Within the CNS, PLTP is highly expressed by neurons, astrocytes, microglia, oligodendrocytes, BBB endothelial cells, choroid plexus ependymal cells and can be found both in brain tissue and CSF in human and animals [57-61]. Within CSF, PLTP is associated with apoE-containing lipoproteins where it actively participates in phospholipid transport [13, 62, 63] with activity corresponding to 15% of plasma levels in humans [62] and 23% of plasma levels in rabbits [59]. Functionally, PLTP has been reported to regulate apoE expression and secretion by astrocytes [63] and participate in neuronal cell signalling [64].

In plasma, CETP catalyses the bi-directional transfer of cholesterol esters from HDL in exchange for triglycerides from VLDL and LDL, thereby reducing circulating HDL concentration and increasing its size [65]. CETP can potentially diffuse through the BCSFB and enter the brain from plasma. However, it is not clear whether CETP is produced in the brain. Yamada et al. reported CETP-like immunoreactivity in astrocytes in healthy human brain [51]. Albers et al. have suggested that CETP is locally produced in the brain, as they were able to detect CETP in human CSF samples at concentrations higher than what would be expected from simple diffusion of proteins across the BCSFB [66]. However, Demeester et al. were unable to detect CETP in human CSF and CETP mRNA in the human brain [13]. A few other studies have also not detected CETP mRNA in the CNS of rabbits and cynomolgus monkeys [59, 67]. Undoubtedly, more research on the production and the role of CETP in the CNS of healthy individuals is needed.

### 2.5. Receptors involved in lipoprotein uptake and turnover

Lipoprotein uptake and delivery of lipids into target cells of the CNS is regulated by the low density lipoprotein receptor (LDLR) family [68]. The four major apoE receptors in the CNS are LDLR, lipoprotein receptor related protein-1 (LRP1), very low density lipoprotein receptor (VLDLR), and apolipoprotein E receptor 2 (apoER2) [69]. Of these, LDLR is the only receptor that has apoE as its only known ligand in the CNS [69]. LDLR and LRP1 levels are inversely correlated with brain apoE levels as deletion or overexpression of these receptors in mice increases or decreases brain apoE levels, respectively [70-73]. VLDLR and apoER2 also serve as essential receptors for the neuromodulatory ligand Reelin, which is involved in long term potentiation, learning and memory [74-76]. Like apoE, clusterin can also bind to VLDLR and apoER2 to regulate Reelin signaling (Table 1) [77]. LDLR, LRP1, VLDLR and apoER2 are all expressed on neurons, which have a high LRP1:LDLR ratio. LRP1 and LDLR are also found on astrocytes, which have a low LRP1:LDLR ratio, and LRP1 and VLDLR are found on microglia [78-81]. Solubilized forms of these receptors, generated via ectodomain shedding or splice variants lacking the transmembrane domain, possibly contribute to negative feedback and inhibition of lipoprotein uptake [82]. Of note, the lipoprotein related protein 2 (LRP2), also known as megalin, and the neuronal sortilin- related receptor (SORL1 receptor) are also additional apoE receptors expressed in the CNS [83, 84].

## 3. Alterations to lipids and lipoproteins in Alzheimer's disease

The neuropathology of AD is defined by the presence of amyloid plaques and neurofibrillary tangles (NTFs), which are composed of deposited amyloid-beta (Aβ) peptides and filamentous hyperphosphorylated tau, respectively [85]. In addition to parenchymal amyloid plaques, most AD patients also have accumulation of amyloid in cerebral blood vessels, known as cerebral amyloid angiopathy (CAA) [14, 86]. Furthermore, neuronal degeneration and dysfunction, the brains of AD patients are often marked by significant signs of chronic inflammation, oxidative stress and vascular dysfunction. Not surprisingly, apolipoproteins, the lipids they carry, and the transporters responsible for their lipidation may be intimately involved in each step of the disease. In particular, the interrelationship between cerebrovascular dysfunction and AD is increasingly appreciated. Epidemiological, clinical, neuropathological and pathophysiological evidence shows that several cardiovascular risk factors also increase AD risk, including age, sex, hypertension, dyslipidemia, and type II diabetes [87-90]. Dementia progresses more rapidly in patients with cerebral infarcts [90- 93] and infarction and other forms of brain injury may potentiate AD pathophysiology [94- 96]. Importantly, many of these cardiovascular risk factors include aspects of dysfunctional lipid and lipoprotein metabolism, which likely occurs at the vessel wall. However, compared to the wealth of knowledge about lipid and lipoprotein physiology in large peripheral vessels, little is known about the mechanisms by which vascular risk factors for AD may impair the function of cerebral vessels. Importantly, BBB dysfunction may contribute to inflammatory processes in the CNS, where exacerbated inflammatory responses or failure to resolve inflammatory reactions are increasingly recognized to play important roles in AD pathogenesis [97].

### 3.1. Changes in brain lipid composition and their direct effects in AD

One often overlooked neuropathological observation initially reported by Alois Alzheimer is the presence of adipose inclusions in the brain, which Alzheimer defined as "extraordinarily strong accumulation of lipoid material in the ganglion cells, glia and vascular wall cells, and the particularly numerous fibril-forming glia cells in the cortex and, indeed, in the entire central nervous system" [98]. Almost all major classes of lipids have some correlation with AD pathogenesis [99]. A recent review by Kosicek and Hecimovic reported that the *post-mortem* brain levels of phosphatidylinositol, phosphatidylethanolamine, ethanolamine plasmalogen, and sulfatide are decreased in AD, while the levels of ceramide are increased [100]. Though not as extensively studied, it has been reported that CSF levels of ceramide are increased, while the levels of sulfatide are decreased in AD [101, 102]. Furthermore, studies by Soderberg et al. and Tully et al. report lower levels of n-3 and n-6 polyunsaturated fatty acids, which are major components of phospholipids, in AD brain compared to healthy controls [103, 104]. Changes to the levels of these lipid classes affects not only the structural properties of the membranes, but also numerous signaling and trafficking pathways that are heavily involved in the normal functioning of the cells in the CNS [99, 105].

Changes to CNS lipid composition can also influence the production of Aβ peptides. As the generation of these peptides involves several lipid-associated steps, including intracellular trafficking and inter-membrane proteolytic cleavage, it is not surprising that, in addition to genetic changes that alter Aβ production, there are also indirect, lipid- dependent changes that can affect production of Aβ. Aβ peptides are derived via sequential proteolytic processing of the amyloid precursor protein (APP) by β-secretase and γ- secretase. This leads to liberation of Aβ peptides 38-46 amino acids in length into the extracellular space [106-108]. Of these, Aβ40 and Aβ42 are quantitatively the most important for amyloid deposition [109]. In healthy brains, the vast majority of APP is processed by $\alpha$-secretase, followed by γ-secretase cleavage, which prevents toxic Aβ peptide generation [110]. All of the enzymes involved in APP processing are transmembrane proteins, raising the hypothesis that the lipid composition and lipid organization in the membrane may affect Aβ production [111]. Numerous *in vitro* studies have focused on determining the role of specific lipid classes in APP processing. For example, it has been shown that reducing membrane cholesterol lowers the levels and activity of β-secretase and reduces γ- secretase activity, decreasing Aβ production [99, 112]. Altered cholesterol content in lipid rafts, regions in the cellular membrane enriched with cholesterol and sphingolipids, affects the localization of enzymes involved in Aβ production, which can lead to changes in amyloidogenic APP processing [99]. Moreover, sphingolipids have been reported to regulate γ-secretase activity [99, 113, 114]. Interestingly, expression of familial presenilin (PS) mutations, which are mutations in components of the γ-secretase complex, affects sphingolipid metabolism, suggesting an interplay of genetics and lipid metabolism in the context of APP processing. Furthermore, *in vitro* elevation of ceramide, which is composed of sphingosine and fatty acids, increases β-secretase stability and promotes Aβ biogenesis [115].

The production of Aβ peptides is not unique to AD pathology, but a constitutive process that is a product of normal cell metabolism throughout life, confirmed by its secretion from primary cells in culture and its presence in the plasma and CSF of healthy individuals [108, 116, 117]. Therefore, it is possible that disrupted Aβ homeostasis, either via increased production or impaired degradation and clearance, leads to its net accumulation in the brain, triggering subsequent neurotoxicity. Aβ production is clearly enhanced in cases of familial early onset AD (<60 years of age), which account for 2-3% of the AD population [118]. In contrast to familial early-onset AD cases, the vast majority of AD subjects who develop cognitive impairment in late life have no genetically-determined net increase in Aβ production. For these late-onset AD patients, who account for up to 99% of the AD population [119], aging, environmental factors, or other genetic-related impairments in Aβ degradation and clearance are thought to lead to the net accumulation of Aβ within the CNS [120-122].

### 3.2. Apolipoproteins and AD pathogenesis

Of the apolipoproteins present in the CNS, *APOE* has the most established genetic association with AD, influencing the risk, progression, and pathology of the disease (Table 1). The *APOE4* allele is a robust risk factor for late-onset AD and is found in 40-60% of AD subjects depending on ethnicity (the prevalence is lower in Asian compared to Northern European populations) even though its carrier frequency in the human population is approximately 15-20% [123-125]. *APOE4* increases AD risk by 3-fold when inherited in a single copy and greater than 9-fold in homozygous individuals. *APOE4* also accelerates the age of onset of AD [123, 126, 127]. A wealth of pre-clinical and clinical evidence has demonstrated that *APOE4* is associated with earlier and more extensive Aβ and amyloid deposition, which is currently believed to result from a net impairment of Aβ degradation and clearance from the CNS [120, 128]. ApoE affects Aβ metabolism through multiple mechanisms, including transport of Aβ across the BBB, modulation of interstitial fluid (ISF) and CSF clearance pathways, effects on BBB integrity, and modulating the growth of Aβ oligomers and fibrils [129, 130]. Some studies suggest that the risk and severity of CAA is also increased in *APOE4* carriers [131, 132]. Intriguingly, a patient with an ablative mutation in *APOE* was recently described to have no detectable impairment in cognitive, neurological and retinal function, with normal levels of CSF Aβ and tau despite very high plasma cholesterol levels [133], suggesting that apoE may have non-essential functions in the human brain and eye. This observation reflects the prediction made from *Apoe*-deficient mice, which also have greatly increased plasma cholesterol levels and exhibit greatly reduced Aβ retention in the CNS [134-137].

In addition to modulating Aβ, apoE may also be involved in tau phosphorylation. In neurons, hyperphosphorylation of the microtubule-associated protein tau by kinases, including GSK-3β and CDK5, causes the dissociation and aggregation of tau to ultimately form neurofibrillary tangles [138]. Under conditions of stress or injury, neurons have been reported to synthesize and process apoE4 to produce neurotoxic C-terminal fragments. Release of these fragments into the neuronal cytosol has been reported to enhance tau phosphorylation and formation of NFT-like structures [139, 140].

ApoE4 has additional deleterious consequences. Compared to apoE3, apoE4 is less effective at mediating cholesterol transport in the brain; human knock-in *APOE4* homozygous mice show reduced total cholesterol and phospholipids compared to wild type mice [81, 141]. The *APOE4* allele has also been implicated in impaired synaptic integrity, as human *APOE4* transgenic mice show lower levels of excitatory synaptic activity that declines to levels comparable to *Apoe* knockout mice by 7 months of age [142]. ApoE4 has also been reported to reduce apoER2 expression at the neuronal surface, impairing the ability of Reelin to enhance synaptic glutamate receptor activity [143].

ApoE plays an integral role in inflammatory processes in the brain. Inflammation of the brain's glial supporting cells, known as neuroinflammation, is a prominent feature AD [144] and contributes to neuronal damage. In response to Aβ or lipopolysaccharide (LPS), LRP1-mediated glial cell activation increases apoE, which can limit the inflammatory response by signaling though LDL receptors to suppress c-Jun N-terminal kinase signaling [145, 146]. There is also evidence that isoform-specific apoE modulation of the innate immune response can modulate Aβ deposition [147]. Consistent with apoE having an anti- inflammatory role, *Apoe*-deficient mice have elevated proinflammatory cytokines in the liver [148]. Importantly, isoform specific effects appear to determine the extent of cytokine induction and may also modulate progression and resolution of CNS inflammation. In mice, apoE4 has reduced ability to suppress the inflammatory response induced by LPS treatment [149] and in the EFAD model (5 familial AD mutations in the presence of human *APOE*), microglial activation in response to Aβ is augmented by the *APOE4* genotype [150]. Indeed, *Apoe*-deficient mice show a similar activation of the inflammatory response to human *APOE4* knock-in mice following LPS injection, implying that apoE4 may lack the anti- inflammatory functions of the other apoE isoforms [151]. Consistent with these findings, non- steroidal anti-inflammatory drugs are associated with a reduced risk of AD only in participants with an *APOE4* allele [152].

According to the AlzGene database, *CLU* is the third most highly associated susceptibility locus for AD following *APOE* and bridging integrator 1 (*BINI*) (www.alzgene.org). In 2009, two independent GWAS studies identified the C allele of the rs11136000 SNP in the *CLU* gene, which occurs in 88% of Caucasians, to confer a modest risk of AD development (odds ratio (OR) 1.16), whereas inheritance of the T allele is protective (OR 0.86) in Caucasians [153, 154]. Although these findings have been replicated in, and confirmed for, Caucasians of European ancestry, the association of *CLU* polymorphisms and AD risk has not been replicated in African-American, Hispanic, or Arab populations [27, 155]. Since this discovery, estensive work has been conducted in an attempt to delineate the mechanism(s) by which the rs11136000 SNP confers AD risk. Inheritance of the TT versus TC versus CC allele appears to result in either no change [156, 157] or a very subtle 8% decrease [158] of plasma clusterin levels in AD and mild cognitive impairment (MCI) patients, with small 10-17% decreases of plasma clusterin observed in cognitively normal aged-matched controls with the TT allele [156, 158]. Despite minimal effects on circulating clusterin levels with the T allele, inheritance of the C allele of the rs11136000 SNP is associated with both structural and functional changes in the CNS. In young (aged 20-30 years) cognitively normal adults, each copy of the C allele of the rs11136000 SNP is associated with lower white matter integrity [159], decreased coupling and connectivity between the hippocampus and prefrontal cortex during memory processing tasks [160], and neural hyperactivity under emotional working paradigms [161], indicative of early structural and functional abnormalities that may leave the brain more vulnerable to disease during aging. In the elderly, independent of dementia status, the CC allele is significantly associated with longitudinal increases in ventricular volume over a 2 year period [162], and increased resting regional cerebral blood flow in the hippocampus and right anterior cingulate cortex, regions which are important for memory function and default mode network activity, over an 8-year period [163]. Further, the protective T allele is associated with a reduced rate of conversion from MCI to AD (OR 0.25) [164], while the detrimental C allele is correlated with a significantly faster rate of decline in verbal but not visual memory performance in MCI and AD patients [163]. Lastly, with respect to CSF biomarkers, the *CLU* C allele is associated with significantly lower CSF Aβ42 in a Finnish [165] but not American cohort [166], with no association found for either total or phosphorylated tau.

Although the specific mechanisms by which an individual SNP in *CLU* may confer disease risk are not well understood, there are well recognized global changes to clusterin mRNA and protein expression both in the plasma and CNS that are associated with AD pathology and clinical presentation [27]. In non-demented elderly controls and patients with subjective memory complaints, CSF clusterin is positively associated with CSF total and phosphorylated tau [167] and an elevated atrophy rate in the entorhinal cortex of older non- demented adults with low CSF Aβ42 [168]. Whereas older studies did not detect significant differences in CSF clusterin between cognitively normal aged matched controls and AD subjects [25, 169], newer studies that utilize higher sensitivity methods have reported up to a 25% increase of CSF clusterin in AD subjects [170, 171], suggesting that increased CNS clusterin may be detrimental. Within brain tissue, clusterin mRNA is increased after correcting for neuronal loss [172, 173], whereas protein levels are reportedly increased by 40-180% depending on the brain region [172, 174-177]. Within the AD brain, clusterin strongly co-stains with dystrophic neurites, neuropil threads, and intracellular NFT [176, 178, 179], with minimal to moderate co-localization observed with mature amyloid plaques [176, 178, 180, 181] and cerebrovascular amyloid [180]. Unlike the CNS, multiple studies have detected no difference between plasma clusterin levels in non-demented controls, MCI, and AD subjects [157, 182-185]. However, increased baseline plasma clusterin levels are suggestive of increased prevalence and severity of AD pathology and presentation, including brain atrophy, amyloid deposition and worsened cognitive function, with a more rapid clinical progression [186-188].

A mechanistic involvement of clusterin in AD pathology is also supported by *in vivo* preclinical studies (Table 1) [27]. Clusterin appears to be directly involved in neuronal health and Aβ metabolism via a variety of mechanisms. In transgenic AD mice, genetic ablation of clusterin results in a reduction of mature fibrillar amyloid deposits and the dystrophic neurites that are associated with them [189]. Supporting this, a recent study found that co- incubation of Aβ with clusterin leads to a 60% decrease in oligomeric and 42% decrease in fibrillar Aβ binding and uptake by primary microglia, and a 72% reduction in binding and uptake of oligomeric Aβ by primary astrocytes, suggesting that clusterin can impede Aβ degradation by local glia [190]. *In vitro* and *in vivo*, clusterin may also mediate Aβ toxicity and tau phosphorylation via dickkopf-1-driven induction of the Wnt-PCP-JNK pathway [191]. In contrast, other studies have found a beneficial role of clusterin in facilitating Aβ clearance across the BBB via LRP-2 [192] and binding to and sequestering Aβ oligomers, thereby reducing their potential toxicity [193]. Clusterin also participates in various aspects of cell signaling. *In vitro*, clusterin signals via Reelin by binding to apoER2 and VLDLR thereby increasing cell proliferation and neuroblast chain formation in the subventricular zone [77]. Clearly, more research is necessary to fully understand the pathways by which clusterin is involved in brain function and the pathogenesis of AD.

Although apoA-I is relatively abundant in CSF and brain tissue, the physiological roles of apoA-I containing lipoprotein particles in the CNS, their potential influence on AD risk and pathology, and whether they affect AD pathogenesis through actions from one or both sides of the BBB remains unknown [14]. The most established data regarding apoA-I and AD are human epidemiological studies examining the interaction between serum apoA-I and HDL-cholesterol levels with AD risk (Table 1). At mid-life, high serum apoA-I levels resulted in a significantly lower risk (hazard ratio (HR) 0.25) of dementia later in life, [194] while high levels of serum HDL cholesterol (> 55 mg/dL) in cognitively normal elderly was associated with a significantly reduced risk (HR 0.4) of AD even after adjusting for *APOE* genotype and vascular risk factors such as heart disease, diabetes, obesity, hypertension, and lipid lowering treatment [195]. Recently, Reed et al. demonstrated that low plasma HDL cholesterol and apoA-I were associated with and predicted higher amyloid Pittsburgh compound B binding independent of *APOE4* in cognitively normal and MCI elderly subjects [196]. There also appears to be a consistent 20-30% reduction in serum apoA-I in late-onset AD subjects compared to age-matched controls [197-199], with levels of serum apoA-I positively correlating to cognitive function [199, 200]. Further, in symptomatic AD patients, plasma apoA-I levels are negatively correlated with measures of brain atrophy, including hippocampal and whole brain volume and mean entorhinal thickness [186]. Alterations to CSF apoA-I are less clear, potentially due to the small number of studies or sample size, whereas two studies reported a decrease of CSF apoA-I in AD subjects [15, 201], two other studies reported no change [13, 202]. Prospective studies designed and powered to assess the levels, and perhaps more importantly, the function of both plasma and CSF apoA-I-HDL with respect to AD onset and progression are needed to determine if apoA-I-HDL potentially contributes to AD pathology.

Although questions remain about the importance of apoA-I to AD in humans, studies in preclinical AD mouse models support a role for apoA-I in removing amyloid selectively from the cerebral vasculature, leading to reduced neuroinflammation and maintenance of cognitive function (Table 1). Specifically, genetic loss of *Apoa1* is associated with increased CAA, greater inflammation, and exacerbated cognitive impairment, whereas transgenic overexpression of human *APOA1* from its endogenous promoter (driving expression from only hepatocytes and enterocytes) prevented AD-related cognitive decline and reduced both CAA and glial activation in symptomatic APP/PS1 mice [203, 204]. Given the known roles of apoA-I-containing HDL in regulating vascular endothelial health, reducing inflammation and oxidative stress, coupled with the relative contributions of these pathologies to AD, it will be paramount to fully elucidate the function of apoA-I in the CNS and evaluate its therapeutic potential [14].

Although the roles of other CNS apolipoproteins in AD pathogenesis are not as extensively studied, apoD, apoC-I, apoA-IV, and apoC-III may play a role. The most significant change due to aging is observed in gene expression levels of *APOD* [205]; CSF and hippocampal apoD are elevated in AD [206] and correlated with disease severity [207]. ApoC-I colocalizes with Aβ plaques in human AD brain [208] and apoC-I has been suggested to influence neuroinflammation in AD [209]. The *APOC1* gene is also considered as an AD susceptibility locus, as the H2 polymorphism of *APOCI* is in linkage disequilibrium with *APOE4* [209-211]. Furthermore, heterozygosity of the *APOA4* (360:His) allele is more common in AD patients [212]. In APP transgenic mice, *Apoa4* deficiency increases Aβ load, enhances neuronal loss, accelerates cognitive dysfunction and increases mortality [213]. Lastly, apoC-III has recently been reported to be associated with Aβ levels in the periphery and is of possible interest for use as an early biomarker for AD [214].

### 3.3. Cholesterol and phospholipid transporters in AD

There is a growing body of pre-clinical and clinical evidence that supports the involvement of ABCA1, and recently ABCA7, in the pathogenesis of AD [215]. In mice, ABCA1-mediated lipidation of apoE correlates with a net increase in Aβ clearance [216]. For example, total body deficiency of *Abca1* markedly decreases soluble apoE and increases amyloid plaque-associated insoluble apoE, decreases plasma and CSF apoA-I, and increases Aβ deposits in both parenchymal and vascular compartments, with no net change in APP production or processing [217-220]. Recently, Fitz et al. demonstrated that haploinsufficiency of *Abca1* significantly exacerbated cognitive deficits, increased Aβ and amyloid deposits, and reduced Aβ clearance in ISF of *APOE4* but not *APOE3* APP/PS1 *Abca1-/+* mice, suggesting a particularly deleterious state of poorly-lipidated apoE4 compared to apoE3 [221]. Of interest, the presence of apoE4 with *Abca1* hemizygosity leads to a modest but statistically significant decrease in CNS apoE (~10%), decreased CNS and plasma apoA-I by approximately 50 and 20%, respectively, and decreased plasma Aβ42 and HDL cholesterol, with a strong inverse correlation between plasma HDL cholesterol levels and amyloid burden [221]. Both genetic and pharmacological approaches that increase brain ABCA1 activity also increase functional CNS apoE [40, 222] and improve learning and memory with [222-227] or without [228-232] changes in Aβ and/or amyloid burden. Importantly, ABCA1 was required to observe an improvement in cognitive function in APP/PS1 mice treated with the LXR agonist GW3965, suggesting that ABCA1 lipidation of lipid-poor apolipoproteins is essential for cognitive function [229]. It is important to note, however, that these manipulations will affect ABCA1-mediated lipidation of apoE in the brain as well as ABCA1-mediated lipidation of apoA-I in the periphery and potentially the CNS, of which the relative contributions are unknown.

The association of *ABCA1* genetic variants and AD risk in human subjects is not as clear despite more than a dozen studies [216]. In 2013, a meta-analysis was conducted on 13 independent studies totaling 6034 controls and 6214 AD patients that examined whether the *ABCA1* variants R219K rs2230806, I883M rs4149313 and R1587K rs2230808 were associated with AD risk. No significant association was found even after adjusting by ethnicity and sample size [233]. This is consistent with *ABCA1* failing to appear in GWAS [216]. It is important to note, however, that most of the *ABCA1* gene variants in heterozygous patients translate to a relatively small reduction in plasma HDL cholesterol that may or may not increase the relative risk of ischemic heart disease [234, 235], raising the caveat that these variants may not be severe enough to impact brain physiology. As Tangier Disease, in which patients completely lack functional ABCA1, is extremely rare and most patients die before 70 years of age, it is not known whether human ABCA1 deficiency is associated with neuropathological changes relevant to AD [236].

In contrast to ABCA1, numerous independent GWAS have identified associations between multiple *ABCA7* SNPs and AD risk [237-244]. ABCA7 expression has been reported to be increased in the brains of AD subjects, with the magnitude of the increase correlating with greater cognitive decline [239, 241]. In 2011, the first two major SNPs of *ABCA7*, rs2764650 [244] and rs3752246 [237], were associated with increased risk of late-onset AD. Two subsequent GWAS found that the rs2764650 SNP was significantly associated with increased neuritic plaque burden [242, 243]. However, both Larch et al. and Vasquez et al. found that the minor allele of the rs2764650 SNP conferred protection from AD by delaying onset and decreasing disease duration, despite increased ABCA7 expression, whereas another study found that rs2764650 neither altered ABCA7 expression or AD risk [238]. In African Americans, the *ABCA7* rs115550680 SNP was shown to increase AD risk by 1.79 even after adjusting for *APOE* genotype, which itself conferred a relative risk of 2.31 [240]. With more *ABCA7* SNPs identified by GWAS to confer AD risk [238], it will be increasingly important to identify the functional consequences of *ABCA7* polymorphisms. In transgenic APP mice, total body loss of *Abca7* increases hippocampal Aβ and amyloid burden with no changes in APP processing or brain levels of ABCA1, apoE, LDLR, or markers of neurodegeneration or synaptic loss [245]. However, increased Aβ and amyloid did not significantly impair any measure of cognitive function, including spatial memory, object recognition, short-term recognition, or fear conditioning [245]. Intriguingly, bone marrow derived macrophages obtained from *Abca7-/-* mice displayed a 50% reduction in Aβ uptake compared to wild type controls, suggesting that phagocytosis may be compromised; however, there were no change to either the number or distribution of microglia or macrophages within the brain parenchyma in AD *Abca7-/-* mice [245].

Despite high expression in the brain, ABCG1 does not appear to have a marked role in AD pathogenesis, as ABCG1 overexpression in AD mice does not significantly change Aβ or amyloid burden [246]. Although a recent GWAS study reported that *ABCG1* SNPs were correlated with neuritic plaque burden in AD subjects [243], the relative risk of *ABCG1* variants has yet to be confirmed.

### 3.4. LCAT, PLTP and CETP in AD

Although better characterized with respect to their involvement in atherosclerosis, research is emerging regarding the potential role of the lipoprotein modifying enzymes LCAT, PLTP and CETP in AD [53, 65, 247]. One early study in a small group of symptomatic AD patients suggested that CSF LCAT activity was reduced by 50% compared to cognitively normal age-matched controls [13], raising the possibility that aging may influence LCAT activity or LCAT activity may influence AD pathogenesis. Stukas et al. recently tested this hypothesis in mice and found that the abundance and activity of LCAT in liver, cortex and plasma is unaltered by aging or the presence of amyloid deposits [14]. Furthermore, total loss of *Lcat* does not impact apoE levels or lipidation, or Aβ or amyloid metabolism in symptomatic APP/PS1 mice, despite a 70-90% decrease in circulating and CNS levels of apoA-I [14]. These results suggest that CNS lipoproteins need not be in a mature spherical form containing cholesterol esters to participate normally in Aβ metabolism.

PLTP may also be involved in the pathogenesis of AD. Intriguingly, whereas PLTP synthesis by neurons and glia is increased in the early stages of AD [62], its levels, and more importantly, its activity are reduced in brain tissue and CSF of AD patients in later stages [57, 63]. In mice, deletion of *Pltp* increases cerebral oxidative stress, elevates Aβ42, reduces synaptophysin expression, increases BBB permeability and decreases expression of tight junction proteins under basal conditions [61, 248]. Further, intracerebroventricular injection of an oligomeric Aβ peptide leads to exacerbated cognitive impairment in *Pltp-/-* mice compared to wild-type controls [248]. In aged *Pltp-/-* mice, enhanced cognitive impairment is accompanied by increased cortical Aβ42, APP expression, and both β- and γ-secretase activity with decreases in cortical Aβ40 and apoE [249]. These preclinical studies suggest a role for PLTP not only in phospholipid transport, but Aβ homeostasis, neuronal function, barrier integrity, and oxidative stress.

Another enzyme that plays a central role in lipid homeostasis that can potentially affect dementia outcome is CETP. As reduced CETP activity in humans is associated with reduced cardiovascular disease risk, the functions of CETP in atherosclerosis and the potential of CETP inhibitors for cardiovascular disease have been of intense interest [65]. The *CETP* 405V allele, which results in low plasma CETP levels in *CETP* 405V homozygotes [250], is associated with longevity. However, the direction and the magnitude of this effect is not clear as some studies have found a positive association, some a negative association, and some no association with longevity [251-256]. It has also been shown that in young adults, this allele is associated with higher fractional anisotropy, a measure of myelination in brain's white matter [257]. In older subjects, however, this effect is reversed [257]. Furthermore, genetic studies have proposed a relationship between C629A, I405V, and D442G *CETP* polymorphisms and AD risk. Intriguingly, the effects that are exerted by these polymorphisms may be dependent on the presence of the *APOE4* allele. Rodriguez et al. reported that in *APOE4* carriers, the AA genotype of the C629A *CETP* polymorphism is associated with lower AD risk [258]. It has also been shown that in the Northern Han Chinese population, there is an association between the G allele of the D442G *CETP* polymorphism and lower AD risk, an effect that was abolished in the absence of *APOE4* [259]. Additionally, Murphy et al. reported that in *APOE4* non-carriers, the I allele of the I405V polymorphism is protective, whereas the V allele is associated with higher AD risk [260]. Interestingly, these associations are reversed in *APOE4* carriers [260]. These results are replicated by the Rotterdam study [250]. However, the Einstein Aging Study reported an association between the VV genotype and slower memory decline and AD risk, and a recent meta-analysis by Li et al. reported no association between AD and the 1405V *CETP* polymorphism [253, 261]. Clearly, more research is required to elucidate the specific role of CETP in the brain and its contribution to AD.

### 3.5. ApoE receptors

APP endocytosis is regulated by several members of the lipoprotein receptor family leading to increased or reduced Aβ generation [74]. These receptors are also critical for Aβ clearance. LRP1 can bind Aβ directly or bind apoE-associated Aβ to internalize and transport soluble Aβ across the BBB to plasma for eventual degradation, or mediate degradation within cell lysosomes [262-266]. *APOE* genotype impacts clearance of Aβ-apoE complexes with Aβ-apoE4 having the slowest net clearance rate [267]. Findings in knockout mice imply LDLR may also enhance Aβ clearance [268, 269]. Other apolipoproteins such as clusterin may play a role in mediating Aβ degradation and clearance though the LDLR family of receptors [83]. In addition to Aβ removal, apoE receptors also regulate tau phosphorylation. Reelin signaling through apoER2 and VLDLR inhibits the activity of GSK- 3β and blockade of this pathway increases hyperphosphorylated tau in the brain [270, 271]. Although apoE receptors are clearly implicated in AD pathogenesis by a number of mechanisms, genetic evidence for their role is not robust, despite mutations in *LDLR* being highly associated with hypercholesterolemia in humans [272]. For example, a polymorphism in exon 3 of the *LRP1* gene (rs1799986) has been weakly correlated with increased risk of AD, although subjects with both this *LRP1* allele and a tau polymorphism (*MAPT*, intron 9, rs2471738) have 6.2-fold higher risk of developing AD than those without this genotype [273-275]. A polymorphism in *LRP2* (rs3755166) has also been reported to be associated with AD [276, 277]. By contrast, the neuronal sortilin-related receptor (*SORL1*, also known as *LR11)* is an apoE receptor that has been shown to be significantly associated with AD risk by multiple groups and in a GWAS [278, 279]. SORL1 levels are reduced in AD brains [280] and risk variants that decrease SORL1 expression, particularly in childhood and adolescence, predict increases in amyloid pathology [281].

## 4. Conclusions and future directions

ApoE is the major apolipoprotein produced within the CNS and is intimately involved in the risk, progression, and pathogenesis of AD. Allelic differences in *APOE* appear to confer isoform specific effects with respect to Aβ deposition, degradation and clearance, tau phosphorylation, neuronal injury and inflammation. Given its gain of toxic or loss of beneficial function, strategies aimed at increasing functional apoE may be of therapeutic interest, although it is possible that elevated levels of dysfunctional apoE4 may actually be detrimental for *APOE4* carriers. However, as over 50% of AD patients carry at least one *APOE4* allele, development of future therapies must take into account the structural and functional differences of this lipoprotein isoform, and seek to develop ways to either correct or bypass the "dysfunction" of apoE4. Long ignored, the importance of clusterin in CNS health and disease is now rapidly expanding. While clinical evidence is mounting that clusterin may be involved in AD disease risk, severity, and rate of decline both with respect to cognitive function and Aβ metabolism, the mechanism(s) by which clusterin confers these roles is poorly understood. ApoA-I may also influence AD pathology, potentially by modulating cerebrovascular integrity and function by assisting in the removal of Aβ peptides from cerebrovascular smooth muscle cells and decreasing inflammation. Indeed, the known effects of common AD comorbidities such as type II diabetes and hypercholesterolemia, on apoA-I function, should be taken into account in clinical studies on dementia risk and potential therapeutic approaches.

In the cardiovascular field, many preclinical and clinical studies have endeavored to increase the net concentration of circulating HDL to protect against cardiovascular disease. Many of these studies may also have implications for CNS function. However, as some of these approaches, such as the inhibition of CETP, have failed to meet their primary endpoints for cardiovascular disease despite significantly increasing HDL cholesterol levels, the lipoprotein field is now deeply invested in understanding the functional complexities of HDL. Therapeutic interventions aimed at increasing the function of HDL particles and their cargo may be of much greater importance than increasing its net levels, in both the peripheral and CNS compartments. Given the complexity of the HDL proteome and lipidome, it will be critical to divest the same details in the CNS to allow for therapeutic development targeting lipoprotein species.

http://dx.doi.org/10.5772/59808

## Author details

Sophie Stukas, Iva Kulic, Shahab Zareyan and Cheryl L. Wellington*

*Address all correspondence to: wcheryl@mail.ubc.ca

Department of Pathology and Laboratory Medicine, Djavad Mowafaghian Centre for Brain Health, University of British Columbia, Vancouver, British Columbia, Canada

## References

[1] Dietschy JM. Central nervous system: cholesterol turnover, brain development and neurodegeneration. Biological chemistry. 2009 Apr;390(4):287-93.

[2] Lim L, Wenk MR. Neuronal Membrane Lipids – Their Role in the Synaptic Vesicle Cycle. In: Tettamanti GG, G., editor. Handbook of Neurochemistry and Molecular Neurobiology. New York: Springer Science+Business Media; 2009. p. 223 - 38.

[3] Vance JE, Hayashi H. Formation and function of apolipoprotein E-containing lipoproteins in the nervous system. Biochimica et biophysica acta. 2010 Aug;1801(8): 806-18.

[4] Beffert U, Danik M, Krzywkowski P, Ramassamy C, Berrada F, Poirier J. The neurobiology of apolipoproteins and their receptors in the CNS and Alzheimer's disease. Brain research Brain research reviews. 1998 Jul;27(2):119-42.

[5] Pitas RE, Boyles JK, Lee SH, Hui D, Weisgraber KH. Lipoproteins and their receptors in the central nervous system. Characterization of the lipoproteins in cerebrospinal fluid and identification of apolipoprotein B,E(LDL) receptors in the brain. The Journal of biological chemistry. 1987 Oct 15;262(29):14352-60.

[6] Ladu MJ, Reardon C, Van Eldik L, Fagan AM, Bu G, Holtzman D, et al. Lipoproteins in the central nervous system. Annals of the New York Academy of Sciences. 2000 Apr;903:167-75.

[7] LaDu MJ, Gilligan SM, Lukens JR, Cabana VG, Reardon CA, Van Eldik LJ, et al. Nascent astrocyte particles differ from lipoproteins in CSF. Journal of neurochemistry. 1998 May;70(5):2070-81.

[8] Koch S, Donarski N, Goetze K, Kreckel M, Stuerenburg HJ, Buhmann C, et al. Characterization of four lipoprotein classes in human cerebrospinal fluid. Journal of lipid research. 2001 Jul;42(7):1143-51.

[9] Borghini I, Barja F, Pometta D, James RW. Characterization of subpopulations of lipoprotein particles isolated from human cerebrospinal fluid. Biochimica et biophysica acta. 1995 Mar 16;1255(2):192-200.

[10] DeMattos RB, Brendza RP, Heuser JE, Kierson M, Cirrito JR, Fryer J, et al. Purification and characterization of astrocyte-secreted apolipoprotein E and J-containing lipoproteins from wild-type and human apoE transgenic mice. Neurochemistry international. 2001 Nov- Dec;39(5-6):415-25.

[11] Roheim PS, Carey M, Forte T, Vega GL. Apolipoproteins in human cerebrospinal fluid. Proceedings of the National Academy of Sciences of the United States of America. 1979 Sep;76(9):4646-9.

[12] Fan J, Shimizu Y, Chan J, Wilkinson A, Ito A, Tontonoz P, et al. Hormonal modulators of glial ABCA1 and apoE levels. Journal of lipid research. 2013 Nov;54(11): 3139-50.

[13] Demeester N, Castro G, Desrumaux C, De Geitere C, Fruchart JC, Santens P, et al. Characterization and functional studies of lipoproteins, lipid transfer proteins, and lecithin:cholesterol acyltransferase in CSF of normal individuals and patients with Alzheimer's disease. Journal of lipid research. 2000 Jun;41(6):963-74.

[14] Stukas S, Robert J, Wellington CL. High Density Lipoproteins and Cerebrovasular Integrity in Alzheimer's Disease. Cell metabolism. 2014.

[15] Roher AE, Maarouf CL, Sue LI, Hu Y, Wilson J, Beach TG. Proteomics-derived cerebrospinal fluid markers of autopsy-confirmed Alzheimer's disease. Biomarkers : biochemical indicators of exposure, response, and susceptibility to chemicals. 2009 Nov; 14(7):493-501.

[16] Wahrle SE, Shah AR, Fagan AM, Smemo S, Kauwe JS, Grupe A, et al. Apolipoprotein E levels in cerebrospinal fluid and the effects of ABCA1 polymorphisms. Molecular neurodegeneration. 2007;2:7.

[17] Ulrich JD, Burchett JM, Restivo JL, Schuler DR, Verghese PB, Mahan TE, et al. In vivo measurement of apolipoprotein E from the brain interstitial fluid using microdialysis. Molecular neurodegeneration. 2013;8:13.

[18] Fagan AM, Holtzman DM, Munson G, Mathur T, Schneider D, Chang LK, et al. Unique lipoproteins secreted by primary astrocytes from wild type, apoE (-/-), and human apoE transgenic mice. The Journal of biological chemistry. 1999 Oct 15;274(42):30001-7.

[19] Dorey E, Chang N, Liu QY, Yang Z, Zhang W. Apolipoprotein E, amyloid-beta, and neuroinflammation in Alzheimer's disease. Neuroscience bulletin. 2014 Apr;30(2): 317-30.

[20] Hirsch-Reinshagen V, Zhou S, Burgess BL, Bernier L, McIsaac SA, Chan JY, et al. Deficiency of ABCA1 impairs apolipoprotein E metabolism in brain. The Journal of biological chemistry. 2004 Sep 24;279(39):41197-207.

[21] Wahrle SE, Jiang H, Parsadanian M, Legleiter J, Han X, Fryer JD, et al. ABCA1 is required for normal central nervous system ApoE levels and for lipidation of astrocyte-secreted apoE. The Journal of biological chemistry. 2004 Sep 24;279(39):40987-93.

[22] Hatters DM, Peters-Libeu CA, Weisgraber KH. Apolipoprotein E structure: insights into function. Trends in biochemical sciences. 2006 Aug;31(8):445-54.

[23] Liu CC, Kanekiyo T, Xu H, Bu G. Apolipoprotein E and Alzheimer disease: risk, mechanisms and therapy. Nature reviews Neurology. 2013 Feb;9(2):106-18.

[24] de Silva HV, Harmony JA, Stuart WD, Gil CM, Robbins J. Apolipoprotein J: structure and tissue distribution. Biochemistry. 1990 Jun 5;29(22):5380-9.

[25] Lidstrom AM, Hesse C, Rosengren L, Fredman P, Davidsson P, Blennow K. Normal levels of clusterin in cerebrospinal fluid in Alzheimer's disease, and no change after acute ischemic stroke. Journal of Alzheimer's disease : JAD. 2001 Oct;3(5):435-42.

[26] Rizzi F, Coletta M, Bettuzzi S. Chapter 2: Clusterin (CLU): From one gene and two transcripts to many proteins. Advances in cancer research. 2009;104:9-23.

[27] Yu JT, Tan L. The role of clusterin in Alzheimer's disease: pathways, pathogenesis, and therapy. Molecular neurobiology. 2012 Apr;45(2):314-26.

[28] Elshourbagy NA, Boguski MS, Liao WS, Jefferson LS, Gordon JI, Taylor JM. Expression of rat apolipoprotein A-IV and A-I genes: mRNA induction during development and in response to glucocorticoids and insulin. Proceedings of the National Academy of Sciences of the United States of America. 1985 Dec;82(23):8242-6.

[29] Zannis VI, Cole FS, Jackson CL, Kurnit DM, Karathanasis SK. Distribution of apolipoprotein A-I, C-II, C-III, and E mRNA in fetal human tissues. Time-dependent induction of apolipoprotein E mRNA by cultures of human monocyte-macrophages. Biochemistry. 1985 Jul 30;24(16):4450-5.

[30] Karasinska JM, Rinninger F, Lutjohann D, Ruddle P, Franciosi S, Kruit JK, et al. Specific loss of brain ABCA1 increases brain cholesterol uptake and influences neuronal structure and function. The Journal of neuroscience : the official journal of the Society for Neuroscience. 2009 Mar 18;29(11):3579-89.

[31] Stukas S, Robert J, Lee M, Kulic I, Carr M, Tourigny K, et al. Intravenously injected human apolipoprotein A-I rapidly enters the central nervous system via the choroid plexus. Journal of the American Heart Association. Forthcoming 2014.

[32] Kratzer I, Wernig K, Panzenboeck U, Bernhart E, Reicher H, Wronski R, et al. Apolipoprotein A-I coating of protamine-oligonucleotide nanoparticles increases particle uptake and transcytosis in an in vitro model of the blood-brain barrier. Journal of controlled release : official journal of the Controlled Release Society. 2007 Feb 26;117(3):301-11.

[33] Song H, Seishima M, Saito K, Maeda S, Takemura M, Noma A, et al. Apo A-I and apo E concentrations in cerebrospinal fluids of patients with acute meningitis. Annals of clinical biochemistry. 1998 May;35 (Pt 3):408-14.

[34] Navarro A, Tolivia J, Astudillo A, del Valle E. Pattern of apolipoprotein D immunoreactivity in human brain. Neuroscience letters. 1998 Sep 18;254(1):17-20.

[35] Dassati S, Waldner A, Schweigreiter R. Apolipoprotein D takes center stage in the stress response of the aging and degenerative brain. Neurobiology of aging. 2014 Jul; 35(7):1632-42.

[36] Koldamova RP, Lefterov IM, Ikonomovic MD, Skoko J, Lefterov PI, Isanski BA, et al. 22R-hydroxycholesterol and 9-cis-retinoic acid induce ATP-binding cassette transporter A1 expression and cholesterol efflux in brain cells and decrease amyloid beta secretion. The Journal of biological chemistry. 2003 Apr 11;278(15):13244-56.

[37] Kim WS, Rahmanto AS, Kamili A, Rye KA, Guillemin GJ, Gelissen IC, et al. Role of ABCG1 and ABCA1 in regulation of neuronal cholesterol efflux to apolipoprotein E discs and suppression of amyloid-beta peptide generation. The Journal of biological chemistry. 2007 Feb 2;282(5):2851-61.

[38] Panzenboeck U, Balazs Z, Sovic A, Hrzenjak A, Levak-Frank S, Wintersperger A, et al. ABCA1 and scavenger receptor class B, type I, are modulators of reverse sterol transport at an in vitro blood-brain barrier constituted of porcine brain capillary endothelial cells. The Journal of biological chemistry. 2002 Nov 8;277(45):42781-9.

[39] Saint-Pol J, Vandenhaute E, Boucau MC, Candela P, Dehouck L, Cecchelli R, et al. Brain pericytes ABCA1 expression mediates cholesterol efflux but not cellular amyloid-beta peptide accumulation. Journal of Alzheimer's disease : JAD. 2012;30(3): 489-503.

[40] Stukas S, May S, Wilkinson A, Chan J, Donkin J, Wellington CL. The LXR agonist GW3965 increases apoA-I protein levels in the central nervous system independent of ABCA1. Biochimica et biophysica acta. 2012 Mar;1821(3):536-46.

[41] Kim WS, Guillemin GJ, Glaros EN, Lim CK, Garner B. Quantitation of ATP-binding cassette subfamily-A transporter gene expression in primary human brain cells. Neuroreport. 2006 Jun 26;17(9):891-6.

[42] Wang N, Lan D, Gerbod-Giannone M, Linsel-Nitschke P, Jehle AW, Chen W, et al. ATP-binding cassette transporter A7 (ABCA7) binds apolipoprotein A-I and mediates cellular phospholipid but not cholesterol efflux. The Journal of biological chemistry. 2003 Oct 31;278(44):42906-12.

[43] Kim WS, Fitzgerald ML, Kang K, Okuhira K, Bell SA, Manning JJ, et al. Abca7 null mice retain normal macrophage phosphatidylcholine and cholesterol efflux activity despite alterations in adipose mass and serum cholesterol levels. The Journal of biological chemistry. 2005 Feb 4;280(5):3989-95.

[44] Iwamoto N, Abe-Dohmae S, Sato R, Yokoyama S. ABCA7 expression is regulated by cellular cholesterol through the SREBP2 pathway and associated with phagocytosis. Journal of lipid research. 2006 Sep;47(9):1915-27.

[45] Tanaka N, Abe-Dohmae S, Iwamoto N, Fitzgerald ML, Yokoyama S. Helical apolipoproteins of high-density lipoprotein enhance phagocytosis by stabilizing ATP-binding cassette transporter A7. Journal of lipid research. 2010 Sep;51(9):2591-9.

[46] Wang N, Lan D, Chen W, Matsuura F, Tall AR. ATP-binding cassette transporters G1 and G4 mediate cellular cholesterol efflux to high-density lipoproteins. Proceedings of the National Academy of Sciences of the United States of America. 2004 Jun 29;101(26):9774- 9.

[47] Tarr PT, Edwards PA. ABCG1 and ABCG4 are coexpressed in neurons and astrocytes of the CNS and regulate cholesterol homeostasis through SREBP-2. Journal of lipid research. 2008 Jan;49(1):169-82.

[48] Wang N, Yvan-Charvet L, Lutjohann D, Mulder M, Vanmierlo T, Kim TW, et al. ATP- binding cassette transporters G1 and G4 mediate cholesterol and desmosterol efflux to HDL and regulate sterol accumulation in the brain. FASEB journal : official publication of the Federation of American Societies for Experimental Biology. 2008 Apr;22(4):1073-82.

[49] Albers JJ, Marcovina SM, Christenson RH. Lecithin cholesterol acyltransferase in human cerebrospinal fluid: reduced level in patients with multiple sclerosis and evidence of direct synthesis in the brain. International journal of clinical & laboratory research. 1992;22(3):169-72.

[50] Warden CH, Langner CA, Gordon JI, Taylor BA, McLean JW, Lusis AJ. Tissue-specific expression, developmental regulation, and chromosomal mapping of the lecithin: cholesterol acyltransferase gene. Evidence for expression in brain and testes as well as liver. The Journal of biological chemistry. 1989 Dec 25;264(36):21573-81.

[51] Yamada T, Kawata M, Arai H, Fukasawa M, Inoue K, Sato T. Astroglial localization of cholesteryl ester transfer protein in normal and Alzheimer's disease brain tissues. Acta neuropathologica. 1995;90(6):633-6.

[52] Lagrost L, Athias A, Gambert P, Lallemant C. Comparative study of phospholipid transfer activities mediated by cholesteryl ester transfer protein and phospholipid transfer protein. Journal of lipid research. 1994 May;35(5):825-35.

[53] Albers JJ, Vuletic S, Cheung MC. Role of plasma phospholipid transfer protein in lipid and lipoprotein metabolism. Biochimica et biophysica acta. 2012 Mar;1821(3): 345-57.

[54] Calabresi L, Simonelli S, Gomaraschi M, Franceschini G. Genetic lecithin:cholesterol acyltransferase deficiency and cardiovascular disease. Atherosclerosis. 2012 Jun; 222(2):299-306.

[55] Hirsch-Reinshagen V, Donkin J, Stukas S, Chan J, Wilkinson A, Fan J, et al. LCAT synthesized by primary astrocytes esterifies cholesterol on glia-derived lipoproteins. Journal of lipid research. 2009 May;50(5):885-93.

[56] Guyton JR, Miller SE, Martin ME, Khan WA, Roses AD, Strittmatter WJ. Novel large apolipoprotein E-containing lipoproteins of density 1.006-1.060 g/ml in human cerebrospinal fluid. Journal of neurochemistry. 1998 Mar;70(3):1235-40.

[57] Albers JJ, Wolfbauer G, Cheung MC, Day JR, Ching AF, Lok S, et al. Functional expression of human and mouse plasma phospholipid transfer protein: effect of recombinant and plasma PLTP on HDL subspecies. Biochimica et biophysica acta. 1995 Aug 24;1258(1):27-34.

[58] Chirackal Manavalan AP, Kober A, Metso J, Lang I, Becker T, Hasslitzer K, et al. Phospholipid transfer protein is expressed in cerebrovascular endothelial cells and involved in high density lipoprotein biogenesis and remodeling at the blood-brain barrier. The Journal of biological chemistry. 2014 Feb 21;289(8):4683-98.

[59] Gander R, Eller P, Kaser S, Theurl I, Walter D, Sauper T, et al. Molecular characterization of rabbit phospholipid transfer protein: choroid plexus and ependyma synthesize high levels of phospholipid transfer protein. Journal of lipid research. 2002 Apr; 43(4):636-45.

[60] Oslakovic C, Krisinger MJ, Andersson A, Jauhiainen M, Ehnholm C, Dahlback B. Anionic phospholipids lose their procoagulant properties when incorporated into high density lipoproteins. The Journal of biological chemistry. 2009 Feb 27;284(9): 5896-904.

[61] Zhou T, He Q, Tong Y, Zhan R, Xu F, Fan D, et al. Phospholipid transfer protein (PLTP) deficiency impaired blood-brain barrier integrity by increasing cerebrovascular oxidative stress. Biochemical and biophysical research communications. 2014 Mar 7;445(2):352-6.

[62] Vuletic S, Jin LW, Marcovina SM, Peskind ER, Moller T, Albers JJ. Widespread distribution of PLTP in human CNS: evidence for PLTP synthesis by glia and neurons, and increased levels in Alzheimer's disease. Journal of lipid research. 2003 Jun;44(6): 1113-23.

[63] Vuletic S, Peskind ER, Marcovina SM, Quinn JF, Cheung MC, Kennedy H, et al. Reduced CSF PLTP activity in Alzheimer's disease and other neurologic diseases; PLTP induces ApoE secretion in primary human astrocytes in vitro. Journal of neuroscience research. 2005 May 1;80(3):406-13.

[64] Dong W, Albers JJ, Vuletic S. Phospholipid transfer protein reduces phosphorylation of tau in human neuronal cells. Journal of neuroscience research. 2009 Nov 1;87(14): 3176-85.

[65] Kingwell BA, Chapman MJ, Kontush A, Miller NE. HDL-targeted therapies: progress, failures and future. Nature reviews Drug discovery. 2014 Jun;13(6):445-64.

[66] Albers JJ, Tollefson JH, Wolfbauer G, Albright RE, Jr. Cholesteryl ester transfer protein in human brain. International journal of clinical & laboratory research. 1992;21(3):264-6.

[67] Pape ME, Rehberg EF, Marotti KR, Melchior GW. Molecular cloning, sequence, and expression of cynomolgus monkey cholesteryl ester transfer protein. Inverse correlation between hepatic cholesteryl ester transfer protein mRNA levels and plasma high density lipoprotein levels. Arteriosclerosis and thrombosis : a journal of vascular biology / American Heart Association. 1991 Nov-Dec;11(6):1759-71.

[68] Bu G. Apolipoprotein E and its receptors in Alzheimer's disease: pathways, pathogenesis and therapy. Nature reviews Neuroscience. 2009 May;10(5):333-44.

[69] Holtzman DM, Herz J, Bu G. Apolipoprotein E and apolipoprotein E receptors: normal biology and roles in Alzheimer disease. Cold Spring Harbor perspectives in medicine. 2012 Mar;2(3):a006312.

[70] Fryer JD, Demattos RB, McCormick LM, O'Dell MA, Spinner ML, Bales KR, et al. The low density lipoprotein receptor regulates the level of central nervous system human and murine apolipoprotein E but does not modify amyloid plaque pathology in PDAPP mice. The Journal of biological chemistry. 2005 Jul 8;280(27):25754-9.

[71] Kim J, Castellano JM, Jiang H, Basak JM, Parsadanian M, Pham V, et al. Overexpression of low-density lipoprotein receptor in the brain markedly inhibits amyloid deposition and increases extracellular A beta clearance. Neuron. 2009 Dec 10;64(5): 632-44.

[72] Liu Q, Zerbinatti CV, Zhang J, Hoe HS, Wang B, Cole SL, et al. Amyloid precursor protein regulates brain apolipoprotein E and cholesterol metabolism through lipoprotein receptor LRP1. Neuron. 2007 Oct 4;56(1):66-78.

[73] Zerbinatti CV, Wahrle SE, Kim H, Cam JA, Bales K, Paul SM, et al. Apolipoprotein E and low density lipoprotein receptor-related protein facilitate intraneuronal Abeta42 accumulation in amyloid model mice. The Journal of biological chemistry. 2006 Nov 24;281(47):36180-6.

[74] Lane-Donovan C, Philips GT, Herz J. More than Cholesterol Transporters: Lipoprotein Receptors in CNS Function and Neurodegeneration. Neuron. 2014 Aug 20;83(4): 771-87.

[75] Rice DS, Curran T. Role of the reelin signaling pathway in central nervous system development. Annual review of neuroscience. 2001;24:1005-39.

[76] Herz J, Chen Y. Reelin, lipoprotein receptors and synaptic plasticity. Nature reviews Neuroscience. 2006 Nov;7(11):850-9.

[77] Leeb C, Eresheim C, Nimpf J. Clusterin is a ligand for apolipoprotein E receptor 2 (ApoER2) and very low density lipoprotein receptor (VLDLR) and signals via the Reelin- signaling pathway. The Journal of biological chemistry. 2014 Feb 14;289(7): 4161-72.

[78] Christie RH, Chung H, Rebeck GW, Strickland D, Hyman BT. Expression of the very low-density lipoprotein receptor (VLDL-r), an apolipoprotein-E receptor, in the central nervous system and in Alzheimer's disease. Journal of neuropathology and experimental neurology. 1996 Apr;55(4):491-8.

[79] Clatworthy AE, Stockinger W, Christie RH, Schneider WJ, Nimpf J, Hyman BT, et al. Expression and alternate splicing of apolipoprotein E receptor 2 in brain. Neuroscience. 1999 Mar;90(3):903-11.

[80] Moestrup SK, Gliemann J, Pallesen G. Distribution of the alpha 2-macroglobulin receptor/low density lipoprotein receptor-related protein in human tissues. Cell and tissue research. 1992 Sep;269(3):375-82.

[81] Rapp A, Gmeiner B, Huttinger M. Implication of apoE isoforms in cholesterol metabolism by primary rat hippocampal neurons and astrocytes. Biochimie. 2006 May; 88(5):473-83.

[82] Rebeck GW, LaDu MJ, Estus S, Bu G, Weeber EJ. The generation and function of soluble apoE receptors in the CNS. Molecular neurodegeneration. 2006;1:15.

[83] Spuch C, Ortolano S, Navarro C. LRP-1 and LRP-2 receptors function in the membrane neuron. Trafficking mechanisms and proteolytic processing in Alzheimer's disease. Frontiers in physiology. 2012;3:269.

[84] Motoi Y, Aizawa T, Haga S, Nakamura S, Namba Y, Ikeda K. Neuronal localization of a novel mosaic apolipoprotein E receptor, LR11, in rat and human brain. Brain research. 1999 Jul 3;833(2):209-15.

[85] Hyman BT, Phelps CH, Beach TG, Bigio EH, Cairns NJ, Carrillo MC, et al. National Institute on Aging-Alzheimer's Association guidelines for the neuropathologic assessment of Alzheimer's disease. Alzheimer's & dementia : the journal of the Alzheimer's Association. 2012 Jan;8(1):1-13.

[86] Zlokovic BV. Neurovascular pathways to neurodegeneration in Alzheimer's disease and other disorders. Nature reviews Neuroscience. 2011 Dec;12(12):723-38.

[87] de la Torre JC. Alzheimer disease as a vascular disorder: nosological evidence. Stroke; a journal of cerebral circulation. 2002 Apr;33(4):1152-62.

[88] Gorelick PB. Risk factors for vascular dementia and Alzheimer disease. Stroke; a journal of cerebral circulation. 2004 Nov;35(11 Suppl 1):2620-2.

[89] Hayden KM, Zandi PP, Lyketsos CG, Khachaturian AS, Bastian LA, Charoonruk G, et al. Vascular risk factors for incident Alzheimer disease and vascular dementia: the

Cache County study. Alzheimer disease and associated disorders. 2006 Apr-Jun; 20(2):93-100.

[90] Kalaria RN. The role of cerebral ischemia in Alzheimer's disease. Neurobiology of aging. 2000 Mar-Apr;21(2):321-30.

[91] Esiri MM, Nagy Z, Smith MZ, Barnetson L, Smith AD. Cerebrovascular disease and threshold for dementia in the early stages of Alzheimer's disease. Lancet. 1999 Sep 11;354(9182):919-20.

[92] Petrovitch H, Ross GW, Steinhorn SC, Abbott RD, Markesbery W, Davis D, et al. AD lesions and infarcts in demented and non-demented Japanese-American men. Annals of neurology. 2005 Jan;57(1):98-103.

[93] Snowdon DA, Greiner LH, Mortimer JA, Riley KP, Greiner PA, Markesbery WR. Brain infarction and the clinical expression of Alzheimer disease. The Nun Study. Jama. 1997 Mar 12;277(10):813-7.

[94] Honjo K, van Reekum R, Verhoeff NP. Alzheimer's disease and infection: do infectious agents contribute to progression of Alzheimer's disease? Alzheimer's & dementia : the journal of the Alzheimer's Association. 2009 Jul;5(4):348-60.

[95] Kalaria RN, Bhatti SU, Lust WD, Perry G. The amyloid precursor protein in ischemic brain injury and chronic hypoperfusion. Annals of the New York Academy of Sciences. 1993 Sep 24;695:190-3.

[96] Nihashi T, Inao S, Kajita Y, Kawai T, Sugimoto T, Niwa M, et al. Expression and distribution of beta amyloid precursor protein and beta amyloid peptide in reactive astrocytes after transient middle cerebral artery occlusion. Acta neurochirurgica. 2001;143(3):287-95.

[97] Takeda S, Sato N, Morishita R. Systemic inflammation, blood-brain barrier vulnerability and cognitive/non-cognitive symptoms in Alzheimer disease: relevance to pathogenesis and therapy. Frontiers in aging neuroscience. 2014;6:171.

[98] Foley P. Lipids in Alzheimer's disease: A century-old story. Biochimica et biophysica acta. 2010 Aug;1801(8):750-3.

[99] Di Paolo G, Kim TW. Linking lipids to Alzheimer's disease: cholesterol and beyond. Nature reviews Neuroscience. 2011 May;12(5):284-96.

[100] Kosicek M, Hecimovic S. Phospholipids and Alzheimer's disease: alterations, mechanisms and potential biomarkers. International journal of molecular sciences. 2013;14(1):1310-22.

[101] Han X, Fagan AM, Cheng H, Morris JC, Xiong C, Holtzman DM. Cerebrospinal fluid sulfatide is decreased in subjects with incipient dementia. Annals of neurology. 2003 Jul;54(1):115-9.

[102] Satoi H, Tomimoto H, Ohtani R, Kitano T, Kondo T, Watanabe M, et al. Astroglial expression of ceramide in Alzheimer's disease brains: a role during neuronal apoptosis. Neuroscience. 2005;130(3):657-66.

[103] Soderberg M, Edlund C, Kristensson K, Dallner G. Fatty acid composition of brain phospholipids in aging and in Alzheimer's disease. Lipids. 1991 Jun;26(6):421-5.

[104] Tully AM, Roche HM, Doyle R, Fallon C, Bruce I, Lawlor B, et al. Low serum cholesteryl ester-docosahexaenoic acid levels in Alzheimer's disease: a case-control study. The British journal of nutrition. 2003 Apr;89(4):483-9.

[105] Bennett SA, Valenzuela N, Xu H, Franko B, Fai S, Figeys D. Using neurolipidomics to identify phospholipid mediators of synaptic (dys)function in Alzheimer's Disease. Frontiers in physiology. 2013;4:168.

[106] Estus S, Golde TE, Younkin SG. Normal processing of the Alzheimer's disease amyloid beta protein precursor generates potentially amyloidogenic carboxyl-terminal derivatives. Annals of the New York Academy of Sciences. 1992 Dec 31;674:138-48.

[107] Haass C, Selkoe DJ. Cellular processing of beta-amyloid precursor protein and the genesis of amyloid beta-peptide. Cell. 1993 Dec 17;75(6):1039-42.

[108] Seubert P, Vigo-Pelfrey C, Esch F, Lee M, Dovey H, Davis D, et al. Isolation and quantification of soluble Alzheimer's beta-peptide from biological fluids. Nature. 1992 Sep 24;359(6393):325-7.

[109] Masters CL, Selkoe DJ. Biochemistry of amyloid beta-protein and amyloid deposits in Alzheimer disease. Cold Spring Harbor perspectives in medicine. 2012 Jun; 2(6):a006262.

[110] Haass C, Kaether C, Thinakaran G, Sisodia S. Trafficking and proteolytic processing of APP. Cold Spring Harbor perspectives in medicine. 2012 May;2(5):a006270.

[111] Grziwa B, Grimm MO, Masters CL, Beyreuther K, Hartmann T, Lichtenthaler SF. The transmembrane domain of the amyloid precursor protein in microsomal membranes is on both sides shorter than predicted. The Journal of biological chemistry. 2003 Feb 28;278(9):6803-8.

[112] Vetrivel KS, Thinakaran G. Membrane rafts in Alzheimer's disease beta-amyloid production. Biochimica et biophysica acta. 2010 Aug;1801(8):860-7.

[113] Grimm MO, Grimm HS, Patzold AJ, Zinser EG, Halonen R, Duering M, et al. Regulation of cholesterol and sphingomyelin metabolism by amyloid-beta and presenilin. Nature cell biology. 2005 Nov;7(11):1118-23.

[114] Sawamura N, Ko M, Yu W, Zou K, Hanada K, Suzuki T, et al. Modulation of amyloid precursor protein cleavage by cellular sphingolipids. The Journal of biological chemistry. 2004 Mar 19;279(12):11984-91.

[115] Puglielli L, Ellis BC, Saunders AJ, Kovacs DM. Ceramide stabilizes beta-site amyloid precursor protein-cleaving enzyme 1 and promotes amyloid beta-peptide biogenesis. The Journal of biological chemistry. 2003 May 30;278(22):19777-83.

[116] Haass C, Schlossmacher MG, Hung AY, Vigo-Pelfrey C, Mellon A, Ostaszewski BL, et al. Amyloid beta-peptide is produced by cultured cells during normal metabolism. Nature. 1992 Sep 24;359(6393):322-5.

[117] Shoji M, Golde TE, Ghiso J, Cheung TT, Estus S, Shaffer LM, et al. Production of the Alzheimer amyloid beta protein by normal proteolytic processing. Science. 1992 Oct 2;258(5079):126-9.

[118] Tanzi RE. The genetics of Alzheimer disease. Cold Spring Harbor perspectives in medicine. 2012 Oct;2(10).

[119] Mawuenyega KG, Sigurdson W, Ovod V, Munsell L, Kasten T, Morris JC, et al. Decreased clearance of CNS beta-amyloid in Alzheimer's disease. Science. 2010 Dec 24;330(6012):1774.

[120] Kanekiyo T, Xu H, Bu G. ApoE and Abeta in Alzheimer's disease: accidental encounters or partners? Neuron. 2014 Feb 19;81(4):740-54.

[121] Tanzi RE, Moir RD, Wagner SL. Clearance of Alzheimer's Abeta peptide: the many roads to perdition. Neuron. 2004 Sep 2;43(5):605-8.

[122] Wildsmith KR, Holley M, Savage JC, Skerrett R, Landreth GE. Evidence for impaired amyloid beta clearance in Alzheimer's disease. Alzheimer's research & therapy. 2013;5(4):33.

[123] Corder EH, Saunders AM, Strittmatter WJ, Schmechel DE, Gaskell PC, Small GW, et al. Gene dose of apolipoprotein E type 4 allele and the risk of Alzheimer's disease in late onset families. Science. 1993 Aug 13;261(5123):921-3.

[124] Farrer LA, Cupples LA, Haines JL, Hyman B, Kukull WA, Mayeux R, et al. Effects of age, sex, and ethnicity on the association between apolipoprotein E genotype and Alzheimer disease. A meta-analysis. APOE and Alzheimer Disease Meta Analysis Consortium. Jama. 1997 Oct 22-29;278(16):1349-56.

[125] Ward A, Crean S, Mercaldi CJ, Collins JM, Boyd D, Cook MN, et al. Prevalence of apolipoprotein E4 genotype and homozygotes (APOE e4/4) among patients diagnosed with Alzheimer's disease: a systematic review and meta-analysis. Neuroepidemiology. 2012;38(1):1-17.

[126] Rebeck GW, Reiter JS, Strickland DK, Hyman BT. Apolipoprotein E in sporadic Alzheimer's disease: allelic variation and receptor interactions. Neuron. 1993 Oct;11(4): 575- 80.

[127] Strittmatter WJ, Saunders AM, Schmechel D, Pericak-Vance M, Enghild J, Salvesen GS, et al. Apolipoprotein E: high-avidity binding to beta-amyloid and increased frequency of type 4 allele in late-onset familial Alzheimer disease. Proceedings of the

National Academy of Sciences of the United States of America. 1993 Mar 1;90(5): 1977-81.

[128] Verghese PB, Castellano JM, Holtzman DM. Apolipoprotein E in Alzheimer's disease and other neurological disorders. Lancet neurology. 2011 Mar;10(3):241-52.

[129] Garai K, Verghese PB, Baban B, Holtzman DM, Frieden C. The Binding of Apolipoprotein E to Oligomers and Fibrils of Amyloid-beta Alters the Kinetics of Amyloid Aggregation. Biochemistry. 2014 Sep 25.

[130] Zlokovic BV. Cerebrovascular effects of apolipoprotein E: implications for Alzheimer disease. JAMA neurology. 2013 Apr;70(4):440-4.

[131] Chalmers K, Wilcock GK, Love S. APOE epsilon 4 influences the pathological phenotype of Alzheimer's disease by favouring cerebrovascular over parenchymal accumulation of A beta protein. Neuropathology and applied neurobiology. 2003 Jun;29(3): 231-8.

[132] Premkumar DR, Cohen DL, Hedera P, Friedland RP, Kalaria RN. Apolipoprotein E-epsilon4 alleles in cerebral amyloid angiopathy and cerebrovascular pathology associated with Alzheimer's disease. The American journal of pathology. 1996 Jun;148(6): 2083-95.

[133] Mak AC, Pullinger CR, Tang LF, Wong JS, Deo RC, Schwarz JM, et al. Effects of the Absence of Apolipoprotein E on Lipoproteins, Neurocognitive Function, and Retinal Function. JAMA neurology. 2014 Aug 11.

[134] Bales KR, Verina T, Cummins DJ, Du Y, Dodel RC, Saura J, et al. Apolipoprotein E is essential for amyloid deposition in the APP(V717F) transgenic mouse model of Alzheimer's disease. Proceedings of the National Academy of Sciences of the United States of America. 1999 Dec 21;96(26):15233-8.

[135] Kim J, Jiang H, Park S, Eltorai AE, Stewart FR, Yoon H, et al. Haploinsufficiency of human APOE reduces amyloid deposition in a mouse model of amyloid-beta amyloidosis. The Journal of neuroscience : the official journal of the Society for Neuroscience. 2011 Dec 7;31(49):18007-12.

[136] Bien-Ly N, Gillespie AK, Walker D, Yoon SY, Huang Y. Reducing human apolipoprotein E levels attenuates age-dependent Abeta accumulation in mutant human amyloid precursor protein transgenic mice. The Journal of neuroscience : the official journal of the Society for Neuroscience. 2012 Apr 4;32(14):4803-11.

[137] Holtzman DM, Fagan AM, Mackey B, Tenkova T, Sartorius L, Paul SM, et al. Apolipoprotein E facilitates neuritic and cerebrovascular plaque formation in an Alzheimer's disease model. Annals of neurology. 2000 Jun;47(6):739-47.

[138] Geschwind DH. Tau phosphorylation, tangles, and neurodegeneration: the chicken or the egg? Neuron. 2003 Oct 30;40(3):457-60.

[139] Brecht WJ, Harris FM, Chang S, Tesseur I, Yu GQ, Xu Q, et al. Neuron-specific apolipoprotein e4 proteolysis is associated with increased tau phosphorylation in brains of transgenic mice. The Journal of neuroscience : the official journal of the Society for Neuroscience. 2004 Mar 10;24(10):2527-34.

[140] Mahley RW, Huang Y. Apolipoprotein e sets the stage: response to injury triggers neuropathology. Neuron. 2012 Dec 6;76(5):871-85.

[141] Hamanaka H, Katoh-Fukui Y, Suzuki K, Kobayashi M, Suzuki R, Motegi Y, et al. Altered cholesterol metabolism in human apolipoprotein E4 knock-in mice. Human molecular genetics. 2000 Feb 12;9(3):353-61.

[142] Klein RC, Mace BE, Moore SD, Sullivan PM. Progressive loss of synaptic integrity in human apolipoprotein E4 targeted replacement mice and attenuation by apolipoprotein E2. Neuroscience. 2010 Dec 29;171(4):1265-72.

[143] Chen Y, Durakoglugil MS, Xian X, Herz J. ApoE4 reduces glutamate receptor function and synaptic plasticity by selectively impairing ApoE receptor recycling. Proceedings of the National Academy of Sciences of the United States of America. 2010 Jun 29;107(26):12011- 6.

[144] Alzheimer A, Stelzmann RA, Schnitzlein HN, Murtagh FR. An English translation of Alzheimer's 1907 paper, "Uber eine eigenartige Erkankung der Hirnrinde". Clinical anatomy. 1995;8(6):429-31.

[145] LaDu MJ, Shah JA, Reardon CA, Getz GS, Bu G, Hu J, et al. Apolipoprotein E and apolipoprotein E receptors modulate A beta-induced glial neuroinflammatory responses. Neurochemistry international. 2001 Nov-Dec;39(5-6):427-34.

[146] Pocivavsek A, Mikhailenko I, Strickland DK, Rebeck GW. Microglial low-density lipoprotein receptor-related protein 1 modulates c-Jun N-terminal kinase activation. Journal of neuroimmunology. 2009 Sep 29;214(1-2):25-32.

[147] Keene CD, Cudaback E, Li X, Montine KS, Montine TJ. Apolipoprotein E isoforms and regulation of the innate immune response in brain of patients with Alzheimer's disease. Current opinion in neurobiology. 2011 Dec;21(6):920-8.

[148] Grainger DJ, Reckless J, McKilligin E. Apolipoprotein E modulates clearance of apoptotic bodies in vitro and in vivo, resulting in a systemic proinflammatory state in apolipoprotein E-deficient mice. Journal of immunology. 2004 Nov 15;173(10): 6366-75.

[149] Lynch JR, Tang W, Wang H, Vitek MP, Bennett ER, Sullivan PM, et al. APOE genotype and an ApoE-mimetic peptide modify the systemic and central nervous system inflammatory response. The Journal of biological chemistry. 2003 Dec 5;278(49): 48529-33.

[150] Rodriguez GA, Tai LM, LaDu MJ, Rebeck GW. Human APOE4 increases microglia reactivity at Abeta plaques in a mouse model of Abeta deposition. Journal of neuroinflammation. 2014;11:111.

[151] Zhu Y, Nwabuisi-Heath E, Dumanis SB, Tai LM, Yu C, Rebeck GW, et al. APOE genotype alters glial activation and loss of synaptic markers in mice. Glia. 2012 Apr; 60(4):559-69.

[152] Szekely CA, Breitner JC, Fitzpatrick AL, Rea TD, Psaty BM, Kuller LH, et al. NSAID use and dementia risk in the Cardiovascular Health Study: role of APOE and NSAID type. Neurology. 2008 Jan 1;70(1):17-24.

[153] Harold D, Abraham R, Hollingworth P, Sims R, Gerrish A, Hamshere ML, et al. Genome-wide association study identifies variants at CLU and PICALM associated with Alzheimer's disease. Nature genetics. 2009 Oct;41(10):1088-93.

[154] Lambert JC, Heath S, Even G, Campion D, Sleegers K, Hiltunen M, et al. Genome-wide association study identifies variants at CLU and CR1 associated with Alzheimer's disease. Nature genetics. 2009 Oct;41(10):1094-9.

[155] Jun G, Naj AC, Beecham GW, Wang LS, Buros J, Gallins PJ, et al. Meta-analysis confirms CR1, CLU, and PICALM as alzheimer disease risk loci and reveals interactions with APOE genotypes. Archives of neurology. 2010 Dec;67(12):1473-84.

[156] Mullan GM, McEneny J, Fuchs M, McMaster C, Todd S, McGuinness B, et al. Plasma clusterin levels and the rs11136000 genotype in individuals with mild cognitive impairment and Alzheimer's disease. Current Alzheimer research. 2013 Nov;10(9): 973-8.

[157] Thambisetty M, Simmons A, Velayudhan L, Hye A, Campbell J, Zhang Y, et al. Association of plasma clusterin concentration with severity, pathology, and progression in Alzheimer disease. Archives of general psychiatry. 2010 Jul;67(7):739-48.

[158] Schurmann B, Wiese B, Bickel H, Weyerer S, Riedel-Heller SG, Pentzek M, et al. Association of the Alzheimer's disease clusterin risk allele with plasma clusterin concentration. Journal of Alzheimer's disease : JAD. 2011;25(3):421-4.

[159] Braskie MN, Jahanshad N, Stein JL, Barysheva M, McMahon KL, de Zubicaray GI, et al. Common Alzheimer's disease risk variant within the CLU gene affects white matter microstructure in young adults. The Journal of neuroscience : the official journal of the Society for Neuroscience. 2011 May 4;31(18):6764-70.

[160] Erk S, Meyer-Lindenberg A, Opitz von Boberfeld C, Esslinger C, Schnell K, Kirsch P, et al. Hippocampal function in healthy carriers of the CLU Alzheimer's disease risk variant. The Journal of neuroscience : the official journal of the Society for Neuroscience. 2011 Dec 7;31(49):18180-4.

[161] Lancaster TM, Baird A, Wolf C, Jackson MC, Johnston SJ, Donev R, et al. Neural hyperactivation in carriers of the Alzheimer's risk variant on the clusterin gene. Europe-

an neuropsychopharmacology : the journal of the European College of Neuropsychopharmacology. 2011 Dec;21(12):880-4.

[162] Roussotte FF, Gutman BA, Madsen SK, Colby JB, Thompson PM, Alzheimer's Disease Neuroimaging I. Combined effects of Alzheimer risk variants in the CLU and ApoE genes on ventricular expansion patterns in the elderly. The Journal of neuroscience : the official journal of the Society for Neuroscience. 2014 May 7;34(19): 6537-45.

[163] Thambisetty M, Beason-Held LL, An Y, Kraut M, Nalls M, Hernandez DG, et al. Alzheimer risk variant CLU and brain function during aging. Biological psychiatry. 2013 Mar 1;73(5):399-405.

[164] Rodriguez-Rodriguez E, Sanchez-Juan P, Vazquez-Higuera JL, Mateo I, Pozueta A, Berciano J, et al. Genetic risk score predicting accelerated progression from mild cognitive impairment to Alzheimer's disease. Journal of neural transmission. 2013 May; 120(5):807-12.

[165] Elias-Sonnenschein LS, Helisalmi S, Natunen T, Hall A, Paajanen T, Herukka SK, et al. Genetic loci associated with Alzheimer's disease and cerebrospinal fluid biomarkers in a Finnish case-control cohort. PloS one. 2013;8(4):e59676.

[166] Kauwe JS, Cruchaga C, Karch CM, Sadler B, Lee M, Mayo K, et al. Fine mapping of genetic variants in BIN1, CLU, CR1 and PICALM for association with cerebrospinal fluid biomarkers for Alzheimer's disease. PloS one. 2011;6(2):e15918.

[167] Jongbloed W, Herrebout MA, Blankenstein MA, Veerhuis R. Quantification of clusterin in paired cerebrospinal fluid and plasma samples. Annals of clinical biochemistry. 2014 Sep;51(Pt 5):557-67.

[168] Desikan RS, Thompson WK, Holland D, Hess CP, Brewer JB, Zetterberg H, et al. The role of clusterin in amyloid-beta-associated neurodegeneration. JAMA neurology. 2014 Feb;71(2):180-7.

[169] Harr SD, Uint L, Hollister R, Hyman BT, Mendez AJ. Brain expression of apolipoproteins E, J, and A-I in Alzheimer's disease. Journal of neurochemistry. 1996 Jun;66(6): 2429-35.

[170] Nilselid AM, Davidsson P, Nagga K, Andreasen N, Fredman P, Blennow K. Clusterin in cerebrospinal fluid: analysis of carbohydrates and quantification of native and glycosylated forms. Neurochemistry international. 2006 Jun;48(8):718-28.

[171] Sihlbom C, Davidsson P, Sjogren M, Wahlund LO, Nilsson CL. Structural and quantitative comparison of cerebrospinal fluid glycoproteins in Alzheimer's disease patients and healthy individuals. Neurochemical research. 2008 Jul;33(7):1332-40.

[172] Baig S, Palmer LE, Owen MJ, Williams J, Kehoe PG, Love S. Clusterin mRNA and protein in Alzheimer's disease. Journal of Alzheimer's disease : JAD. 2012;28(2): 337-44.

[173] May PC, Johnson SA, Poirier J, Lampert-Etchells M, Finch CE. Altered gene expression in Alzheimer's disease brain tissue. The Canadian journal of neurological sciences Le journal canadien des sciences neurologiques. 1989 Nov;16(4 Suppl):473-6.

[174] Bertrand P, Poirier J, Oda T, Finch CE, Pasinetti GM. Association of apolipoprotein E genotype with brain levels of apolipoprotein E and apolipoprotein J (clusterin) in Alzheimer disease. Brain research Molecular brain research. 1995 Oct;33(1):174-8.

[175] Chen LH, Kao PY, Fan YH, Ho DT, Chan CS, Yik PY, et al. Polymorphisms of CR1, CLU and PICALM confer susceptibility of Alzheimer's disease in a southern Chinese population. Neurobiology of aging. 2012 Jan;33(1):210 e1-7.

[176] Lidstrom AM, Bogdanovic N, Hesse C, Volkman I, Davidsson P, Blennow K. Clusterin (apolipoprotein J) protein levels are increased in hippocampus and in frontal cortex in Alzheimer's disease. Experimental neurology. 1998 Dec;154(2):511-21.

[177] Oda T, Pasinetti GM, Osterburg HH, Anderson C, Johnson SA, Finch CE. Purification and characterization of brain clusterin. Biochemical and biophysical research communications. 1994 Nov 15;204(3):1131-6.

[178] Martin-Rehrmann MD, Hoe HS, Capuani EM, Rebeck GW. Association of apolipoprotein J-positive beta-amyloid plaques with dystrophic neurites in Alzheimer's disease brain. Neurotoxicity research. 2005;7(3):231-42.

[179] McGeer PL, Kawamata T, Walker DG. Distribution of clusterin in Alzheimer brain tissue. Brain research. 1992 May 8;579(2):337-41.

[180] Howlett DR, Hortobagyi T, Francis PT. Clusterin associates specifically with Abeta40 in Alzheimer's disease brain tissue. Brain pathology. 2013 Nov;23(6):623-32.

[181] Kida S, Weller RO, Zhang ET, Phillips MJ, Iannotti F. Anatomical pathways for lymphatic drainage of the brain and their pathological significance. Neuropathology and applied neurobiology. 1995 Jun;21(3):181-4.

[182] Hughes TM, Lopez OL, Evans RW, Kamboh MI, Williamson JD, Klunk WE, et al. Markers of cholesterol transport are associated with amyloid deposition in the brain. Neurobiology of aging. 2014 Apr;35(4):802-7.

[183] Silajdzic E, Minthon L, Bjorkqvist M, Hansson O. No diagnostic value of plasma clusterin in Alzheimer's disease. PloS one. 2012;7(11):e50237.

[184] Thambisetty M, An Y, Kinsey A, Koka D, Saleem M, Guntert A, et al. Plasma clusterin concentration is associated with longitudinal brain atrophy in mild cognitive impairment. NeuroImage. 2012 Jan 2;59(1):212-7.

[185] L IJ, Dekker LJ, Koudstaal PJ, Hofman A, Sillevis Smitt PA, Breteler MM, et al. Serum clusterin levels are not increased in presymptomatic Alzheimer's disease. Journal of proteome research. 2011 Apr 1;10(4):2006-10.

[186] Hye A, Riddoch-Contreras J, Baird AL, Ashton NJ, Bazenet C, Leung R, et al. Plasma proteins predict conversion to dementia from prodromal disease. Alzheimer's & dementia : the journal of the Alzheimer's Association. 2014 Jul 3.

[187] Schrijvers EM, Koudstaal PJ, Hofman A, Breteler MM. Plasma clusterin and the risk of Alzheimer disease. Jama. 2011 Apr 6;305(13):1322-6.

[188] Thambisetty M. Do extracellular chaperone proteins in plasma have potential as Alzheimer's disease biomarkers? Biomarkers in medicine. 2010 Dec;4(6):831-4.

[189] DeMattos RB, O'Dell M A, Parsadanian M, Taylor JW, Harmony JA, Bales KR, et al. Clusterin promotes amyloid plaque formation and is critical for neuritic toxicity in a mouse model of Alzheimer's disease. Proceedings of the National Academy of Sciences of the United States of America. 2002 Aug 6;99(16):10843-8.

[190] Mulder SD, Nielsen HM, Blankenstein MA, Eikelenboom P, Veerhuis R. Apolipoproteins E and J interfere with amyloid-beta uptake by primary human astrocytes and microglia in vitro. Glia. 2014 Apr;62(4):493-503.

[191] Killick R, Ribe EM, Al-Shawi R, Malik B, Hooper C, Fernandes C, et al. Clusterin regulates beta-amyloid toxicity via Dickkopf-1-driven induction of the wnt-PCP-JNK pathway. Molecular psychiatry. 2014 Jan;19(1):88-98.

[192] Bell RD, Sagare AP, Friedman AE, Bedi GS, Holtzman DM, Deane R, et al. Transport pathways for clearance of human Alzheimer's amyloid beta-peptide and apolipoproteins E and J in the mouse central nervous system. Journal of cerebral blood flow and metabolism : official journal of the International Society of Cerebral Blood Flow and Metabolism. 2007 May;27(5):909-18.

[193] Narayan P, Meehan S, Carver JA, Wilson MR, Dobson CM, Klenerman D. Amyloid-beta oligomers are sequestered by both intracellular and extracellular chaperones. Biochemistry. 2012 Nov 20;51(46):9270-6.

[194] Saczynski JS, White L, Peila RL, Rodriguez BL, Launer LJ. The relation between apolipoprotein A-I and dementia: the Honolulu-Asia aging study. American journal of epidemiology. 2007 May 1;165(9):985-92.

[195] Reitz C, Tang MX, Schupf N, Manly JJ, Mayeux R, Luchsinger JA. Association of higher levels of high-density lipoprotein cholesterol in elderly individuals and lower risk of late-onset Alzheimer disease. Archives of neurology. 2010 Dec;67(12):1491-7.

[196] Reed B, Villeneuve S, Mack W, DeCarli C, Chui HC, Jagust W. Associations between serum cholesterol levels and cerebral amyloidosis. JAMA neurology. 2014 Feb;71(2): 195- 200.

[197] Kawano M, Kawakami M, Otsuka M, Yashima H, Yaginuma T, Ueki A. Marked decrease of plasma apolipoprotein AI and AII in Japanese patients with late-onset nonfamilial Alzheimer's disease. Clinica chimica acta; international journal of clinical chemistry. 1995 Aug 14;239(2):209-11.

[198] Kuriyama M, Takahashi K, Yamano T, Hokezu Y, Togo S, Osame M, et al. Low levels of serum apolipoprotein A I and A II in senile dementia. The Japanese journal of psychiatry and neurology. 1994 Sep;48(3):589-93.

[199] Shih YH, Tsai KJ, Lee CW, Shiesh SC, Chen WT, Pai MC, et al. Apolipoprotein C-III is an Amyloid-beta-Binding Protein and an Early Marker for Alzheimer's Disease. Journal of Alzheimer's disease : JAD. 2014 Mar 31.

[200] Merched A, Xia Y, Visvikis S, Serot JM, Siest G. Decreased high-density lipoprotein cholesterol and serum apolipoprotein AI concentrations are highly correlated with the severity of Alzheimer's disease. Neurobiology of aging. 2000 Jan-Feb;21(1):27-30.

[201] Castano EM, Roher AE, Esh CL, Kokjohn TA, Beach T. Comparative proteomics of cerebrospinal fluid in neuropathologically-confirmed Alzheimer's disease and non-demented elderly subjects. Neurological research. 2006 Mar;28(2):155-63.

[202] Song H, Saito K, Seishima M, Noma A, Urakami K, Nakashima K. Cerebrospinal fluid apo E and apo A-I concentrations in early- and late-onset Alzheimer's disease. Neuroscience letters. 1997 Aug 15;231(3):175-8.

[203] Lefterov I, Fitz NF, Cronican AA, Fogg A, Lefterov P, Kodali R, et al. Apolipoprotein A-I deficiency increases cerebral amyloid angiopathy and cognitive deficits in APP/PS1DeltaE9 mice. The Journal of biological chemistry. 2010 Nov 19;285(47):36945-57.

[204] Lewis TL, Cao D, Lu H, Mans RA, Su YR, Jungbauer L, et al. Overexpression of human apolipoprotein A-I preserves cognitive function and attenuates neuroinflammation and cerebral amyloid angiopathy in a mouse model of Alzheimer disease. The Journal of biological chemistry. 2010 Nov 19;285(47):36958-68.

[205] de Magalhaes JP, Curado J, Church GM. Meta-analysis of age-related gene expression profiles identifies common signatures of aging. Bioinformatics. 2009 Apr 1;25(7):875-81.

[206] Terrisse L, Poirier J, Bertrand P, Merched A, Visvikis S, Siest G, et al. Increased levels of apolipoprotein D in cerebrospinal fluid and hippocampus of Alzheimer's patients. Journal of neurochemistry. 1998 Oct;71(4):1643-50.

[207] Glockner F, Ohm TG. Hippocampal apolipoprotein D level depends on Braak stage and APOE genotype. Neuroscience. 2003;122(1):103-10.

[208] Abildayeva K, Berbee JF, Blokland A, Jansen PJ, Hoek FJ, Meijer O, et al. Human apolipoprotein C-I expression in mice impairs learning and memory functions. Journal of lipid research. 2008 Apr;49(4):856-69.

[209] Cudaback E, Li X, Yang Y, Yoo T, Montine KS, Craft S, et al. Apolipoprotein C-I is an APOE genotype-dependent suppressor of glial activation. Journal of neuroinflammation. 2012;9:192.

[210] Poduslo SE, Neal M, Herring K, Shelly J. The apolipoprotein CI A allele as a risk factor for Alzheimer's disease. Neurochemical research. 1998 Mar;23(3):361-7.

[211] Drigalenko E, Poduslo S, Elston R. Interaction of the apolipoprotein E and CI loci in predisposing to late-onset Alzheimer's disease. Neurology. 1998 Jul;51(1):131-5.

[212] Csaszar A, Kalman J, Szalai C, Janka Z, Romics L. Association of the apolipoprotein A-IV codon 360 mutation in patients with Alzheimer's disease. Neuroscience letters. 1997 Jul 25;230(3):151-4.

[213] Cui Y, Huang M, He Y, Zhang S, Luo Y. Genetic ablation of apolipoprotein A-IV accelerates Alzheimer's disease pathogenesis in a mouse model. The American journal of pathology. 2011 Mar;178(3):1298-308.

[214] Shih YH, Tsai KJ, Lee CW, Shiesh SC, Chen WT, Pai MC, et al. Apolipoprotein C-III is an amyloid-beta-binding protein and an early marker for Alzheimer's disease. Journal of Alzheimer's disease : JAD. 2014;41(3):855-65.

[215] Pahnke J, Langer O, Krohn M. Alzheimer's and ABC transporters - new opportunities for diagnostics and treatment. Neurobiology of disease. 2014 Apr 16.

[216] Koldamova R, Fitz NF, Lefterov I. ATP-binding cassette transporter A1: From metabolism to neurodegeneration. Neurobiology of disease. 2014 May 17.

[217] Hirsch-Reinshagen V, Maia LF, Burgess BL, Blain JF, Naus KE, McIsaac SA, et al. The absence of ABCA1 decreases soluble ApoE levels but does not diminish amyloid deposition in two murine models of Alzheimer disease. The Journal of biological chemistry. 2005 Dec 30;280(52):43243-56.

[218] Wahrle SE, Jiang H, Parsadanian M, Hartman RE, Bales KR, Paul SM, et al. Deletion of Abca1 increases Abeta deposition in the PDAPP transgenic mouse model of Alzheimer disease. The Journal of biological chemistry. 2005 Dec 30;280(52):43236-42.

[219] Koldamova R, Staufenbiel M, Lefterov I. Lack of ABCA1 considerably decreases brain ApoE level and increases amyloid deposition in APP23 mice. The Journal of biological chemistry. 2005 Dec 30;280(52):43224-35.

[220] Lefterov I, Fitz NF, Cronican A, Lefterov P, Staufenbiel M, Koldamova R. Memory deficits in APP23/Abca1+/- mice correlate with the level of Abeta oligomers. ASN neuro. 2009;1(2).

[221] Fitz NF, Cronican AA, Saleem M, Fauq AH, Chapman R, Lefterov I, et al. Abca1 deficiency affects Alzheimer's disease-like phenotype in human ApoE4 but not in ApoE3- targeted replacement mice. The Journal of neuroscience : the official journal of the Society for Neuroscience. 2012 Sep 19;32(38):13125-36.

[222] Lefterov I, Bookout A, Wang Z, Staufenbiel M, Mangelsdorf D, Koldamova R. Expression profiling in APP23 mouse brain: inhibition of Abeta amyloidosis and in-

flammation in response to LXR agonist treatment. Molecular neurodegeneration. 2007;2:20.

[223] Koldamova RP, Lefterov IM, Staufenbiel M, Wolfe D, Huang S, Glorioso JC, et al. The liver X receptor ligand T0901317 decreases amyloid beta production in vitro and in a mouse model of Alzheimer's disease. The Journal of biological chemistry. 2005 Feb 11;280(6):4079-88.

[224] Riddell DR, Zhou H, Comery TA, Kouranova E, Lo CF, Warwick HK, et al. The LXR agonist TO901317 selectively lowers hippocampal Abeta42 and improves memory in the Tg2576 mouse model of Alzheimer's disease. Molecular and cellular neurosciences. 2007 Apr;34(4):621-8.

[225] Jiang Q, Lee CY, Mandrekar S, Wilkinson B, Cramer P, Zelcer N, et al. ApoE promotes the proteolytic degradation of Abeta. Neuron. 2008 Jun 12;58(5):681-93.

[226] Fitz NF, Cronican A, Pham T, Fogg A, Fauq AH, Chapman R, et al. Liver X receptor agonist treatment ameliorates amyloid pathology and memory deficits caused by high-fat diet in APP23 mice. The Journal of neuroscience : the official journal of the Society for Neuroscience. 2010 May 19;30(20):6862-72.

[227] Cramer PE, Cirrito JR, Wesson DW, Lee CY, Karlo JC, Zinn AE, et al. ApoE-directed therapeutics rapidly clear beta-amyloid and reverse deficits in AD mouse models. Science. 2012 Mar 23;335(6075):1503-6.

[228] Vanmierlo T, Rutten K, Dederen J, Bloks VW, van Vark-van der Zee LC, Kuipers F, et al. Liver X receptor activation restores memory in aged AD mice without reducing amyloid. Neurobiology of aging. 2011 Jul;32(7):1262-72.

[229] Donkin JJ, Stukas S, Hirsch-Reinshagen V, Namjoshi D, Wilkinson A, May S, et al. ATP-binding cassette transporter A1 mediates the beneficial effects of the liver X receptor agonist GW3965 on object recognition memory and amyloid burden in amyloid precursor protein/presenilin 1 mice. The Journal of biological chemistry. 2010 Oct 29;285(44):34144- 54.

[230] Fitz NF, Castranio EL, Carter AY, Kodali R, Lefterov I, Koldamova R. Improvement of Memory Deficits and Amyloid-beta Clearance in Aged APP23 Mice Treated with a Combination of Anti-Amyloid-beta Antibody and LXR Agonist. Journal of Alzheimer's disease: JAD. 2014 Mar 18.

[231] Fitz NF, Cronican AA, Lefterov I, Koldamova R. Comment on "ApoE-directed therapeutics rapidly clear beta-amyloid and reverse deficits in AD mouse models". Science. 2013 May 24;340(6135):924-c.

[232] Tesseur I, Lo AC, Roberfroid A, Dietvorst S, Van Broeck B, Borgers M, et al. Comment on "ApoE-directed therapeutics rapidly clear beta-amyloid and reverse deficits in AD mouse models". Science. 2013 May 24;340(6135):924-e.

[233] Wang XF, Cao YW, Feng ZZ, Fu D, Ma YS, Zhang F, et al. Quantitative assessment of the effect of ABCA1 gene polymorphism on the risk of Alzheimer's disease. Molecular biology reports. 2013 Feb;40(2):779-85.

[234] Frikke-Schmidt R, Nordestgaard BG, Stene MC, Sethi AA, Remaley AT, Schnohr P, et al. Association of loss-of-function mutations in the ABCA1 gene with high-density lipoprotein cholesterol levels and risk of ischemic heart disease. Jama. 2008 Jun 4;299(21):2524-32.

[235] Clee SM, Kastelein JJ, van Dam M, Marcil M, Roomp K, Zwarts KY, et al. Age and residual cholesterol efflux affect HDL cholesterol levels and coronary artery disease in ABCA1 heterozygotes. The Journal of clinical investigation. 2000 Nov;106(10): 1263-70.

[236] Rader DJ, deGoma EM. Approach to the patient with extremely low HDL-cholesterol. The Journal of clinical endocrinology and metabolism. 2012 Oct;97(10):3399-407.

[237] Naj AC, Jun G, Beecham GW, Wang LS, Vardarajan BN, Buros J, et al. Common variants at MS4A4/MS4A6E, CD2AP, CD33 and EPHA1 are associated with late-onset Alzheimer's disease. Nature genetics. 2011 May;43(5):436-41.

[238] Allen M, Zou F, Chai HS, Younkin CS, Crook J, Pankratz VS, et al. Novel late-onset Alzheimer disease loci variants associate with brain gene expression. Neurology. 2012 Jul 17;79(3):221-8.

[239] Karch CM, Jeng AT, Nowotny P, Cady J, Cruchaga C, Goate AM. Expression of novel Alzheimer's disease risk genes in control and Alzheimer's disease brains. PloS one. 2012;7(11):e50976.

[240] Reitz C, Jun G, Naj A, Rajbhandary R, Vardarajan BN, Wang LS, et al. Variants in the ATP-binding cassette transporter (ABCA7), apolipoprotein E 4,and the risk of late-onset Alzheimer disease in African Americans. Jama. 2013 Apr 10;309(14):1483-92.

[241] Vasquez JB, Fardo DW, Estus S. ABCA7 expression is associated with Alzheimer's disease polymorphism and disease status. Neuroscience letters. 2013 Nov 27;556:58-62.

[242] Shulman JM, Chen K, Keenan BT, Chibnik LB, Fleisher A, Thiyyagura P, et al. Genetic susceptibility for Alzheimer disease neuritic plaque pathology. JAMA neurology. 2013 Sep 1;70(9):1150-7.

[243] Beecham GW, Hamilton K, Naj AC, Martin ER, Huentelman M, Myers AJ, et al. Genome-Wide Association Meta-analysis of Neuropathologic Features of Alzheimer's Disease and Related Dementias. PLoS genetics. 2014 Sep;10(9):e1004606.

[244] Hollingworth P, Harold D, Sims R, Gerrish A, Lambert JC, Carrasquillo MM, et al. Common variants at ABCA7, MS4A6A/MS4A4E, EPHA1, CD33 and CD2AP are associated with Alzheimer's disease. Nature genetics. 2011 May;43(5):429-35.

[245] Kim WS, Li H, Ruberu K, Chan S, Elliott DA, Low JK, et al. Deletion of Abca7 increases cerebral amyloid-beta accumulation in the J20 mouse model of Alzheimer's disease. The Journal of neuroscience : the official journal of the Society for Neuroscience. 2013 Mar 6;33(10):4387-94.

[246] Burgess BL, Parkinson PF, Racke MM, Hirsch-Reinshagen V, Fan J, Wong C, et al. ABCG1 influences the brain cholesterol biosynthetic pathway but does not affect amyloid precursor protein or apolipoprotein E metabolism in vivo. Journal of lipid research. 2008 Jun;49(6):1254-67.

[247] Rousset X, Shamburek R, Vaisman B, Amar M, Remaley AT. Lecithin cholesterol acyltransferase: an anti- or pro-atherogenic factor? Current atherosclerosis reports. 2011 Jun;13(3):249-56.

[248] Desrumaux C, Pisoni A, Meunier J, Deckert V, Athias A, Perrier V, et al. Increased amyloid-beta peptide-induced memory deficits in phospholipid transfer protein (PLTP) gene knockout mice. Neuropsychopharmacology : official publication of the American College of Neuropsychopharmacology. 2013 Apr;38(5):817-25.

[249] Wang H, Yu Y, Chen W, Cui Y, Luo T, Ma J, et al. PLTP deficiency impairs learning and memory capabilities partially due to alteration of amyloid-beta metabolism in old mice. Journal of Alzheimer's disease : JAD. 2014;39(1):79-88.

[250] Arias-Vasquez A, Isaacs A, Aulchenko YS, Hofman A, Oostra BA, Breteler M, et al. The cholesteryl ester transfer protein (CETP) gene and the risk of Alzheimer's disease. Neurogenetics. 2007 Aug;8(3):189-93.

[251] Barzilai N, Atzmon G, Schechter C, Schaefer EJ, Cupples AL, Lipton R, et al. Unique lipoprotein phenotype and genotype associated with exceptional longevity. Jama. 2003 Oct 15;290(15):2030-40.

[252] Cellini E, Nacmias B, Olivieri F, Ortenzi L, Tedde A, Bagnoli S, et al. Cholesteryl ester transfer protein (CETP) I405V polymorphism and longevity in Italian centenarians. Mechanisms of ageing and development. 2005 Jun-Jul;126(6-7):826-8.

[253] Li Q, Huang P, He QC, Lin QZ, Wu J, Yin RX. Association between the CETP polymorphisms and the risk of Alzheimer's disease, carotid atherosclerosis, longevity, and the efficacy of statin therapy. Neurobiology of aging. 2014 Jun;35(6):1513 e13-23.

[254] Novelli V, Viviani Anselmi C, Roncarati R, Guffanti G, Malovini A, Piluso G, et al. Lack of replication of genetic associations with human longevity. Biogerontology. 2008 Apr;9(2):85-92.

[255] Sun L, Hu CY, Shi XH, Zheng CG, Huang ZZ, Lv ZP, et al. Trans-ethnical shift of the risk genotype in the CETP I405V with longevity: a Chinese case-control study and meta- analysis. PloS one. 2013;8(8):e72537.

[256] Yang JK, Gong YY, Xie L, Yang Y, Xu LY, Zhang YP. Association study of promoter polymorphisms in the CETP gene with longevity in the Han Chinese population. Molecular biology reports. 2014 Jan;41(1):325-9.

[257] Warstadt NM, Dennis EL, Jahanshad N, Kohannim O, Nir TM, McMahon KL, et al. Serum cholesterol and variant in cholesterol-related gene CETP predict white matter microstructure. Neurobiology of aging. 2014 Nov;35(11):2504-13.

[258] Rodriguez E, Mateo I, Infante J, Llorca J, Berciano J, Combarros O. Cholesteryl ester transfer protein (CETP) polymorphism modifies the Alzheimer's disease risk associated with APOE epsilon4 allele. Journal of neurology. 2006 Feb;253(2):181-5.

[259] Chen Y, Jia L, Wei C, Wang F, Lv H, Jia J. Association between polymorphisms in the apolipoprotein D gene and sporadic Alzheimer's disease. Brain research. 2008 Oct 3;1233:196-202.

[260] Murphy EA, Roddey JC, McEvoy LK, Holland D, Hagler DJ, Jr., Dale AM, et al. CETP polymorphisms associate with brain structure, atrophy rate, and Alzheimer's disease risk in an APOE-dependent manner. Brain imaging and behavior. 2012 Mar; 6(1):16-26.

[261] Sanders AE, Wang C, Katz M, Derby CA, Barzilai N, Ozelius L, et al. Association of a functional polymorphism in the cholesteryl ester transfer protein (CETP) gene with memory decline and incidence of dementia. Jama. 2010 Jan 13;303(2):150-8.

[262] Deane R, Wu Z, Sagare A, Davis J, Du Yan S, Hamm K, et al. LRP/amyloid beta- peptide interaction mediates differential brain efflux of Abeta isoforms. Neuron. 2004 Aug 5;43(3):333-44.

[263] Kanekiyo T, Cirrito JR, Liu CC, Shinohara M, Li J, Schuler DR, et al. Neuronal clearance of amyloid-beta by endocytic receptor LRP1. The Journal of neuroscience : the official journal of the Society for Neuroscience. 2013 Dec 4;33(49):19276-83.

[264] Shibata M, Yamada S, Kumar SR, Calero M, Bading J, Frangione B, et al. Clearance of Alzheimer's amyloid-ss(1-40) peptide from brain by LDL receptor-related protein-1 at the blood-brain barrier. The Journal of clinical investigation. 2000 Dec;106(12): 1489-99.

[265] Tamamizu-Kato S, Cohen JK, Drake CB, Kosaraju MG, Drury J, Narayanaswami V. Interaction with amyloid beta peptide compromises the lipid binding function of apolipoprotein E. Biochemistry. 2008 May 6;47(18):5225-34.

[266] Van Uden E, Mallory M, Veinbergs I, Alford M, Rockenstein E, Masliah E. Increased extracellular amyloid deposition and neurodegeneration in human amyloid precursor protein transgenic mice deficient in receptor-associated protein. The Journal of neuroscience : the official journal of the Society for Neuroscience. 2002 Nov 1;22(21): 9298-304.

[267] Deane R, Sagare A, Hamm K, Parisi M, Lane S, Finn MB, et al. apoE isoform-specific disruption of amyloid beta peptide clearance from mouse brain. The Journal of clinical investigation. 2008 Dec;118(12):4002-13.

[268] Cao D, Fukuchi K, Wan H, Kim H, Li L. Lack of LDL receptor aggravates learning deficits and amyloid deposits in Alzheimer transgenic mice. Neurobiology of aging. 2006 Nov;27(11):1632-43.

[269] Castellano JM, Deane R, Gottesdiener AJ, Verghese PB, Stewart FR, West T, et al. Low-density lipoprotein receptor overexpression enhances the rate of brain-to-blood Abeta clearance in a mouse model of beta-amyloidosis. Proceedings of the National Academy of Sciences of the United States of America. 2012 Sep 18;109(38):15502-7.

[270] Beffert U, Morfini G, Bock HH, Reyna H, Brady ST, Herz J. Reelin-mediated signaling locally regulates protein kinase B/Akt and glycogen synthase kinase 3beta. The Journal of biological chemistry. 2002 Dec 20;277(51):49958-64.

[271] Ohkubo N, Lee YD, Morishima A, Terashima T, Kikkawa S, Tohyama M, et al. Apolipoprotein E and Reelin ligands modulate tau phosphorylation through an apolipoprotein E receptor/disabled-1/glycogen synthase kinase-3beta cascade. FASEB journal : official publication of the Federation of American Societies for Experimental Biology. 2003 Feb;17(2):295-7.

[272] Ridker PM. LDL cholesterol: controversies and future therapeutic directions. Lancet. 2014 Aug 16;384(9943):607-17.

[273] Beffert U, Arguin C, Poirier J. The polymorphism in exon 3 of the low density lipoprotein receptor-related protein gene is weakly associated with Alzheimer's disease. Neuroscience letters. 1999 Jan 4;259(1):29-32.

[274] Sanchez-Guerra M, Combarros O, Infante J, Llorca J, Berciano J, Fontalba A, et al. Case-control study and meta-analysis of low density lipoprotein receptor-related protein gene exon 3 polymorphism in Alzheimer's disease. Neuroscience letters. 2001 Dec 4;316(1):17-20.

[275] Vazquez-Higuera JL, Mateo I, Sanchez-Juan P, Rodriguez-Rodriguez E, Pozueta A, Infante J, et al. Genetic interaction between tau and the apolipoprotein E receptor LRP1 Increases Alzheimer's disease risk. Dementia and geriatric cognitive disorders. 2009;28(2):116-20.

[276] Vargas T, Bullido MJ, Martinez-Garcia A, Antequera D, Clarimon J, Rosich-Estrago M, et al. A megalin polymorphism associated with promoter activity and Alzheimer's disease risk. American journal of medical genetics Part B, Neuropsychiatric genetics : the official publication of the International Society of Psychiatric Genetics. 2010 Jun 5;153B(4):895-902.

[277] Wang LL, Pan XL, Wang Y, Tang HD, Deng YL, Ren RJ, et al. A single nucleotide polymorphism in LRP2 is associated with susceptibility to Alzheimer's disease in the

Chinese population. Clinica chimica acta; international journal of clinical chemistry. 2011 Jan 30;412(3-4):268-70.

[278] Miyashita A, Koike A, Jun G, Wang LS, Takahashi S, Matsubara E, et al. SORL1 is genetically associated with late-onset Alzheimer's disease in Japanese, Koreans and Caucasians. PloS one. 2013;8(4):e58618.

[279] Rogaeva E, Meng Y, Lee JH, Gu Y, Kawarai T, Zou F, et al. The neuronal sortilin- related receptor SORL1 is genetically associated with Alzheimer disease. Nature genetics. 2007 Feb;39(2):168-77.

[280] Scherzer CR, Offe K, Gearing M, Rees HD, Fang G, Heilman CJ, et al. Loss of apolipoprotein E receptor LR11 in Alzheimer disease. Archives of neurology. 2004 Aug; 61(8):1200-5.

[281] Felsky D, Szeszko P, Yu L, Honer WG, De Jager PL, Schneider JA, et al. The SORL1 gene and convergent neural risk for Alzheimer's disease across the human lifespan. Molecular psychiatry. 2013 Oct 29.

Chapter 6

# Free Cholesterol — A Double-Edge Sword in Alzheimer Disease

José C. Fernández-Checa

Additional information is available at the end of the chapter

http://dx.doi.org/10.5772/59935

## 1. Introduction

Alzheimer's disease (AD) is a progressive neurodegenerative disorder that accounts for most of dementia cases in elder people. The main features of AD include a progressive deterioration of intellectual functions, most prominently memory impairment, loss of language ability, and cognitive deficits. Motor defects appear in the late phases of the disease and basic activities of daily living are gradually compromised as the pathology progresses to advanced phases, and are often accompanied by psychosis and agitation [1, 2]. The hallmarks of the disease include the accumulation of amyloid-β peptide (Aβ) inside neurons and in the extracellular brain space, and the intracellular formation of neurofibrillary tangles (NFTs) composed of hyper-phosphorylated tau protein, loss of synapses at specific brain sites as well as the degeneration of cholinergic neurons from the basal forebrain [3]. The prevalence of AD is about 8–10 % of the population over 65 years of age, which increases 2-fold every 5 years afterwards [4, 5]. This high rate prevalence together with the increase in life expectancy, point to AD as one of the most serious health concerns wordlwide, whose incidence is expected to tiple in the next 2-3 decades unless more effective therapies are available [6].

The identification of new targets for the development of more effective therapeutic approaches requires a better understanding of the molecular pathways leading to AD. In this regard, both genetic and environmental factors are increasingly recognized to contribute to the development of AD, which occurs in two forms. The sporadic form of the disease, which affects people over 65 years of age and accounts for the vast mayority of AD cases. In a small proportion (6–8 %), the disease is inherited as an autosomal dominant trait and appears as an early onset in people younger than 65 years of age. Mutations within three genes, the amyloid precursor protein (APP) gene on chromosome 21, the presenilin 1 (PSEN1) gene on chromosome 14, and the presenilin 2 (PSEN2) gene on chromosome 1, have been identified as the main cause of early onset familial AD [7-10]. While these findings are key for our understanding of the pathogenesis of familial AD, these mutations account for 30–50% of all autosomal dominant early onset cases.

In the last years, it has become increasingly recognized that cholesterol plays a significant role in AD. The first evidence of the importance of cholesterol was the discovery that the ε4 allele of the cholesterol transport protein apolipoprotein E (ApoE) is associated with a higher risk of developing both familial and sporadic AD and modulates the age of AD onset [11-14]. Despite these findings, the impact and causal role of cholesterol in AD remains controversial (see below), as exemplified by the inconsistent outcome of statins in modulating AD risk and progression, which calls for the need for large-scale trials to document whether statins and cholesterol modification regulate or modify the course of AD [15, 16]. Emerging data, however, position the small pool of cholesterol in mitochondria as a key player in AD by determining the susceptibility of neurons to Aβ neuroinflammation, synaptotoxicity and neurotoxicity and as a culprit of cognitive decline by depleting specific mitochondrial antioxidant defense mechanisms. In this review, we will briefly summarize the role of cholesterol in AD, focusing not only in the evidence that cholesterol may foster the amiloidogenic processing of APP and the generation of Aβ peptide, but most importantly, recent findings indicate that cholesterol trafficking to mitochondria stands as a novel critical factor that sensitizes to Aβ-induced neuroinflammation and neurotoxicity, emerging as a potential target for intervention.

## 2. The involvement of Aβ and cholesterol in AD

### 2.1. The role of Aβ in AD

Since Aβ was first identified as a component of amyloid plaques, increasing evidence has suggested that Aβ is a major player in AD pathogenesis. According to the amyloid cascade hypothesis, the dysregulation of APP metabolism and Aβ deposition are primary events in the onset of the disease [17, 18]. The Aβ 1–42 and Aβ 1–40 peptides are the major forms found in amyloid plaques, which are generated by proteolytic cleavage of APP. These plaques are predominantly found in areas affected by neurodegeneration, such as entorhinal cortex, amygdala, neocortex, and particularly, hippocampus [19, 20]. While the number of plaques usually does not correlate with the severity of dementia, clinical correlation between elevated Aβ deposition in the brain and cognitive decline has been reported [21]. As described below, several lines of evidence suggest that overproduction and/or reduced clearance of Aβ peptides are key to amyloid aggregation, which contributes to the development of NFTs and neurodegeneration in AD pathology. Intraneuronal Aβ can derive by either APP cleavage within neuronal endocytic compartments, as well as by Aβ internalization from the extracellular space. Both sources are of relevance in the formation of the pool of Aβ involved in neurodegeneration. Intraneuronal Aβ accumulation is one of the earliest pathological events in humans and in animal models of AD, which correlates with early abnormalities in long term potentiation (LTP), cognitive dysfunctions and precedes the formation of amyloid plaques and NFTs formation and the neurodegeneration in animal models in which intracellular Aβ and neuronal loss have been reported [22-26]. Furthermore, Aβ plaques could generate from the death of neurons that contained elevated amounts of Aβ and this release can account for the loss of intraneuronal Aβ immunoreactivity in areas of plaque formation [24, 27, 28]. Moreover, recent findings indicated that internalized Aβ elicits fibrillization in the multivesicular bodies (MVBs), which after reaching the plasma membrane, cause cell death and the release of amyloid structures into the extracellular space, indicating that exosomes derived from MVBs could release part of the intracellular pool of Aβ to contribute to the extracellular Aβ pool [29, 30]. The contribution of intracellular Aβ to neuronal death has been well documented in cortical neurons from brains of AD and Down syndrome patients that undergo apoptosis after accumulation of Aβ42 [31, 32]. In addition, microinjection of Aβ1-42 or cDNA-expressing cytosolic Aβ1-42 induces cell death in primary human neurons, while neuronal loss associated with intracellular accumulation of Aβ has been described in a transgenic APP(SL)PS1KI mouse that closely mimics the development of AD-related neuropathological features of AD [33, 34]. Intracellular Aβ accumulation has been associated with neuritic and synaptic pathology and transgenic mice harboring constructs that target Aβ intracellularly developed neurodegeneration [35-37]. Furthermore, antibodies against Aβ reduced intraneuronal Aβ accumulation prevented synaptotoxicity and reversed cognitive impairment in triple transgenic mice [22, 38]. Finally, a coding mutation (A673TT) in APP has been recently shown to protect against AD and age-related cognitive decline in elderly Icelanders [39]. This mutation that affects the aspartyl protease β-site in APP significantly reduces the formation of amyloidogenic peptides, strongly indicating that reducing the β-cleavage of APP protect against the disease. Thus, although targeting Aβ may be a rationale approach to prevent or treat AD progression, recent findings have unfolded the diversity of Aβ structures revealed by the immune response to fibrillar Aβ [40]. This outcome may account for the failure of single therapeutic monoclonal antibodies against Aβ in the treatment of AD.

### 2.2. Amiloidogenic processing of APP and Aβ generation

Amiloidogenic processing of APP yields toxic Aβ peptides (Fig 1). In this pathway, the β- and γ-secretases cleave APP at the N- and C-termini of the Aβ peptide, respectively. APP, β - secretase, PS1 and Aβ are all present in lipid rafts, which are enriched in cholesterol and glycosphingolipids. This led to the suggestion that APP in lipid rafts is primarily processed via the β-secretase, and APP outside of ratfs is processed via the α-secretase pathway. β-secretase has been characterized as a membrane-bound aspartic protease termed beta-site APP-cleaving enzyme 1 (BACE1), while γ-secretase is a complex comprised of presenilin-1 or -2, nicastrin, anterior pharynx-defective 1 (Aph-1) and presenilin enhancer 2 (Pen-2) [41]. β-arrestin 2, is a novel member of the γ-secretase complex that physically associates with the Aph-1α subunit of the γ-secretase complex and redistributes the complex toward detergent-resistant membranes, increasing the catalytic activity of the complex [42]. Moreover, β-arrestin 2 expression is elevated in individuals with AD and its overexpression leads to an increase in Aβ peptide generation, whereas genetic silencing of Arrb2 (encoding β-arrestin 2) reduces generation of Aβ in cell cultures and in Arrb2-/- mice. In addition to its amyloidogenic processing by β- and γ-secretases, APP can be cleaved within the Aβ domain by α-secretase. This non-amyloidogenic processing prevents the deposition of intact Aβ peptide and results in the release of a large soluble ectodomain, sAPP$\alpha$, from the cell, which has neuroprotective and memory-enhancing effects. Members of the ADAMs, a disintegrin and metalloprotease family of proteases, have been shown to possess $\alpha$-secretase activity [43].

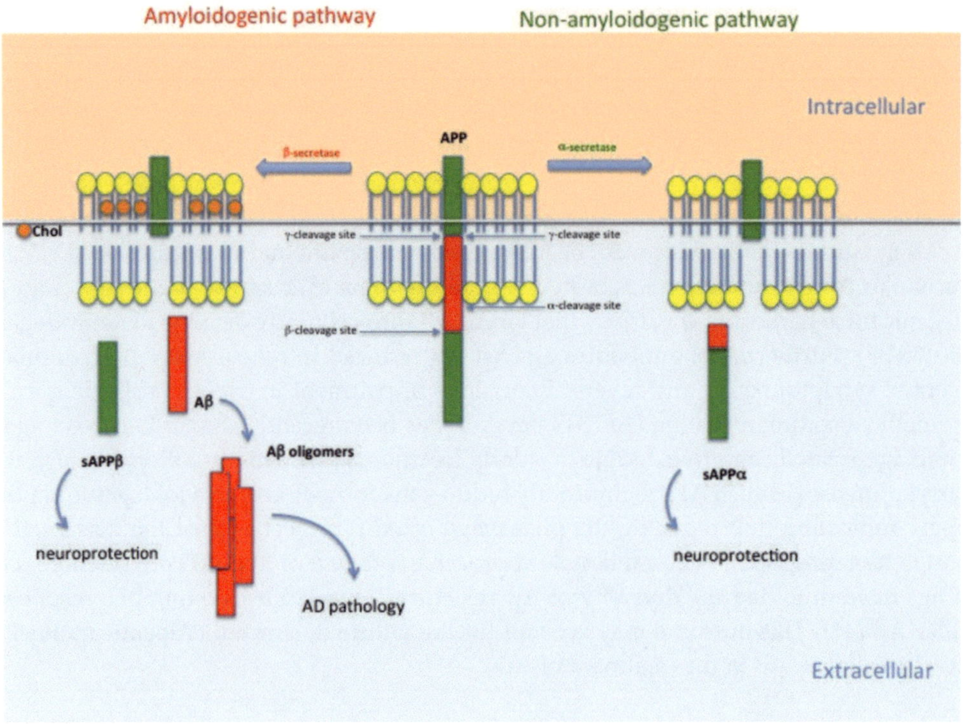


**Figure 1.** Role of membrane cholesterol in amyloidogenesis. β- and γ-secretases cleave APP at the N- and C-termini of the Aβ peptide, respectively. APP, β-secretase, PS1 and Aβ are all present in lipid rafts, which are enriched in cholesterol and glycosphingolipids. Therefore, APP in lipid rafts is primarily processed via the β-secretase, and APP outside of ratfs is processed via the $\alpha$-secretase pathway. In the former, β-secretase-mediated Aβ peptides oligomerize and accumulate in plaques contributing to the neurotoxicity of AD.

Besides its extracellular deposition, current evidence indicates the processing and targeting of APP and Aβ to intracellular sites, including mitochondria [44]. Moreover, levels of mitochondrial APP are higher in affected brain areas and in subjects with advanced disease symptons [45]. Immunoelectron microscopy analyses indicated the association of APP with mitochondrial protein translocation components, TOM40 and TIM23, which correlated with decreased import of respiratory chain subunits *in vitro*, decreased cytochrome oxidase activity, increased ROS generation and impaired mitochondrial reducing capacity [45].

### 2.3. The role of cholesterol in AD: facts and controversies

Cholesterol is an essential component of membrane bilayers that regulate strucutral and functional properties and, hence, a pleiotropic number of cell functions and in the intracellular trafficking of proteins [46]. Cholesterol is required for synapse formation, biogenesis of synaptic vesicles and regulation of neurotransmitter release and the precursor of steroid hormones and oxysterols, which are critical intermediates in many metabolic pathways [47-49]. Cholesterol homeostasis is altered in AD; however, whether cholesterol levels are upregulated or downregulated in AD remains to be established. The pathogenic processing of APP into toxic Aβ fragments is known to occur in cholesterol-enriched membrane domains of the plasma membrane, called lipid rafts. The first evidence that cholesterol may impact Aβ production in the brain came from observations that dietary cholesterol increases amyloid production in rabbit hippocampal neurons [50]. Work in mice genetically modified to deposit cerebral Aβ demonstrated that a cholesterol-enriched diet resulted in increased Aβ deposition and increased amyloid plaque formation [51], and these observations were confirmed in subsequent studies in mice fed diets enriched in cholesterol [52-55]. As discussed below, very little cholesterol is transferred from the periphery to the brain due to the impermeability of the blood brain barrier (BBB), so the observations of diet-induced cholesterol-mediated Aβ deposition in neurons are puzzling. A potential explanation for these findings is the fact that BBB permeability is impaired in AD [56, 57]. Exploiting the relative detergent insolubility of lipid rafts, there has been evidence indicating the localization of APP, the $\alpha$-, β- and $\gamma$-secretases in rafts [58, 59]. In addition, the activities of BACE1 and $\gamma$-secretase are stimulated by lipid components of rafts, in particular glycosphingolipids and cholesterol. Consistent with these findings supporting a role for cholesterol in AD pathogenesis, high cholesterol levels have been shown to correlate with Aβ deposition and the risk of developing AD [60-62]. Patients taking the cholesterol-lowering drug statins have a lower incidence of the disease [62, 63]. Besides ApoE, other genes encoding proteins involved in cholesterol homeostasis, including cholesteol 24-hydroxylase (CYP46A1), the acyl-coenzyme A:cholesterol acyltransferase (ACAT), the cholesterol efflux transporters ABCA1 and ABCA7, and the lipopotrein-receptor-related protein (LRP) have been linked to the risk, development or progression of AD [64-68]. Despite this experimental and epidemiological evidence, the role of increased cholesterol in AD is controversial with findings showing the opposite. For instance, earlier studies indicated that hippocampal membranes of AD brains showed a reduced fluidity in the hydrocarbon core region compared to control subjects that correlated with the cholesterol content in AD samples [69]. Moreover, reduced cholesterol levels and cholesterol/phospholipids mole ratio have been reported in the temporal gyrus but unaffected in the cerebellum of AD patients with respect to controls [70]. Decreased 24-hydroxycholesterol levels that correlated with lower lathosterol content was reported in the frontal and occipital cortex of patients with AD compared to subjects controls [71]. In addition, cholesterol levels were slightly increased in frontal cortex gray matter in AD patients with the ApoE4 genotype compared with ApoE4 control subjects [72]. Finally, neuronal membrane cholesterol loss has been shown to enhance Aβ generation in hippocampal membranes from AD patients exhibiting increased colocalization of BACE1 and APP [73], and hippocampal membranes from the brain of AD patients contain less membrane cholesterol than control [74]. Furthermore, it has been reported that inhibition of the mevalonate pathway increased production of Aβ and amyloid plaques [75]. Prospective cohort studies have failed to demonstrate the protective effect of statins on dementia, while others reports did not replicate the Aβ lowering effect of statins in the cerebrospinal fluid [76-81]. In addition to these findings arguing against the correlation between increased brain cholesterol and AD, there is evidence that both cholesterol and Aβ reciprocally regulate each other and that Aβ impacts negatively in cholesterol synthesis, in part, by inhibiting stero-regulated element binding proteins-2 (SREBP-2) cleavage [82, 83]. Interestingly, the consequent decrease in protein prenylation contributes to Aβ-induced neuronal death, which is reversed by exogenous supply of isoprenoids. Further work is needed to ascertain whether the intracelular distribution rather than the levels of brain cholesterol levels may correlate with disease severity.

## 3. Regulation of cholesterol metabolism in the brain

### 3.1. De novo cholesterol synthesis

Compared with other organs, the brain is the highest cholesterol-containing organ, which is present mainly in unsterified form. Most of the free cholesterol pool is localized predominantly in specialized membranes (myelin) and to a lesser extent in neurons and glial cells. Experimental evidence indicates that brain cholesterol is independent of serum cholesterol levels, as the BBB is impermeable to circulating cholesterol, which determines that both neurons and glial cells synthesize cholesterol *de novo*. Oligodendrocytes control the synthesis of myelin and therefore have the highest capacity to synthesize cholesterol, followed by astrocytes [84, 85]. Cholesterol is synthesized from acetate in a multistep cascade that requires oxygen and energy. The precursor acetyl-CoA is first converted to 3-hydroxy-3-methylglutaryl-CoA (HMG-CoA) and then to mevalonate (Fig. 2). The phosphorylation of mevalonate yields 5-pyrophosphomevalonate, which is converted to isopentenyl pyrophosphate (IPP). IPP can be reversibly transformed to dimethylallyl pyrophosphate (DMAPP), and the combination of both IPP and DMAPP yields the 10-carbon isoprenoid geranyl pyrophosphate (GPP). The sequential addition of 1 or 2 more IPP units to GPP generates the 15-carbon and the 20-carbon isoprenoids farnesyl pyrophosphate (FPP) and the geranylgeranyl pyrophosphate (GGPP), respectively. FPP branches into the non-sterol pathways, which contributes to the generation of other derivatives such as ubiquinol, dolichol, and the sterol pathway via conversion into squalene by squalene synthase, which catalyzes the first committed step in cholesterol synthesis. The rate-limiting step of cholesterol biosynthesis is the conversion of HMG-CoA to mevalonate catalyzed by the HMG-CoA reductase (HMGCR), which is bound to endoplasmic reticulum (ER). Cholesterol levels control HMGCR through several mechanisms. First, high cholesterol exerts a feedback inhibition by activating HMGCR ubiquitination and subsequent proteasomal degradation. Moreover, HMGCR expression is regulated by ER-bound transcription factor SREBP-2, which in turn is controlled by a sterol-sensitive SREBP cleavage-activating protein (SCAP) [86]. In the presence of sterols, full-length SREBP-2 is restricted to the ER. Upon sterol depletion, SREBP-2 interacts with SCAP and is transported from the ER to the Golgi apparatus, where SREBP-2 is cleaved by two proteases and the released N terminus domain acts as a transcription factor to subsequently enhance the levels of HMGCR [86, 87]. Thus, ER plays a key role in the supply of endogenous cholesterol synthesis, which operates to meet demand for cell cholesterol.

http://dx.doi.org/10.5772/59935

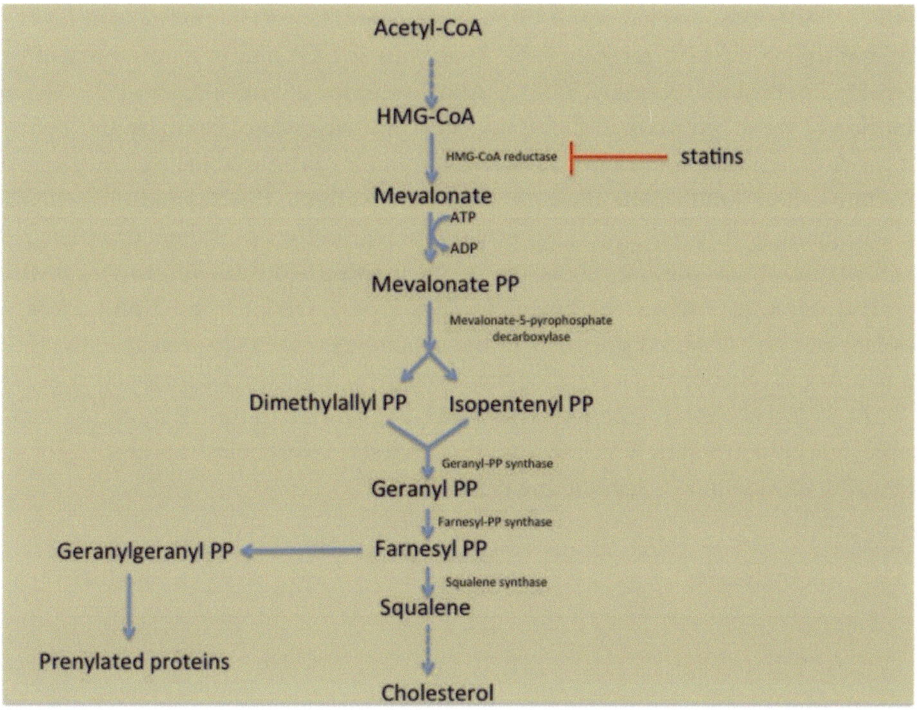


**Figure 2.** Cholesterol synthesis in the mevalonate pathway. Cholesterol is synthesized from acetate in a multistep cascade that requires oxygen and energy. The precursor acetyl-CoA is first converted to 3-hydroxy-3-methylglutaryl-CoA (HMG-CoA) and then to mevalonate. This pathway also generates isoprenoids. Farnesyl pyrophosphate (FPP) branches into the non-sterol pathways, which contributes to the generation of other derivatives such as ubiquinol, dolichol, and the sterol pathway via conversion into squalene by squalene synthase, which catalyzes the first committed step in cholesterol synthesis. The rate-limiting step of cholesterol biosynthesis is the conversion of HMG-CoA to mevalonate catalyzed by the HMG-CoA reductase (HMGCR), which is the target of statins. Statins hence will not only block cholesterol synthesis but also isoprenoids and other non-sterols, which may account for the pleiotropic effects of statins.

### 3.2. Cholesterol storage and transport

In contrast to developing neurons, which synthesize most of the cholesterol required for growth and synaptogenesis, mature neurons depend on the availability of exogenous cholesterol derived from astrocytes (Figure 3). This process not only ensures steady supply of cholesterol to neurons but also spares energy, as ATP hydrolysis is required to synthesize cholesterol de novo [88]. Besides de novo synthesis, astrocytes can also internalize and recycle the cholesterol released from degenerating nerve terminals and deliver it back to neurons [89]. The transport of cholesterol from astrocytes to neurons requires binding to one of the variants of ApoE, the most prevalent lipoprotein in the central nervous system. In this process, cholesterol first forms a complex with ApoE, which is then secreted in a process involving ABCA1 and ABCG1 transporters [90, 91]. Using cultured cerebellar murine astroglia cells, it has been shown that partially lipidated apoE, secreted directly by glia, is likely to be the major extracellular acceptor of cholesterol released from glia in a process mediated by ABCG1 rather than ABCA1 [91]. The secreted ApoE–cholesterol complex is then internalized into neurons predominantly via the LDL receptor (LDLR) as well as LRP, and to a minor extent by very-low-density lipoprotein receptor (VLDL), ApoE receptor 2, and megalin [92]. The specific contribution of these receptors in the uptake of ApoE-cholesterol complex and hence in the maintenance of neuronal cholesterol homeostasis remains to be established. Once internalized the receptor-bound ApoE–cholesterol complex is delivered to the late endosomes/lysosomes where acid lipase hydrolyses the cholesterol esters within the lipoprotein complex, resulting in the release of intracellular free cholesterol. This unesterified cholesterol subsequently exits the late endosomes/lysosomes via Niemann–Pick type C (NPC) 1 and 2 protein-dependent mechanism and is distributed primarily to the plasma membrane as well as to the ER, which serves as a negative feedback sensor for the cholesterol homeostasis genes such as HMGCR and LDLR. Excess cholesterol, on the other hand, is esterified in the ER by ACAT and stored in cytoplasmic lipid droplets, which serves as reserve source of cholesterol needed for synaptic and dendritic formation and remodeling [93, 94].

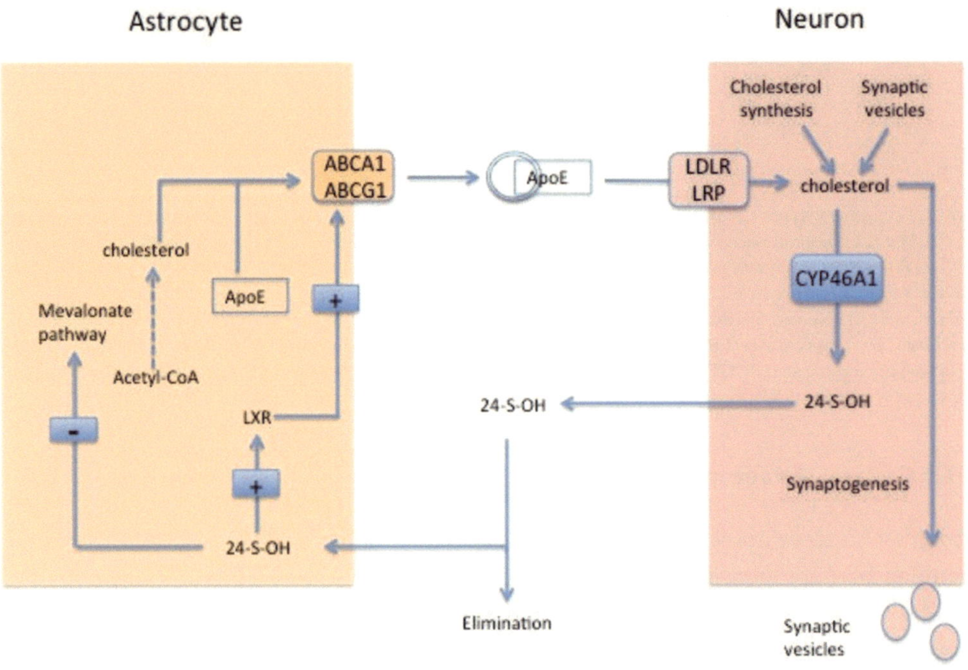


**Figure 3.** Cross talk between astrocytes and neurons in cholesterol homeostasis. Although neurons can synthesize cholesterol de novo in the adult state neurons rely on the delivery of cholesterol from astrocytes, which exhibit a significantly higher rate of de novo cholesterol activity than neurons. Cholesterol packed in ApoE particles assembled in astrocytes are delivered via ABCA1 carrier to neurons. Excess neuronal cholesterol is transformed into the oxysterol 24S-hydroxysterol (24S-OH) by the CYP46A1 which represents the major mechanism for the elimination of brain cholesterol, as it crosses the BBB to the periphery for disposal. Oxysterols activate transcription factor LXRβ isoform, which in turn induces the activation of carriers such as ABCA1 to stimulate trafficking of cholesterol in the form of ApoE to neurons. 24S-OH inhibits the novo cholesterol synthesis in astrocytes.

### 3.3. Cholesterol efflux from the brain

Unlike other organs and epithelial cells, neurons and glial cells do not degrade cholesterol, therefore in order to maintain homeostasis they export cholesterol to the circulation for its disposal by peripheral organs. Two different mechanisms are involved in the elimination of cholesterol from the brain. The major mechanism by which cholesterol is excreted from the brain is by its conversion to 24S-hydroxylcholesterol—an oxidized lipophilic metabolite that can freely cross the BBB [95]. The conversion of free cholesterol to 24S-hydroxycholesterol is mediated by the cytochrome P450-containing enzyme cholesterol 24-hydroxylase, encoded by the Cyp46A1 gene, which is expressed selectively in the brain [96]. High levels of this enzyme are found in certain neuronal cells such as pyramidal neurons of the hippocampus and cortex, Purkinje cells of the cerebellum, thalamic neurons, and in hippocampal and cerebellar interneurons. Interestingly, a minor fraction of cholesterol 24-hydroxylase immunoreactivity has also been detected in glial cells from the brains of AD patients [95]. It is estimated that about 40% of the total cholesterol turnover is mediated by cholesterol 24-hydroxylase [97]. Indeed, deletion of the Cyp46A1 gene encoding cholesterol 24-hydroxylase leads to about 50% reduction in brain cholesterol excretion. This decrease, however, is compensated by the reduction in de novo synthesis, thus suggesting a close relationship between synthesis and metabolism of cholesterol in the brain. The other mechanism of cholesterol elimination, called reverse cholesterol transport pathway, involves translocation of a fraction of brain cholesterol to the blood by membrane transport protein such as ABCA1 [98]. The level of ABCA1 is partly regulated by cholesterol-derived ligand oxysterols (e.g., 24S-hydroxylcholesterol) of the liver X receptor (LXR), which has been shown to influence the transcription of multiple genes involved in cholesterol metabolism [99-101]. There are two known LXR isoforms, LXR$\alpha$ and LHR$\beta$. LXR$\alpha$ expression is mainly limited to the liver, adrenals, intestine and spleen, while LXR$\beta$ is expressed in all tissue types, including the brain. In vivo induction of LXR results in increased expression of ABCA1 and ABCG1, increased cholesterol efflux and a reduction in synaptosomal plasma membrane cholesterol [101]. As such, it is expected that LXR agonists (e.g. T0901317) should lower A$\beta$ levels. However, results with LXR agonists have been inconsistent. For instance, T0901317 has been shown in some studies to decrease A$\beta$, while others reported an increase in A$\beta$42 without chaning A$\beta$40 levels [102]. Hence, it is conceivable that both synthesis and elimination of cholesterol, especially in the adult brain, are not only tightly regulated but also compartmentalized. Astrocytes are responsible for the majority of cholesterol synthesis but contribute relatively little to its elimination, whereas neurons with reduced synthetic ability can eliminate about two thirds of the cholesterol from the brain.

## 4. Intracellular cholesterol and AD

As a key component of membrane bilayers, intracellular cholesterol traffics to different compartments to maintain physical and functional membrane properties. Cholesterol that enters the cell via the endocytic pathway is transported to the ER for processing, while cholesterol synthesized in the ER de novo it is transported to the plasma membrane within a short time frame. Of relevance to AD pathogenesis, in the following sections we will focus on the endo-lysosomal cholesterol and in the small pool of cholesterol in mitochondria and their contribution to AD.

### 4.1. Endo-lysosomal cholesterol

The supply of cholesterol from astrocytes to neurons via receptor-bound ApoE-cholesterol complex relies on the trafficking and subsequent hydrolysis of these complexes in endo/lysosomes. The generated free cholesterol exits lysosomes via NPC1/2 proteins to be distributed to other membrane bilayers. The impact of NPC proteins in intracelular cholesterol homeostasis has been best characterized in the NPC disease, a neurological disorders caused by mutations in NPC1/2 proteins characterized by increased accumulation of cholesterol and other lipids (e.g. glycosphingolipids) in lysosomes in the affected organs, predominantly brain and liver. NPC knockout mice, which mimic the pathology of NPC patients, exhibit increased lysosomal cholesterol in cerebellum, mainly in Purkinje cells, and suffer from progressive motor deterioration and a short life span (typically 8-10 weeks). NPC disease and AD share many parallels including endo/lysosomal abnormalities and APP processing and Aβ accumulation. Previous findings have shown that mutated NPC1 in mice causes the accumulation of Aβ40 and Aβ42, which coincided with accumulation of presenilins in early endocytic compartment [103]. Similar findings have been reported in human NPC1 brain, with accumulation of Aβ ocurring in early endosomes [104]. In CHO cells deficient in NPC1 protein and in cells treated with U18666A, which inhibits NPC1/2, Aβ and presenilin accumulation were found in late endosomes [105]. However, the expression of NPC1 in AD has been poorly characterized. Quite intriguingly, recent findings have reported increased expression of the lysosomal cholesterol transporter NPC1 in AD [106]. NPC1 expression was described to be upregulated at both mRNA and protein levels in the hippocampus and frontal cortex of AD patients compared to controls subjects. However, no difference in NPC1 expression was detected in the cerebellum, a brain region that is relatively spared in AD. Moreover, murine NPC1 mRNA levels increased in the hippocampus of 12-month-old APP/PS1 mice compared to wild type mice. While these findings strongly suggest the lack of lysosomal cholesterol accumulation in AD, endosomal abnormalities have been found in AD that precede amyloid and tau pathology in the neocortex. In addition to the proteolytic processing by secretases, APP and its corresponding C-terminal fragments are also metabolized by lysosomal proteases. SORLA/SORL1 is a unique neuronal sorting receptor for APP that has been causally implicated in sporadic and autosomal dominant familial AD. Brain concentrations of SORLA are inversely correlated with Aβ in mouse models and AD patients. Indeed, transgenic mice overexpressing SORLA exhibit decreased Aβ concentrations in brain [107]. Mechanistically, Aβ binds to the amino-terminal VP10P domain of SORLA and this binding is impaired by a familial AD mutation in SORL1. Although previous studies have shown that lysosomal cholesterol accumulation impairs autophagy by disrupting lysosomal function [108], the lysosomal impairment and subsequent contribution to decreased Aβ degradation in AD may occur through mechanisms independent of cholesterol accumulation in lysosomes. Moreover, sphingosine-1-phosphate (S1P) accumulation by S1P lyase deficiency has recently been shown to impair lysosomal APP metabolism, resulting in increased Aβ accumulation [109]. The intracellular accumulation of S1P interferes with the maturation of cathepsin D and degradation of Lamp2, suggesting a general impairment of lysosomal function and autophagy. Sphingolipids have strong affinity to bind cholesterol and play a role in Alzheimer disease [110]. However, it remains to be established whether increased lysosomal cholesterol may contribute to impaired lysosomal Aβ degradation and if sphingolipids accumulate in lysosomes in AD.

### 4.2. Mitochondrial cholesterol

Unlike plasma membrane, mitochondria are cholesterol-poor organelles. The limited pool of mitochondrial cholesterol plays important physiological roles, such as in the synthesis of steroids in specialized tissues and bile acids in the liver. However, under pathological conditions the unphysiological accumulation of cholesterol in mitochondrial membranes have profound effects in mitochondrial function and antioxidant defense and has emerged as an important factor in liver diseases and neurodegeneration [111-114]. In particular, the transport of cholesterol from the outer to the inner mitochondria is essential for the generation of steroid precursor pregnenolone upon metabolism of cholesterol by the P540 side-chain cleavage enzyme CYP11A1. Availability of cholesterol in mitochondria inner membrane is rate-limiting step in steroidogenesis and is a highly regulated process.

StARD1 is the founding member of a family of lipid transporting proteins that contain StAR-related lipid transfer (START) domains. StARD1 is an outer mitochondrial membrane protein which was first described and best characterized in steroidogenic cells where it plays an essential role in cholesterol transfer to the mitochondrial inner membrane for metabolism by CYP11A1 to generate pregnenolone. Despite similar features with StARD1, other START members cannot replace StARD1 deficiency as global StARD1 knockout mice dye within 10 days due to adrenocortical lipoid hyperplasia [115]. These findings imply that other members of the family cannot functionally replace StARD1, indicating the key role of this member in the regulation of cholesterol trafficking to the mitochondrial inner membrane. Recent findings in APP/PS1 models of AD have indicated the expression of StARD1 in neurons, which correlate with the age-dependent increase in mitochondrial cholesterol [114, 116]. Consistent with these findings in experimental models, enhanced immunocytochemical localization of StARD1 has been described in the pyramidal hippocampal neurons of AD-affected patients [117]. Given the role of StARD1 in the mitochondrial transport of cholesterol and hence in the modulation of mitochondrial cholesterol levels, the increased expression of StARD1 in AD patients, would strongly suggest that mitochondrial cholesterol accumulation may actually occur in patients with AD. Furthermore, the increase in mitochondrial cholesterol in brain mitochondria of Alzheimer's disease was not accompanied by a selective increase in mitochondrial-associated membranes (MAM), a specific membrane domain made of ER and mitochondria bilayers thought to be of relevance in the traffic of lipids, suggesting that StARD1-mediated cholesterol trafficking to mitochondria is independent of MAM. TSPO, a protein particularly abundant in steroidogenic tissues and primarily localized in the mitochondrial outer membrane, has been suggested to play an important role in steroidogenesis via the transport of cholesterol to the mitochondrial inner membrane (IMM) [118, 119]. However, quite interestingly, recent studies using tissue-specific genetic deletion of TSPO demonstrated that TSPO is dispensable for steroidogenesis in Leydig cells [120], questioning the relevance of previous findings on TSPO using pharmacological ligands and inhibitors. These data underscore that TSPO does not play a significant role in the trafficking of cholesterol to IMM, and highlights the relevance of StARD1 in this process. Overall, these findings underscore the accumulation of cholesterol in mitochondrial membranes in patients and models of AD, and quite interestingly, paralell the increase in mitochondrial cholesterol observed in brain and liver mitochondria in NPC, arguing that this pool of cholesterol may be a common nexus in both AD and NPC.

## 5. Mitochondrial cholesterol promotes AD by depleting GSH

In addition to the amyloidogenic effect of cholesterol by fostering Aβ generation from APP, recent data has provided evidence that mitochondrial cholesterol accumulation sensitizes neurons to Aβ-induced neuroinflammation and neurotoxicity by depleting mGSH, effects that are prevented by mGSH replenishment [114, 116]. The mechanism of mitochondrial cholesterol accumulation involves the upregulation of StARD1 induced by Aβ *via* ER stress, confirming previous findings in hepatocytes [121]. Consistent wiht the reported increased expression of StARD1 in pyramidal hippocampal neurons of AD-affected patients, it is likely that this outcome may be accompanied by increased accumulation of cholesterol in mitochondria and subsequent depeltion of mGSH levels [117]. Moreover, a novel mouse model engineered to have enhanced cholesterol synthesis by SREBP-2 overexpression superimposed to APP/PS1 mutations triggered Aβ accumulation and tau pathology [122]. This triple transgenic model exhibited increased mitochondrial cholesterol loading and mGSH depletion and accelerated Aβ generation by β-secretase activation compared to APP/PS1 mice. Moreover, SREBP-2/APP/PS1 mice displayed synaptotoxicity, cognitive decline, tau hyperphosphorylation and neurofibrillary tangle formation in the absence of mutated tau, indicating that cholesterol, particularly mitochondrial cholesterol, can precipitate Aβ accumulation and tau pathology. Importantly, *in vivo* replenishment of mGSH with cell-permeable GSH monoethyl ester (GSH-EE) attenuated neuropathological features of AD in SREBP-2/APP/PS1 mice. These findings established that mitochondrial cholesterol promotes AD by selective depletion of mGSH stores. Therefore, understanding the molecular mechanisms on this cause-and-effect relationship may be of interest in AD.

The properties of GSH transport in isolated rat brain mitochondria appear to differ from those reported previously other tissues such as liver and kidney, as they were influenced most by inhibitors of the tricarboxylate carrier, citrate, isocitrate, and benzenyl-1,2,3-tricarboxylate [123] Moreover, in mouse brain mitochondria it has been shown that 2-oxoglutarate (OGC) and dicarboxylate (DIC) are both expressed in cortical neurons and astrocytes [124]. In addition, butylmalonate, an inhibitor of DIC, significantly decreased mGSH, suggesting DIC as an important GSH transporter in mouse cerebral cortical mitochondria. Interestingly, a role for UCP2 in the transport of mGSH has been described in neurons, suggesting that the transport of protons back into the matrix by UCP2 may favor the movement of GSH [125]. These studies suggest that multiple IMM anion transporters might be involved in mGSH transport and that they might differ in different cell populations within the brain. However, the fact that mitochondrial cholesterol loading selectively depleted mGSH indicated that this transport function is sensitive to cholesterol-mediated changes in membrane dynamics, similar to what has been reported in liver mitochondria. Indeed, the effect of cholesterol in the regulation of mGSH is mediated by the susceptibility of the OGC to perturbations in membrane dynamics. Functional expression analyses in Xenopus laevis oocytes microinjected with OGC cRNA showed enhanced transport of GSH in isolated mitochondria [126]. Moreover, cholesterol enrichment impairs the transport kinetics of 2-oxoglutarate via the OGC by decreasing mitochondrial membrane fluidity. Restoration of membrane dynamics by the fatty acid analog $A_2C$ improves the activity of OGC and mGSH transport despite cholesterol enrichment. Therefore, strategies aimed to replenish mitochondrial membrane physical properties may be of relevance to AD by replenishing mGSH.

# 6. Regulation of mitochondrial cholesterol

The ER plays an essential role in the integration of multiple metabolic signals and the maintenance of cell homeostasis, particularly protein synthesis and folding. Under stress conditions induced by protein misfolding, the ER triggers an adaptive response called uncoupled protein response (UPR). To resolve ER stress, UPR promotes a decrease in protein synthesis, and an increase in protein degradation and chaperone production for protein folding. Aβ is well known to induce ER stress, which is believed to mediate in part the pathogenesis of AD [127]. Moreover, tauroursodeoxycholic acid (TUDCA), a chemical chaperone that prevents ER stress, has been shown to restore the mGSH pool in alcohol fed rats [128] and ameliorates alcohol-induced ER stress [121]. In line with these findings in liver, we have recently reported that TUDCA and PBA abolish Aβ-induced hepatic ER stress, mitochondrial cholesterol loading and subsequent mGSH depletion [116]. Emerging evidence has demonstrated that StARD1 is a previously unrecognized target of the UPR and ER stress signaling. Indeed, tunicamycin, an ER stress trigger, induces the expression of StARD1 in isolated hepatocytes and this effect is prevented by TUDCA treatment [121]. Moreover, mice fed a high cholesterol diet (HC) exhibited increased expression of StARD1. However, HC feeding downregulates the expression of SREBP-2-regulated target genes, including hydroxymethylglutaryl Co-A reductase, demonstrating that StARD1 is and an ER stress but not SREBP-2 regulated gene. In contrast to StARD1, the role of ER stress in the regulation of StART family members has been limited to StARD5 [129, 130], with conflicting results reported for StARD4 [130, 131]. As the UPR comprises three transducers, namely inositol requiring (IRE) 1$\alpha$, PKR-like ER kinase (PERK), and activating transcription factor (ATF) 6$\alpha$, which are controlled by the master regulator glucose-regulated protein 78 (GRP78 also known as BiP), further work is needed to examine the relative contribution of the involved arms of the UPR in the regulation of StARD1 by Aβ. Besides ER stress, StARD1 activation is regulated at the transcriptional and post-translational levels. In murine steroidogenic cells StARD1 activity and subsequent steroidogenesis increases upon StARD1 phosphorylation at serine residues [132, 133]. Whether or not StARD1 phosphorylation by Aβ regulates mitochondrial cholesterol homeostasis remains to be explored. If so, then the identification of putative kinases that phosphorylate and activate StARD1 may be of potential relevance in AD. The other unresolved question relates as to the mechanism whereby Aβ induces ER stress. As ER $Ca^{2+}$ homeostasis is a key housekeeping mechanism to maintain ER function, it is conceivable that Aβ may disrupt ER $Ca^{2+}$, thereby causing ER stress. Whether Aβ modulates the activity of the ER $Ca^{2+}$ pump SERCA, whose disruption is known to trigger ER stress remains to be investigated.

## 7. Concluding remarks

With an expected increase in cases, AD may represent one of the most important health burdens in the near future worlwide. Therefore the identification of effective therapeutic treatments for AD is of priority for health authorities around the world. Unfortunately our limited understanding of the molecular pathways underlying AD has curved the possibilities to have effective treatments at hand. While cholesterol and in particular hypercholesterolemia has been identified as a risk factor for AD development, the causal effect of cholesterol and the impact of cholesterol-lowering approach in AD still remains controversial. Unexpectedly, evidence in the last five years has indicated that the small pool of cholesterol in mitochondria plays an important role in AD, as its accumulation in mitochondria causes mGSH depletion amplifying the neurotoxic effects of Aβ peptides. Therefore, targeting mGSH may be of therapeutic relevance in AD. However, mGSH is regulated by its transport through mitochondrial inner membrane via specific carriers that are sensitive to changes in mitochondrial membrane properties. Hence the mere increase in cytosolic GSH by GSH prodrugs, such as N-acetylcysteine, may not be effective in restoring mGSH as cytosolic GSH would not be transported into mitochndrial matrix due to cholesterol-mediated disruption in mitochondrial membrane dynamics. Thus, more specific approaches would imply the use of membrane-permeable GSH prodrugs such as GSH ethyl ester, which has been shown to protect against AD in experimental models and is known to cross the BBB. Alternatively, targeting the increase in mitochondrial cholesterol by antagonizing StARD1 may arise as another attractive possiblity in the future. This approach requires a better understanding of the cell biology of StARD1 and in the identification of BBB permeable specific StARD1inhibitors. We are looking forward to these and other more exciting discoveries to start controlling the onset and progression of this devastating disease.

## Acknowledgements

This chapter is dedicated to the many patients, past and present that suffer AD, and very especially to my mother.

The work was supported by CIBEREHD, Fundació la Maratǒ de TV3 and Grants PI11/0325 (META) from the Instituto de Salud Carlos III and Grant SAF2012-34831 from Plan Nacional de I+D, Spain; and the Center Grant P50-AA-11999 (Research Center for Liver and Pancreatic Diseases) funded by NIAAA/NIH. I want to thank the people in my lab who have made major contributions to unveil the role of mitochondrial cholesterol in Alzheimer, in particular Drs. Anna Fernandez, Carmen Garcia-Ruiz, Elisabet Barbero-Camps and Anna Colell.

## Author details

José C. Fernández-Checa[1,2,3]

Address all correspondence to: checa229@yahoo.com

1 Department of Cell Death and Proliferation, Instituto Investigaciones Biomedicas de Barcelona, CSIC, Barcelona, and Liver Unit-Hospital Clinic-IDIBAPS, Spain

2 Centro de Investigación Biomédica en Red (CIBERehd), Barcelona, Spain

3 University of Southern California Research Center for Alcohol Liver and Pancreatic Diseases and Cirrhosis, Keck School of Medicine, USC, Los Angeles, CA, USA

## References

[1] Katzov H, Chalmers K, Palmgren J, Andreasen N, Johansson B, Cairns NJ et al (2004) Genetic variants of ABCA1 modify Alz- heimer disease risk and quantitative traits related to beta-amyloid metabolism. Hum Mutat 23(4):358–367

[2] Whitehouse PJ (1997) Genesis of Alzheimer's disease. Neurology 48(5 Suppl 7):S2–S7

[3] Selkoe, D.J. 2001. Alzheimer's disease: genes, proteins, and therapy. Physiol. Rev. 81(2): 741–766.

[4] Cummings JL (2004) Alzheimer's disease. N Engl J Med 351 (1):56–67

[5] Bertram L, Tanzi RE (2005) The genetic epidemiology of neuro- degenerative disease. J Clin Invest 115(6):1449–1457

[6] Minati, L., Edginton, T., Grazia Bruzzone, M., and Giaccone, G. 2009. Current concepts in Alzheimer's disease: a multidisciplinary review. Am. J. Alzheimers Dis. Other Demen. 24(2): 95–121.

[7] Bertram L, McQueen MB, Mullin K, Blacker D, Tanzi RE (2007) Systematic meta-analyses of Alzheimer disease genetic associa- tion studies: the AlzGene database. Nat Genet 39(1):17–23

[8] Holmes C (2002) Genotype and phenotype in Alzheimer's disease. Br J Psychiatry 180:131–134

[9] St George-Hyslop PH, Petit A (2005) Molecular biology and genetics of Alzheimer's disease. C R Biol 328(2):119–130

[10] Tanzi RE, Bertram L (2005) Twenty years of the Alzheimer's disease amyloid hypothesis: a genetic perspective. Cell 120 (4):545–555

[11] Corder, E.H., Saunders, A.M., Strittmatter, W.J., Schmechel, D.E., Gaskell, P.C., Small, G.W., et al. 1993. Gene dose of apolipoprotein E type 4 allele and the risk of Alzheimer's disease in late onset families. Science, 261(5123): 921–923.

[12] Strittmatter, W.J., Saunders, A.M., Schmechel, D., Pericak-Vance, M., Enghild, J., Salvesen, G.S., and Roses, A.D. 1993. Apolipoprotein E: high-avidity binding to beta-amyloid and increased frequency of type 4 allele in late-onset familial Alzheimer disease. Proc. Natl. Acad. Sci. U.S.A. 90(5): 1977–1981.

[13] Poirier, J., Bertrand, P., Poirier, J., Kogan, S., Gauthier, S., Poirier, J., et al. 1993. Apolipoprotein E polymorphism and Alzheimer's disease. Lancet, 342(8873): 697–699.

[14] Chartier-Harlin, M.-C., Parfitt, M., Legrain, S., Pérez-Tur, J., Brousseau, T., Evans, A., et al. 1994. Apolipoprotein E, 3 4 allele as a major risk factor for sporadic early and late-onset forms of Alzheimer's disease: analysis of the 19q13.2 chromosomal region. Hum. Mol. Genet. 3(4): 569–574.

[15] Mendoza-Oliva A, Zepeda A, Arias C. The Complex Actions of Statins in Brain and their Relevance for Alzheimer's Disease Treatment: an Analytical Review. Curr Alzheimer Res. 2014 Oct 1

[16] Opie L.H. Can dementia be lessened by statins. The Lancet 384: 953, 2014.

[17] Hardy, J., and Allsop, D. 1991. Amyloid deposition as the central event in the aetiology of Alzheimer's disease. Trends Pharmacol. Sci. 12(10): 383–388.

[18] Hardy, J.A., and Higgins, G.A. 1992. Alzheimer's disease: the amyloid cascade hypothesis. Science, 256(5054): 184–185.

[19] Clippingdale AB, Wade JD, Barrow CJ (2001) The amyloid-beta peptide and its role in Alzheimer's disease. J Pept Sci 7(5):227–249

[20] Dickson DW (1997) The pathogenesis of senile plaques. J Neuro- pathol Exp Neurol 56(4):321–339

[21] Naslund J, Haroutunian V, Mohs R, Davis KL, Davies P, Greengard P et al (2000) Correlation between elevated levels of amyloid beta- peptide in the brain and cognitive decline. JAMA 283(12):1571– 1577

[22] Billings, L.M., Oddo, S., Green, K.N., McGaugh, J.L., and LaFerla, F.M. 2005. Intraneuronal Ab causes the onset of early Alzheimer's disease-related cognitive deficits in transgenic mice. Neuron, 45 (5): 675–688.

[23] D'Andrea, M.R., Nagele, R.G., Wang, H.Y., Peterson, P.A., and Lee, D.H. 2001. Evidence that neurones accumulating amyloid can undergo lysis to form amyloid plaques in Alzheimer's disease. Histopathology, 38(2): 120–134.

[24] Gouras, G.K., Tsai, J., Naslund, J., Vincent, B., Edgar, M., Checler, F., et al. 2000. Intraneuronal Ab42 accumulation in human brain. Am. J. Pathol. 156(1): 15–20.

[25] Oddo, S., Caccamo, A., Shepherd, J.D., Murphy, M.P., Golde, T.E., Kayed, R., et al. 2003. Triple-transgenic model of Alzheimer's disease with plaques and tangles: intracellular Ab and synaptic dysfunction. Neuron, 39(3): 409–421.

[26] Wirths, O., Multhaup, G., and Bayer, T.A. 2004. A modified beta- amyloid hypothesis: intraneuronal accumulation of the beta- amyloid peptide–the first step of a fatal cascade. J. Neurochem. 91(3): 513–520.

[27] Glabe, C. 2001. Intracellular mechanisms of amyloid accumulation and pathogenesis in Alzheimer's disease. J. Mol. Neurosci. 17(2):137–145.

[28] Bahr, B.A., Hoffman, K.B., Yang, A.J., Hess, U.S., Glabe, C.G., and Lynch, G. 1998. Amyloid beta protein is internalized selectively by hippocampal field CA1 and causes neurons to accumulate amyloidogenic carboxyterminal fragments of the amyloid pre- cursor protein. J. Comp. Neurol. 397(1): 139–147.

[29] Friedrich, R.P., Tepper, K., Ronicke, R., Soom, M., Westermann, M., Reymann, K., et al. 2010. Mechanism of amyloid plaque formation suggests an intracellular basis of Ab pathogenicity. Proc. Natl. Acad. Sci. U.S.A. 107(5): 1942–1947.

[30] Rajendran, L., Honsho, M., Zahn, T.R., Keller, P., Geiger, K.D., Verkade, P., and Simons, K. 2006. Alzheimer's disease beta- amyloid peptides are released in association with exosomes. Proc. Natl. Acad. Sci. U.S.A. 103(30): 11172–11177.

[31] Busciglio, J., Pelsman, A., Wong, C., Pigino, G., Yuan, M., Mori, H., and Yankner, B.A. 2002. Altered metabolism of the amyloid beta precursor protein is associated with mitochondrial dysfunction in Down's syndrome. Neuron, 33(5): 677–688.

[32] Chui, D.H., Dobo, E., Makifuchi, T., Akiyama, H., Kawakatsu, S., Petit, A., et al. 2001. Apoptotic neurons in Alzheimer's disease frequently show intracellular Ab42 labeling. J. Alzheimers Dis. 3 (2): 231–239.

[33] Zhang, Y., McLaughlin, R., Goodyer, C., and LeBlanc, A. 2002. Selective cytotoxicity of intracellular amyloid beta peptide 1–42 through p53 and Bax in cultured primary human neurons. J. Cell Biol. 156(3): 519–529.

[34] Casas, C., Sergeant, N., Itier, J.M., Blanchard, V., Wirths, O., van der Kolk, N., et al. 2004. Massive CA1/2 neuronal loss with intraneuronal and N-terminal truncated Ab42 accumulation in a novel Alzheimer transgenic model. Am. J. Pathol. 165(4): 1289– 1300.

[35] LaFerla, F.M., Tinkle, B.T., Bieberich, C.J., Haudenschild, C.C., and Jay, G. 1995. The Alzheimer's Ab peptide induces neurodegenera- tion and apoptotic cell death in transgenic mice. Nat. Genet. 9(1): 21–30.

[36] Takahashi, R.H., Milner, T.A., Li, F., Nam, E.E., Edgar, M.A., Yamaguchi, H., et al. 2002. Intraneuronal Alzheimer Ab42 accumulates in multivesicular bodies and is associated with synaptic pathology. Am. J. Pathol. 161(5): 1869–1879.

[37] Almeida, C.G., Tampellini, D., Takahashi, R.H., Greengard, P., Lin, M.T., Snyder, E.M., and Gouras, G.K. 2005. Beta-amyloid accumulation in APP mutant neurons reduces PSD-95 and GluR1 in synapses. Neurobiol. Dis. 20(2): 187–198.

[38] Tampellini, D., Magrane, J., Takahashi, R.H., Li, F., Lin, M.T., Almeida, C.G., and Gouras, G.K. 2007. Internalized antibodies to the Ab domain of APP reduce neuronal Ab and protect against synaptic alterations. J. Biol. Chem. 282(26): 18895–18906.

[39] Jonsson, T., Atwal, J. K., Steinberg, S., Snaedal, J., Jonsson, P. V., Bjornsson, S., et al. (2012). A mutation in APP protects against Alzheimer's disease and age-related cognitive decline. *Nature* 488, 96–99.

[40] Hatami A, Albay R 3rd, Monjazeb S, Milton S, Glabe C., Monoclonal Antibodies Against Aβ42 Fibrils Distinguish Multiple Aggregation State Polymorphisms in vitro and in Alzheimer's Disease Brain. J.Biol. Chem, October 3 2014

[41] Haass, C. (2004). Take five – BACE and the gamma-secretase quartet con- duct Alzheimer's amyloid beta-peptide generation. *EMBO J.* 23, 483–488.

[42] Thathiah, A., Horre, K., Snellinx, A., Vandewyer, E., Huang, Y., Ciesielska, M., et al. (2013). beta-arrestin 2 regulates Abeta generation and gamma-secretase activity in Alzheimer's disease. *Nat. Med.* 19, 43–49.

[43] Hooper, N. M., and Turner, A. J. (2002). The search for alpha-secretase and its potential as a therapeutic approach to Alzheimer s disease. *Curr. Med. Chem.* 9, 1107–1119.

[44] Lin, M. T., and Beal, M. F. (2006). Alzheimer's APP mangles mitochondria. *Nat. Med.* 12, 1241–1243.

[45] Devi, L., Prabhu, B. M., Galati, D. F., Avadhani, N. G., and Anandatheerthavarada, H. K. (2006). Accumulation of amyloid precursor protein in the mitochondrial import channels of human Alzheimer's disease brain is associated with mitochon- drial dysfunction. *J. Neurosci.* 26, 9057–9068.

[46] Maxfield FR, Tabas I. Role of choleserol and lipid organization in disease. Nature 438:612-621, 2005.

[47] Goritz, C., Mauch, D.H., and Pfrieger, F.W. 2005. Multiple mechanisms mediate cholesterol-induced synaptogenesis in a CNS neuron. Mol. Cell. Neurosci. 29(2): 190–201.

[48] Pfrieger, F.W. 2003. Cholesterol homeostasis and function in neurons of the central nervous system. Cell. Mol. Life Sci. 60(6): 1158– 1171.

[49] Thiele, C., Hannah, M.J., Fahrenholz, F., and Huttner, W.B.2000. Cholesterol binds to synaptophysin and is required for biogenesis of synaptic vesicles. Nat. Cell Biol.2(1): 42–49.

[50] Sparks DL, Scheff SW, Hunsaker JC 3rd, Liu H, Landers T, Gross DR. Induction of Alzheimer-like beta-amyloid immunoreactivity in the brains of rabbits with dietary cholesterol.Exp Neurol. 1994 Mar;126(1):88-94

[51] Refolo LM, Malester B, LaFrancois J, Bryant-Thomas T, Wang R, Tint GS, Sambamurti K, Duff K, Pappolla MA. Hypercholesterolemia accelerates the Alzheimer's amyloid pathology in a transgenic mouse model.Neurobiol Dis. 2000 Aug;7(4):321-31

[52] Thirumangalakudi L, Prakasam A, Zhang R, Bimonte-Nelson H, Sambamurti K, Kindy MS, Bhat NR. High cholesterol-induced neuroinflammation and amyloid precursor protein processing correlate with loss of working memory in mice.J Neurochem. 2008 Jul;106(1):475-85.

[53] Oksman M, Iivonen H, Hogyes E, Amtul Z, Penke B, Leenders I, Broersen L, Lütjohann D, Hartmann T, Tanila H. Impact of different saturated fatty acid, polyunsaturated fatty acid and cholesterol containing diets on beta-amyloid accumulation in APP/PS1 transgenic mice. Neurobiol Dis. 2006 Sep;23(3):563-72.

[54] Shie FS, Jin LW, Cook DG, Leverenz JB, LeBoeuf RC. Diet-induced hypercholesterolemia enhances brain A beta accumulation in transgenic mice.Neuroreport. 2002 Mar 25;13(4):455-9

[55] Levin-Allerhand JA, Lominska CE, Smith JD. Increased amyloid- levels in APPSWE transgenic mice treated chronically with a physiological high-fat high-cholesterol diet.J Nutr Health Aging. 2002;6(5):315-9.

[56] Ujiie M, Dickstein DL, Carlow DA, Jefferies WA. Blood-brain barrier permeability precedes senile plaque formation in an Alzheimer disease model. Microcirculation. 2003 Dec;10(6):463-70.

[57] Winkler EA, Sagare AP, Zlokovic BV. The pericyte: a forgotten cell type with important implications for Alzheimer's disease? Brain Pathol. 2014 Jul;24(4):371-86

[58] Wahrle, S., Das, P., Nyborg, A.C., McLendon, C., Shoji, M., Kawarabayashi, T., et al. 2002. Cholesterol-dependent gamma- secretase activity in buoyant cholesterol-rich membrane micro- domains. Neurobiol. Dis. 9(1): 11–23.

[59] Vetrivel, K.S., and Thinakaran, G. 2010. Membrane rafts in Alzheimer's disease beta-amyloid production. Biochim. Biophys. Acta, 1801(8): 860–867.

[60] Anstey, K. J., Lipnicki, D. M., and Low, L. F. (2008). Cholesterol as a risk factor for dementia and cognitive decline: a systematic review of prospec- tive studies with meta-analysis. *Am. J. Geriatr. Psychiatry* 16, 343–354.

[61] Notkola, I. L., Sulkava, R., Pekkanen, J., Erkinjuntti, T., Ehnholm, C., Kivinen, P., et al. (1998). Serum total cholesterol, apolipoprotein E epsilon 4 allele, and Alzheimer's disease. *Neuroepidemiology* 17, 14–20.

[62] Wolozin, B., Kellman, W., Ruosseau, P., Celesia, G. G., and Siegel, G. (2000). Decreased prevalence of Alzheimer disease associated with 3-hydroxy- 3-methyglutaryl coenzyme A reductase inhibitors. *Arch. Neurol.* 57, 1439–1443.

[63] Martins, I.J., Berger, T., Sharman, M.J., Verdile, G., Fuller, S.J., and Martins, R.N. 2009. Cholesterol metabolism and transport in the pathogenesis of Alzheimer's disease. J. Neurochem. 111(6): 1275– 1308.

[64] Burns MP, Igbavboa U, Wang L, Wood WG, Duff K. Cholesterol distribution, not total levels, correlate with altered amyloid precursor protein processing in statin-treated mice. Neuromolecular Med. 2006;8(3):319-28

[65] Chan SL, Kim WS, Kwok JB, Hill AF, Cappai R, Rye KA, Garner B. ATP-binding cassette transporter A7 regulates processing of amyloid precursor protein in vitro. J Neurochem. 2008 Jul;106(2):793-804.

[66] Kim WS, Weickert CS, Garner B. Role of ATP-binding cassette transporters in brain lipid transport and neurological disease. J Neurochem. 2008 Mar;104(5):1145-66.

[67] DiPaolo G, Kim TW. Linking lipids to Alzheimer's disease: cholesterol and beyond. Nat Rev Neurosci. 2011 May;12(5):284-96

[68] Urano Y, Ochiai S, Noguchi N. Suppression of amyloid-β production by 24S-hydroxycholesterol via inhibition of intracellular amyloid precursor protein trafficking. FASEB J. 2013 Oct;27(10):4305-15.

[69] Eckert GP, Cairns NJ, Maras A, Gattaz WF, Müller WE. Cholesterol modulates the membrane-disordering effects of beta-amyloid peptides in the hippocampus: specific changes in Alzheimer's disease. Dement Geriatr Cogn Disord. 2000 Jul-Aug;11(4): 181-6.

[70] Mason RP, Shoemaker WJ, Shajenko L, Chambers TE, Herbette LG. Evidence for changes in the Alzheimer's disease brain cortical membrane structure mediated by cholesterol. Neurobiol Aging. 1992 May-Jun;13(3):413-9.

[71] Heverin M, Bogdanovic N, Lütjohann D, Bayer T, Pikuleva I, Bretillon L, Diczfalusy U, Winblad B, Björkhem I. Changes in the levels of cerebral and extracerebral sterols in the brain of patients with Alzheimer's disease. J Lipid Res 2004 Jan;45(1):186-93.

[72] Sparks DL. Coronary artery disease, hypertension, ApoE, and cholesterol: a link to Alzheimer's disease? Ann N Y Acad Sci. 1997 Sep 26;826:128-46.

[73] Abad-Rodriguez J, Ledesma MD, Craessaerts K, Perga S, Medina M, Delacourte A, Dingwall C, De Strooper B, Dotti CG. Neuronal membrane cholesterol loss enhances amyloid peptide generation. J Cell Biol. 2004 Dec 6;167(5):953-60.

[74] Ledesma MD, Abad-Rodriguez J, Galvan C, Biondi E, Navarro P, Delacourte A, Dingwall C, Dotti CG. Raft disorganization leads to reduced plasmin activity in Alzheimer's disease brains. EMBO Rep. 2003 Dec;4(12):1190-6.

[75] Cole SL, Grudzien A, Manhart IO, Kelly BL, Oakley H, Vassar R. Statins cause intracellular accumulation of amyloid precursor protein, beta-secretase-cleaved fragments, and amyloid beta-peptide via an isoprenoid-dependent mechanism. J Biol Chem. 2005 May 13;280(19):18755-70.

[76] Li G, Higdon R, Kukull WA, Peskind E, Van Valen Moore K, Tsuang D, van Belle G, McCormick W, Bowen JD, Teri L, Schellenberg GD, Larson EB. Statin therapy and risk of dementia in the elderly: a community-based prospective cohort study. Neurology. 2004 Nov 9;63(9):1624-8.

[77] Rea TD, Breitner JC, Psaty BM, Fitzpatrick AL, Lopez OL, Newman AB, Hazzard WR, Zandi PP, Burke GL, Lyketsos CG, Bernick C, Kuller LH. Statin use and the risk of incident dementia: the Cardiovascular Health Study.Arch Neurol. 2005 Jul;62(7): 1047-51.

[78] Zandi PP, Sparks DL, Khachaturian AS, Tschanz J, Norton M, Steinberg M, Welsh-Bohmer KA, Breitner JC; Cache County Study investigators. Do statins reduce risk of incident dementia and Alzheimer disease? The Cache County Study. Arch Gen Psychiatry. 2005 Feb;62(2):217-24.

[79] Carlsson CM, Gleason CE, Hess TM, Moreland KA, Blazel HM, Koscik RL, Schreiber NT, Johnson SC, Atwood CS, Puglielli L, Hermann BP, McBride PE, Stein JH, Sager MA, Asthana S. Effects of simvastatin on cerebrospinal fluid biomarkers and cognition in middle-aged adults at risk for Alzheimer's disease. J Alzheimers Dis. 2008 Mar;13(2):187-97.

[80] Hoglund K, Thelen KM, Syversen S, Sjogren M, von Bergmann K, Wallin A, Vanmechelen E, Vanderstichele H, Lutjohann D, Blennow K. The effect of simvastatin treatment on the amyloid precursor protein and brain cholesterol metabolism in patients with Alzheimer's disease. Dement Geriatr Cogn Disord. 2005;19(5-6):256-65.

[81] Riekse RG, Li G, Petrie EC, Leverenz JB, Vavrek D, Vuletic S, Albers JJ, Montine TJ, Lee VM, Lee M, Seubert P, Galasko D, Schellenberg GD, Hazzard WR, Peskind ER. Effect of statins on Alzheimer's disease biomarkers in cerebrospinal fluid. J Alzheimers Dis. 2006 Dec;10(4):399-406.

[82] Posse de Chaves E. Reciprocal regulation of cholesterol and beta amyloid at the subcellular level in Alzheimer’s disease. Can J Physiol Pharmacol 90: 753-764, 2012.

[83] Mohamed A, Saavedra L, Di Pardo A, Sipione S, Posse de Chaves E. β-amyloid inhibits protein prenylation and induces cholesterol sequestration by impairing SREBP-2 cleavage. J Neurosci. 2012 May 9;32(19):6490-500.

[84] Bjorkhem I, Meaney S (2004) Brain cholesterol: long secret life behind a barrier. Arterioscler Thromb Vasc Biol 24(5):806–815

[85] Dietschy JM, Turley SD (2004) Thematic review series: brain Lipids. Cholesterol metabolism in the central nervous system during early development and in the mature animal. J Lipid Res 45(8):1375–1397

[86] Goldstein JL, DeBose-Boyd RA, Brown MS. Protein sensors for membrane sterols. Cell. 2006 Jan 13;124(1):35-46

[87] Jo Y, DeBose-Boyd RA. Control of cholesterol synthesis through regulated ER-associated degradation of HMG CoA reductase. Crit Rev Biochem Mol Biol. 2010 Jun;45(3): 185-98.

[88] Pfrieger FW. Cholesterol homeostasis and function in neurons of the central nervous system.Cell Mol Life Sci. 2003 Jun;60(6):1158-71.

[89] Jurevics H, Morell P. Cholesterol for synthesis of myelin is made locally, not imported into brain. J Neurochem 64: 895-901, 1995.

[90] Wahrle SE, Jiang H, Parsadanian M, Legleiter J, Han X, Fryer JD, Kowalewski T, Holtzman DM. ABCA1 is required for normal central nervous system ApoE levels and for lipidation of astrocyte-secreted apoE. J Biol Chem. 2004 Sep 24;279(39): 40987-93.

[91] Karten B, Campenot RB, Vance DE, Vance JE. Expression of ABCG1, but not ABCA1, correlates with cholesterol release by cerebellar astroglia. J Biol Chem. 2006 Feb 17;281(7):4049-57

[92] Herz J. Apolipoprotein E receptors in the nervous system. Curr Opin Lipidol. 2009 Jun;20(3):190-6.

[93] Poirier J. Apolipoprotein E and cholesterol metabolism in the pathogenesis and treatment of Alzheimer's disease.Trends Mol Med. 2003 Mar;9(3):94-101.

[94] Puglielli L, Konopka G, Pack-Chung E, Ingano LA, Berezovska O, Hyman BT, Chang TY, Tanzi RE, Kovacs DM. Acyl-coenzyme A: cholesterol acyltransferase modulates the generation of the amyloid beta-peptide. Nat Cell Biol. 2001 Oct;3(10):905-12.

[95] Bogdanovic N, Bretillon L, Lund EG, Diczfalusy U, Lannfelt L, Winblad B, Russell DW, Björkhem I. On the turnover of brain cholesterol in patients with Alzheimer's disease. Abnormal induction of the cholesterol-catabolic enzyme CYP46 in glial cells. Neurosci Lett. 2001 Nov 13;314(1-2):45-8.

[96] Lung EG, Guileyardo JM, Rusell DW. cDNA cloning of cholesterol 24-hydroxylase, a mediator of cholesterol homeostasis in the brain. Proc Natl Acad Sci. USA 96: 7238-43, 1999.

[97] Lund EG, Xie C, Kotti T, Turley SD, Dietschy JM, Russell DW. Knockout of the cholesterol 24-hydroxylase gene in mice reveals a brain-specific mechanism of cholesterol turnover. J Biol Chem. 2003 Jun 20;278(25):22980-8.

[98] Kim WS, Rahmanto AS, Kamili A, Rye KA, Guillemin GJ, Gelissen IC, Jessup W, Hill AF, Garner B.Role of ABCG1 and ABCA1 in regulation of neuronal cholesterol efflux to apolipoprotein E discs and suppression of amyloid-beta peptide generation. J Biol Chem 282: 2851-2861, 2007.

[99] Muscat GE, Wagner BL, Hou J, Tangirala RK, Bischoff ED, Rohde P, Petrowski M, Li J, Shao G, Macondray G, Schulman IG. Regulation of cholesterol homeostasis and lipid metabolism in skeletal muscle by liver X receptors.J Biol Chem. 2002 Oct 25;277(43):40722-8.

[100] Whitney KD, Watson MA, Collins JL, Benson WG, Stone TM, Numerick MJ, Tippin TK, Wilson JG, Winegar DA, Kliewer SA. Regulation of cholesterol homeostasis by the liver X receptors in the central nervous system. Mol Endocrinol. 2002 Jun;16(6): 1378-85.

[101] Eckert GP, Vardanian L, Rebeck GW, Burns MP. Regulation of central nervous system cholesterol homeostasis by the liver X receptor agonist TO-901317. Neurosci Lett. 2007 Aug 9;423(1):47-52.

[102] Burns MP, Rebeck GW. Intracellular cholesterol homeostasis and amyloid precursor protein processing. Biochim Biophys Acta 1801: 853-859, 2010.

[103] Burns M, Gaynor K, Olm V, Mercken M, LaFrancois J, Wang L, Mathews PM, Noble W, Matsuoka Y, Duff K. Presenilin redistribution associated with aberrant cholesterol transport enhances beta-amyloid production in vivo. J Neurosci. 2003 Jul 2;23(13): 5645-9.

[104] Jin LW, Shie FS, Maezawa I, Vincent I, Bird T. Intracellular accumulation of amyloidogenic fragments of amyloid-beta precursor protein in neurons with Niemann-Pick type C defects is associated with endosomal abnormalities. Am J Pathol. 2004 Mar; 164(3):975-85.

[105] Runz H, Rietdorf J, Tomic I, M Bernard, Byereuthe K, Pepperkok R, Hartmann T. Inhibition of intracellular cholesterol transport alters presenilin localization and amyloid precursor protein processing in neuronal cells. J Neurosci 22: 1679-1689.

[106] Kågedal K, Kim WS, Appelqvist H, Chan S, Cheng D, Agholme L, Barnham K, McCann H, Halliday G, Garner B. Increased expression of the lysosomal cholesterol transporter NPC1 in Alzheimer's disease. Biochim Biophys Acta. 2010 Aug;1801(8): 831-8.

[107] Caglayan S, Takagi-Niidome S, Liao F, Carlo AS, Schmidt V, Burgert T, Kitago Y, Füchtbauer EM, Füchtbauer A, Holtzman DM, Takagi J, Willnow TE. Lysosomal sorting of amyloid-β by the SORLA receptor is impaired by a familial Alzheimer's disease mutation. Sci Transl Med. 2014 Feb 12;6(223):223ra20.

[108] Fucho R, Martínez L, Baulies A, Torres S, Tarrats N, Fernandez A, Ribas V, Astudillo AM, Balsinde J, Garcia-Rovés P, Elena M, Bergheim I, Lotersztajn S, Trautwein C, Appelqvist H, Paton AW, Paton JC, Czaja MJ, Kaplowitz N, Fernandez-Checa JC, García-Ruiz C. ASMase regulates autophagy and lysosomal membrane permeabilization and its inhibition prevents early stage non-alcoholic steatohepatitis. J Hepatol. 2014 Nov;61(5):1126-34.

[109] Karaca I, Tamboli IY, Glebov K, Richter J, Fell LH, Grimm MO, Haupenthal VJ, Hartmann T, Gräler MH, van Echten-Deckert G, Walter J. Deficiency of sphingosine-1-phosphate lyase impairs lysosomal metabolism of the amyloid precursor protein. J Biol Chem. 2014 Jun 13;289(24):16761-72.

[110] Van Echten-Deckert G, Walter J. Sphingolipids: critical players in Alzheimer's disease. Prog Lipid Res 51: 378-93, 2012.

[111] Garcia-Ruiz C, Mari M, Colell A, Morales A, Montero J, Terrones O, Basañez G, Fernandez-Checa JC Mitochondrial cholesterol in health and disease. Histol Histopathol 24: 117-32, 2009

[112] Bosch M, Marí M, Herms A, Fernández A, Fajardo A, Kassan A, Giralt A, Colell A, Balgoma D, Barbero E, González-Moreno E, Matias N, Tebar F, Balsinde J, Camps M, Enrich C, Gross SP, García-Ruiz C, Pérez-Navarro E, Fernández-Checa JC, Pol A. Caveolin-1 deficiency causes cholesterol-dependent mitochondrial dysfunction and apoptotic susceptibility. Curr Biol. 2011 Apr 26;21(8):681-6.

[113] Colell A, Fernández A, Fernández-Checa JC. Mitochondria, cholesterol and amyloid beta peptide: a dangerous trio in Alzheimer disease. J Bioenerg Biomembr. 2009 Oct; 41(5):417-23.

[114] Fernandez A, Llacuna L, Fernandez-Checa JC, Colell A. Mitochondrial cholesterol loading exacerbates amyloid beta peptide-induced inflamation and neurotoxicity. J Neurosci 2009; 29: 6394-405.

[115] Caron KM, Soo SC, Wetsel WC, Stocco DM, Clark BJ, Parker KL. argeted disruption of the mouse gene encoding steroidogenic acute regulatory protein provides insights into congenital lipoid adrenal hyperplasia. Proc Natl Acad Sci U S A. 1997 Oct 14;94(21):11540-5.

[116] Barbero-Camps E, Fernández A, Baulies A, Martinez L, Fernández-Checa JC, Colell A. Endoplasmic reticulum stress mediates amyloid β neurotoxicity via mitochondrial cholesterol trafficking. Am J Pathol. 2014 Jul;184(7):2066-81.

[117] Webber KM, Stocco DM, Casadesus G, Bowen RL, Atwood CS, Previll LA, Harris PL, Zhu X, Perry G, Smith MA. Steroidogenic acute regulatory protein (StAR): evidence

of gonadotropin-induced steroidogenesis in Alzheimer disease. Mol Neurodegener 1:14, 2006.

[118] Papadopoulos, V., and Miller, W. L. (2012). Role of mitochondria in steroido- genesis. *Best Pract. Res. Clin. Endocrinol. Metab.* 26, 771–790.

[119] Miller, W. L. (2013). Steroid hormone synthesis in mitochondria. *Mol. Cell. Endocrinol.* 379, 62–73.

[120] Morohaku, K., Pelton, S. H., Daugherty, D. J., Butler, W. R., Deng, W., and Selvaraj, V. (2014). Translocator protein/peripheral benzodiazepine receptor is not required for steroid hormone biosynthesis. *Endocrinology* 155, 89–97.

[121] Fernandez A, Matias N, Fucho R, Ribas V, Von Montfort C, Nuño N, Baulies A, Martinez L, Tarrats N, Mari M, Colell A, Morales A, Dubuquoy L, Mathurin P, Bataller R, Caballeria J, Elena M, Balsinde J, Kaplowitz N, Garcia-Ruiz C, Fernandez-Checa JC. ASMase is required for chronic alcohol induced hepatic endoplasmic reticulum stress and mitochondrial cholesterol loading. J Hepatol. 2013 Oct;59(4):805-13.

[122] Barbero-Camps E, Fernández A, Martínez L, Fernández-Checa JC, Colell A. APP/PS1 mice overexpressing SREBP-2 exhibit combined Aβ accumulation and tau pathology underlying Alzheimer's disease. Hum Mol Genet. 2013 Sep 1;22(17):3460-76.

[123] Wadey, A. L., Muyderman, H., Kwek, P. T., and Sims, N. R. (2009). Mitochon- drial glutathione uptake: characterization in isolated brain mitochondria and astrocytes in culture. *J. Neurochem.* 109(Suppl. 1), 101–108.

[124] Kamga, C. K., Zhang, S. X., and Wang, Y. (2010). Dicarboxylate carrier-mediated glutathione transport is essential for reactive oxygen species homeostasis and normal respiration in rat brain mitochondria. *Am. J. Physiol. Cell Physiol.* 299, C497–C505.

[125] de Bilbao, F., Arsenijevic, D., Vallet, P., Hjelle, O. P., Ottersen, O. P., Bouras, C., etal. (2004). Resistance to cerebral ischemic injury in UCP2 knockout mice: evidence for a role of UCP2 as a regulator of mitochondrial glutathione levels. *J. Neurochem.* 89, 1283–1292.

[126] O. Coll, A. Colell, C. García-Ruiz, N. Kaplowitz, J.C. Fernández-Checa. Sensitivity of the 2-oxoglutarate carrier to alcohol intake contributes to mitochondrial glutathione depletion. Hepatology, 38 (2003), pp. 692–702

[127] Ferreiro E, Resende R, Costa R, Oliveira CR, Pereira CM. An endoplasmic-reticulum-specific apoptotic pathway is involved in prion and amyloid-beta peptides neurotoxicity. Neurobiol Dis. 2006 Sep;23(3):669-78.

[128] Colell A, Coll O, García-Ruiz C, París R, Tiribelli C, Kaplowitz N, Fernández-Checa JC. Tauroursodeoxycholic acid protects hepatocytes from ethanol-fed rats against tumor necrosis factor-induced cell death by replenishing mitochondrial glutathione. Hepatology. 2001 Nov;34(5):964-71.

[129] R.E. Soccio, R.M. Adams, K.N. Maxwell, J.L. Breslow, Differential gene regulation of StarD4 and StarD5 cholesterol transfer proteins. Activation of StarD4 by sterol regulatory element-binding protein-2 and StarD5 by endoplasmic reticulum stress, J. Biol. Chem. 280 (2005) 19410–19418.

[130] D. Rodriguez-Agudo, M. Calderon-Dominguez, M.A. Medina, S. Ren, G. Gil, W. M. Pandak, ER stress increases StarD5 expression by stabilizing its mRNA and leads to relocalization of its protein from the nucleus to the membranes, J. Lipid Res. 53 (2012) 2708–2715.

[131] S. Yamada, T. Yamaguchi, A. Hosoda, T. Iwawaki, K. Kohno, Regulation of human STARD4 gene expression under endoplasmic reticulum stress, Biochem. Biophys. Res. Commun. 343 (2006) 1079–1085.

[132] P.R. Manna, J.W. Soh, D.M. Stocco, The involvement of specific PKC iso- enzymes in phorbol ester-mediated regulation of steroidogenic acute reg- ulatory protein expression and steroid synthesis in mouse Leydig cells, Endocrinology 152 (2011) 313–325.

[133] F. Arakane, S.R. King, Y. Du, C.B. Kallen, L.P. Walsh, H. Watari, D.M. Stocco, J. F. Strauss, Phosphorylation of steroidogenic acute regulatory protein (StAR) modulates its steroidogenic activity, J. Biol. Chem. 272 (1997) 32656–32662.

Chapter 7

# The Mevalonate Pathway in Alzheimer's Disease — Cholesterol and Non-Sterol Isoprenoids

Amany Mohamed, Kevan Smith and Elena Posse de Chaves

Additional information is available at the end of the chapter

http://dx.doi.org/10.5772/59904

## 1. Introduction

The brain is a lipid-rich organ, with approximately 50% of its dry mass constituted by lipids [1]. The main lipid in the brain is cholesterol. The human brain represents only 2% of the total body mass but contains 25% of the total body cholesterol [2, 3]. Therefore, it is not surprising that lipids have important functions in the brain and that dysregulation of brain lipid metabolism has been linked to brain diseases, in particular Alzheimer's disease (AD). The interest in understanding the link between lipids and AD pathology has increased dramatically since the 1990s, when it was discovered that the isoform 4 (ε4) of the cholesterol transport protein apolipoprotein E, is a major risk factor for AD development [4]. Since then an important body of evidence derived from genetic, epidemiological, and biochemical studies has identified the role of cholesterol in many critical aspects of AD neuropathology. The finding that a number of genes involved in cholesterol homeostasis represent susceptibility loci for sporadic or late-onset AD (reviewed in [5-9]), and the evidence that alterations in cholesterol homeostasis are significant in regulation of Aβ production, formation of amyloid plaques, tau hyperphosphorylation, Aβ toxicity, and other mechanisms (reviewed in [5, 10-12]) highlight the importance of the dysregulation of cholesterol homeostasis in AD. [7, 9, 13-20]. Cholesterol homeostasis disturbances in AD may be both consequences of the neurodegenerative process and contributors to the pathogenesis.

## 2. Cholesterol homeostasis in the brain

Cholesterol homeostasis is the balance between synthesis and uptake, and efflux and metabolism. In the brain, this process acquires peculiar characteristics because of differences in the ability of neurons and glia to perform each of these processes (Figure 1).

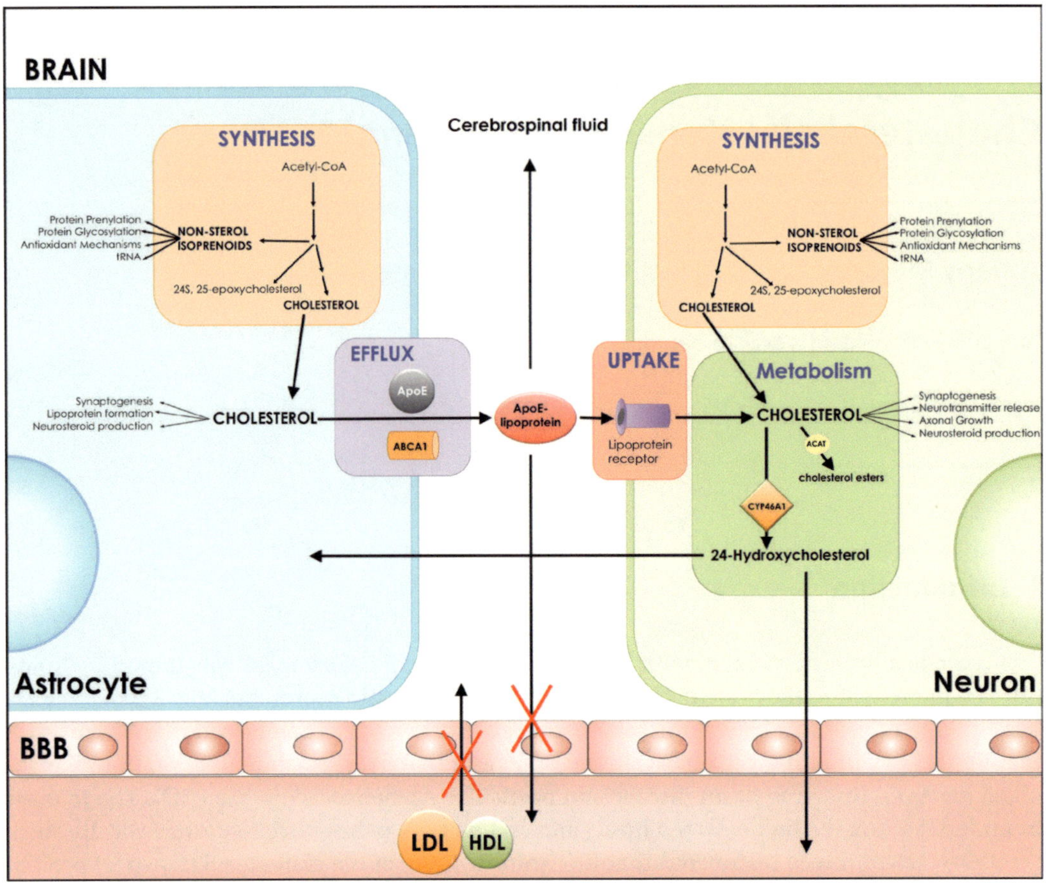


**Figure 1.** Cholesterol homeostasis in the brain. Cellular cholesterol is synthesized from acetyl-CoA in a multistep mevalonate pathway. Cholesterol and Apo-E synthesized in astrocytes are secreted in an ABCA1-dependent process, forming discoidal lipoprotein particles, which can be further lipidated. Brain lipoproteins are delivered to the CSF. Apo-E is a ligand for LDLR family members, which mediate neuronal lipoprotein uptake, thereby providing a supply of cholesterol to neurons. Excess cholesterol is metabolized to 24-hydroxycholesterol, which crosses the BBB and passes into the circulation. A small part of cholesterol (~1%) is esterified by ACAT. Only insignificant amounts of plasma HDL or LDL cross the BBB under normal conditions.

Cholesterol synthesis is crucial in the brain because the brain is separated from the peripheral pool of cholesterol by the blood brain barrier (BBB), which, under normal conditions, is impermeable to plasma lipoproteins [2, 3]. Thus, brain cholesterol originates almost exclusively from *de novo* biosynthesis through the mevalonate pathway. Cholesterol synthesis *in situ* in the brain is very active in order to meet the brain demands. Cholesterol is essential for normal synaptogenesis and plays important roles in axonal development, neurotransmitter release and neurosteroid production [2, 21]. Brain cholesterol synthesis is sufficient to meet the demands during development and in adult life, although this local synthesis decreases with age [22]. Genetic defects in enzymes involved in cholesterol synthesis cause severe neurological abnormalities underscoring the importance of endogenous cholesterol synthesis for normal brain function [23, 24]. The identity of the cells responsible for cholesterol synthesis in the adult brain is still a matter of debate. Neurons have a lower rate of cholesterol synthesis than astrocytes [25] and outsource cholesterol from astrocytes to form and maintain axons, dendrites and synapses [21, 26, 27]. In fact, based on the discovery that suppression of cholesterol synthesis in vivo in adult cerebellar neurons did not affect the viability of the neurons or the shape and density of synapses [28], it was suggested that neurons do not require autonomous cholesterol synthesis and are minor contributors to adult brain cholesterol synthesis [28]. However, *in situ* hybridization demonstrated that transcripts of several enzymes involved in cholesterol synthesis localize specifically to neurons in pyramidal and granular layers of mouse hippocampus [29], indicating that some adult neurons maintain the ability to synthesize cholesterol. Yet, there is ample evidence that brain neurons utilize cholesterol derived from astrocytes. Astrocytes provide cholesterol to neurons via apolipoprotein-mediated efflux and formation of HDL-like particles containing apoE [27]. Adenosine triphosphate-binding cassette (ABC) transporters, mainly ABCA1, mediate lipidation of nascent lipoproteins [30]. Neurons import cholesterol via lipoprotein receptor-mediated endocytosis [31]. Astrocyte-secreted lipoproteins are delivered to the CSF but they don't cross the BBB [32, 33].

Neurons convert excess cholesterol into a more polar metabolite that crosses the BBB, 24 (S) hydroxycholesterol (24-HC) by the enzyme cholesterol 24-hydroxylase (CYP46A1) [34, 35]. CYP46A1 is selectively expressed in the brain [36], in particular in pyramidal neurons of the hippocampus and cortex and in Purkinje cells in cerebellum, but not in astrocytes [25, 37]. 24-HC is a very important regulator of the mevalonate pathway (Section 3). In addition, 24-HC regulates cholesterol efflux in astrocytes [38]. Cholesterol also undergoes esterification catalyzed by the enzyme acyl CoA-cholesterol acyltransferase (ACAT) [39]. Although cholesterol esterification is not a major metabolic process in the brain, and cholesterol esters represent only 1% of the total cholesterol content in brains of human [40] and mice [41], ACAT has been identified as a crucial enzyme in AD [42].

Cholesterol-related genes that have been associated with AD encode primarily, components of the glia/neuron cholesterol shuttle processes, including apoE [4, 43], the apolipoprotein clusterin [44], ABCA1 [45-48], CYP46A1 [49-52], several members of the LDL receptor family [53-55], and ACAT [56]. Much less information is available with respect to the genetic association of AD with genes of enzymes of the mevalonate pathway. The few studies available did not provide strong associations. Thus, it is likely that changes in the mevalonate pathway identified in AD are a consequence of the disease. Here we focus on the evidence that indicate that the mevalonate pathway "per se" is affected in AD.

## 3. The mevalonate pathway in the brain and in AD

The brain produces cholesterol and a number of non-sterol isoprenoids such as farnesylpyrophosphate (FPP), geranylgeranylpyrophosphate (GGPP), ubiquinone and dolichol, exclusively through the mevalonate pathway. The mevalonate pathway comprises successive enzymatic reactions that convert acetyl-CoA into the different final sterol and non-sterol products [57, 58]. For the purposes of the discussion we have separated the mevalonate pathway in components: pre-squalene pathway, post-squalene pathway, shunt pathway and non-sterols isoprenoids pathway (Figure 2). The kinetics of the enzymes involved in the mevalonate pathway have been thoroughly studied [58, 59]. Enzymes of the mevalonate pathway are expressed in the brain of rodents and humans [29, 60] and the expression of many of them is developmentally regulated in the brain [61, 62]. Inborn defects in enzymes of the mevalonate pathway result in structural abnormalities of the brain and may be accompanied by neurodevelopmental/behavioral defects [63].

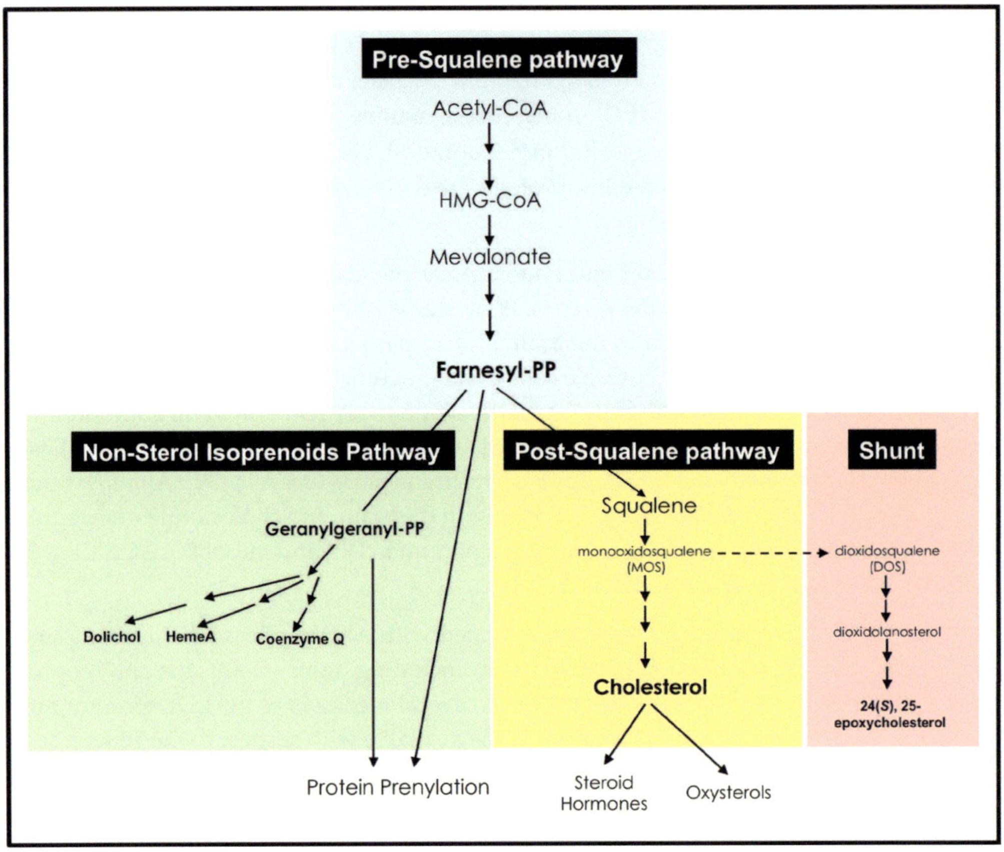


**Figure 2.** The mevalonate pathway. The mevalonate pathway has been divided in different components to facilitate the understanding of its regulation.

There is only limited information of changes in the mevalonate pathway enzymes and lipid intermediates in AD brains, although certain exceptions exist. The lipid products of the mevalonate pathway seem to be regulated highly individually in AD, likely through post-translational modifications of the enzymes and/or changes in levels of substrates. Most of the studies on the mevalonate pathway in AD have focused on cholesterol, although more recent work has also paid attention to the non-sterol isoprenoid branch of the pathway. In this chapter we focused on studies performed in brains and brain cells although there is important evidence that changes in plasma cholesterol levels may be relevant to AD development and/or progression [64]. The interest in understanding the role of the mevalonate pathway in AD increased with the reports that patients taking statins had lower incidence of AD than the general population [13-17, 65]. More recent prospective studies have produced conflicting results on the matter [15-19]. This is still an area of intense research and debate.

The mevalonate pathway is tightly regulated at the transcriptional and post-transcriptional levels to avoid accumulation of cholesterol while maintaining proper supply of non-sterol isoprenoids.

### 3.1. Regulation of the mevalonate pathway by SREBP-2 and LXR

Transcriptional regulation of the mevalonate pathway is mediated by two main transcription factors namely sterol-regulatory element binding protein type-2 (SREBP-2) and liver X receptors (LXR). SREBP-2 belongs to a family of membrane-bound transcription factors that regulate cholesterol and fatty acid homeostasis. Studies in knockout and transgenic mice demonstrated that cholesterol synthesis is preferentially regulated by SREBP-2 [66, 67]. SREBP-2 is synthesized and inserted in the endoplasmic reticulum (ER) as an inactive precursor (P)SREBP-2 [68]. (P)SREBP-2 has two transmembrane helices with the N- and C- terminals projecting into the cytosol [68]. The C-terminus of (P)SREBP-2 interacts with C-terminus of SREBP cleavage-activating protein (SCAP), a sterol-regulated escort protein. SCAP has eight transmembrane helices, of which transmembrane helices 2-6 are defined as a sterol sensing domain [68, 69]. (P)SREBP-2-SCAP complex has to be transported into coat protein complex II (COPII) vesicles that bud from the ER and travel to the Golgi complex [70]. Mice with haploinsufficiency of SCAP in the brain had reduced SREBP-2 processing and reduced SREBP-2 expression. Consequently, reduced SCAP level resulted in decreased expression of many enzymes in the mevalonate pathway and 30% reduction in cholesterol synthesis leading to impaired synaptic transmission and cognitive deficits [71]. At the Golgi, sequential proteolytic cleavage of (P)SREBP-2 by Site-1-protease (S1P) [72] and Site-2-protease (S2P) [73] releases the N-terminal /mature/nuclear SREBP-2 ((M)SREBP-2) that enters the nucleus to regulate gene transcription [66, 68, 74]. In the nucleus, (M)SREBP-2 binds to sterol regulatory elements (SREs) in the promoter of target genes in order to regulate gene expression [68]. SREBPs alone are relatively weak activators of gene expression. Transcriptional activities of SREBPs are highly enhanced by other cofactors such as nuclear factor Y(NF-Y) [75] and specificity protein-1 (sp-1) [76] or by the presence of two SRE motifs as in genes encoding enzymes such as 3-hydroxy-3-methylglutarylCoA reductase (HMGCR), squalene synthase [75] and 24-dihydrocholesterol reductase (DHCR24) [77]. (M)SREBP-2 increases the expression of most enzymes involved in the mevalonate pathway and the expression of LDLR involved in exogenous cholesterol uptake [66, 67]. In addition, SREBP-2 increases the expression of miR33a (encoded by an intron of SREBP-2) and miR128-2. miR33a and miR128-2 block ABCA1 and ABCG1 expression reducing cholesterol efflux [78-84]. High level of (M)SREBP-2 were detected in pyramidal neurons in hippocampus and cerebral neocotex of normal rat brain [85]. The main regulator of SREBP-2 proteolytic processing is cholesterol. When ER cholesterol falls below 5% of total ER lipids (molar basis), SREBP-2 cleavage is activated [86]. On the other hand, when cholesterol accumulates at the ER, it binds to SCAP inducing a conformational change that promotes SCAP binding to ER integral membrane proteins Insulin-Induced gene-1 or 2 (Insig-1 and Insig- 2) [87, 88]. Once bound to Insigs, SCAP is unable to bind to COPII and the SCAP-(P)SREBP-2 complex is not transported to the Golgi leading to reduced SREBP-2 processing [89]. In vitro experiments revealed that cholesterol, and the cholesterol precursors desmosterol and 7-DHC, but not lanosterol or oxysterols are able to change SCAP conformation [87]. Desmosterol and cholesterol bind to SCAP in a similar manner [88, 90, 91]. Oxysterols also reduce SREBP-2 processing but they do so by binding directly to Insigs and not to SCAP [92]. SREBP-2 positively regulates its own expression via binding to SRE in the promoter of its own gene [93]. It also increases expression of specific miRNAs for negative SREBP-2 regulators such as miR-182, which reduce expression of Fbxw7, an E3 ubiquitin ligase involved in nuclear SREBP-2 degradation and miR-96, which targets Insig-2 [94]. Therefore, miR-182 and miR-96 increase SREBP-2 processing, reduce its degradation and consequently enhance its transcriptional activity.

LXRs (LXR$\alpha$ and LXR$\beta$) also play a role in the regulation of the mevalonate pathway by activating or inhibiting expression of enzymes of the mevalonate pathway (reviewed in [95]). LXR are ligand-activated transcription factors belonging to the nuclear hormone receptor superfamily [96, 97]. Expression level of LXR$\alpha$ in the brain is much lower than in the liver, however, LXR$\beta$ is highly expressed in the brain compared to the liver [98]. SREBP-2 and LXR work in harmony in order to regulate the mevalonate pathway. SREBP-2 activation will enhance cholesterol production and consequently oxysterol production, leading to LXR activation and LXR targets expression [99]. On the other hand, LXRs activation enhances cholesterol efflux, reduces cellular cholesterol uptake [100, 101] and suppresses the expression of some enzymes in the post-squalene mevalonate pathway [102]. Consequently, LXR activation will reduce cellular cholesterol level leading to SREBP-2 processing and activation. In accordance, synthetic LXR agonist GW683965A significantly increased SREBP-2, LDLR, and HMGCR expression in astrocytes by indirect mechanims [38]. Moreover, significantly reduced number of SREBP-2 and HMGCR transcripts were detected in brains of LXR$\alpha$ and $\beta$ null mice [103].

### *3.1.1. Transcriptional regulation of the mevalonate pathway by SREBP-2 in AD*

Transcription factor profiling showed no difference in SREBPs between non-demented and AD brain cortical samples [104], however it was not discriminated if the probe was for SREBP-2 or SREBP-1. In autopsied hippocampus of patients with incipient AD, SREBF-1 was found to be elevated [105]. Haploinsufficiency of Scap, a key regulator of SREBP-2, in mice brain resulted in impaired synaptic transmission, as measured by decreased paired pulse facilitation and long-term potentiation; and was associated with behavioral and cognitive changes [71], suggesting that down-regulation of the mevalonate pathway may play an important role in the increased rates of cognitive decline in AD. Studies at the subcellular level suggest that SREBP-2 may be posttranslationally regulated in AD. We demonstrated that oA$\beta_{42}$ inhibit

SREBP-2 maturation in cultured neurons [106]. We also discovered that the levels of (M)SREBP-2 are reduced in the frontal cortex of the AD CRND8 mouse [107], suggesting that the negative regulation of SREBP-2 may also occur *in vivo* in AD. Recently, it was reported that APP also controls neuronal cholesterol synthesis through the SREBP pathway [108]. These studies showed that APP levels inversely correlate with SREBP in mice and man, and demonstrated that inhibition of the mevalonate pathway by APP impairs neuronal activity. The interaction of APP and SREBP-1 in the Golgi prevented the release of mature SREBP-1 and the translocation of SREBP-1 to the nucleus. Our data, on the other hand, indicated that $A\beta_{42}$ did not affect the enzymatic cleavage of SREBP-2 "per se" nor did it block mature SREBP-2 translocation to the nucleus, but impaired the delivery of SREBP-2 to the Golgi preventing cleavage of (P)SREBP-2 [107]. Interestingly, the regulation of SREBP by APP takes place preferentially in neurons. In astrocytes, APP and SREBP1 did not interact nor did APP affect cholesterol biosynthesis, but neuronal expression of APP decreased both HMGCR and cholesterol 24-hydroxylase mRNA levels leading to inhibition of neuronal activity [108].

### 3.2. Pre-squalene pathway

The pre-squalene mevalonate pathway is depicted in Figure 3. Acetoacetyl Co-A is formed from two moles of acetyl Co-A in the presence of acetoacetyl Co-A thiolase. 3-hydroxy-3-methylglutaryl (HMG) Co-A is formed from one mole of acetyl Co-A and acetoacetyl Co-A in the presence of HMG Co-A synthase (HMGS). HMGCR converts HMG Co-A to mevalonic acid [109]. The rate-limiting enzyme of the pathway is HMGCR [110], one of the most highly regulated enzymes in nature [111]. In human brains HMGCR expression was demonstrated in both neurons and glia [112]. Studies in adult mouse brain tissue showed HMGCR expression within cortical, hippocampal, and basal forebrain cholinergic neurons [29, 60]. HMGCR protein and activity are localized in the ER and peroxisomes in the CNS [113] and in other organs. Due to the critical function of this enzyme early in the mevalonate pathway, there are no human syndromes known to be associated with HMGCR loss of function, and mouse embryos homozygous for the Hmgcr knockout allele do not progress beyond the blastocyst stage. On the other hand mice heterozygous for the Hmgcr mutation showed normal development, gross anatomy, and fertility (reviewed in [114]). HMGCR is the target of statins.

The product of HMGCR, mevalonic acid, is phosphorylated sequentially to 5-phosphomevalonate by the enzyme mevalonate kinase (MK) and to 5-pyrophosphomevalonate by phosphomevalonate kinase (PMK). MK is the second essential enzyme of the isoprenoid/cholesterol biosynthetic pathway [115]. Inherited mutations in human MK are correlated with two diseases characterized by neurological dysfunction namely mevalonic aciduria and Hyper-IgD syndrome (reviewed in [114, 116]).

5-Pyrophosphomevalonate is converted to isopentenylpyrophosphate (IPP) by mevalonate diphosphate decarboxylase. IPP is required for synthesis of all further products of the mevalonate pathway [117]. IPP is isomerized to dimethylallyl pyrophosphate (DMPP) in the presence of IPP isomerase (IPPI) [58, 118].

IPP and/or DMPP are required for isopentenylation, which is an essential modification of specialized tRNA that transfers the amino acid selenocysteine ($tRNA^{Sec}$) [119, 120]. Selenopro-

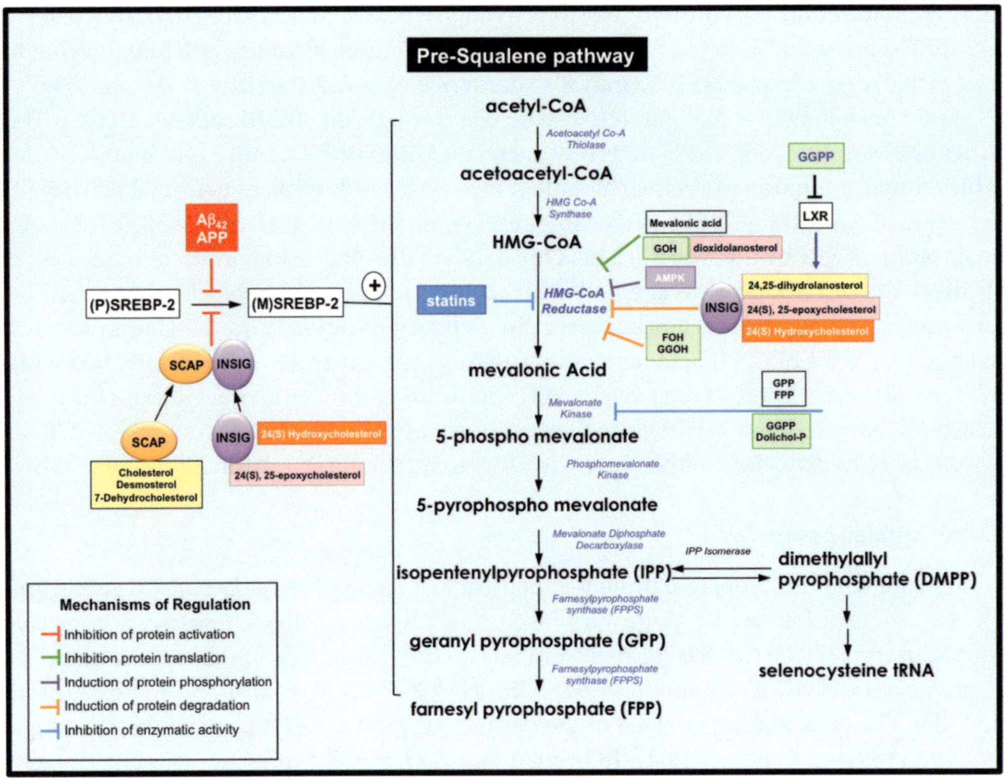


**Figure 3.** The pre-squalene pathway. Schematic representation of the pre-squalene mevalonate pathway and key enzymes regulating FPP synthesis. The rate-limiting enzyme of the pathway is HMGCR. Several regulatory feedback mechanisms exist at the level of many enzymes of the pathway.

teins have been implicated in protein folding, degradation of misfolded membrane proteins, and control of cellular calcium homeostasis, all processes known to be dysfunctional in neurodegenerative diseases [121, 122]. Moreover, neuron-specific ablation of selenoprotein expression causes a neurodevelopmental and neurodegenerative phenotype affecting the cerebral cortex and hippocampus [123]; and impaired expression of selenoproteins in the brain triggers striatal neuronal loss leading to coordination defects in mice [124]. Statins, by reducing production of IPP, interfere with the enzymatic isopentenylation of $tRNA^{Sec}$ and prevent its maturation to a functional tRNA molecule, resulting in the reduction of the expression of selenoproteins [125]. Other functions of IPP include its antinociceptive effect, mediated by inhibition of transient receptor potential (TRP)-channels, TRPV3 and TRPA1 [126]. Interestingly, DMPP has effects on TRP- channels opposites to those of IPP, inducing enhanced acute pain behavior [127].

IPP combines with DMPP to form geranyl pyrophosphate (GPP); and GPP is condensed with another molecule of IPP to yield farnesylpyrophosphate (FPP). GPP and FPP syntheses are catalyzed by farnesylpyrophosphate synthase (FPPS), a prenyltranferase [128-130]. FPP initiates the branches of the pathway that generate cholesterol and non-sterol isoprenoids.

### *3.2.1. Regulation of enzymes of the pre-squalene pathway*

HMGCR is the rate-limiting enzyme of the mevalonate pathway. HMGCR is transcriptionally activated by SREBP-2 [131]. The presence of two SRE motifs in HMGCR promoter leads to a higher level sterol-dependent regulation [75]. Gene regulation by the SREBP pathway is slow and its down-regulation requires several hours to effectively decrease mRNA of target genes [132]. In order to accomplish a rapid (within 1 h) switch off of cholesterol synthesis HMGCR is extensively regulated at the translational and posttranslational levels (Figure 3). HMGCR is post-transcriptionally regulated by alternative splicing/skipping of exon 13 leading to production of a shorter unproductive transcript that encodes an inactive enzyme. In the liver, HMGCR alternative splicing is regulated by sterols (cholesterol and 25-hydroxycholesterol), so sterol accumulation increases the proportion of shorter transcript and vice versa. Interestingly, sterol-mediated alternative splicing of HMGCR occurs faster than sterol-mediated transcriptional inhibition of HMGCR [133]. Mevalonate and certain downstream derivatives such as dioxidolanosterol (a shunt pathway intermediate) and GOH regulate HMGCR mRNA translation reducing its rate of synthesis [134-137]. Mevalonate has been shown to change polysome distribution of HMGCR mRNA leading to inhibition of HMGCR translation at the initiation step [138]. HMGCR is post-translationally regulated via phosphorylation and ubiquitin/proteasomal degradation. Short-term regulation of HMGCR is mediated via phosphorylation by AMPK and dephosphorylation by PP2A (protein phosphatase 2A). HMGCR exists in the cell in both unphosphorylated (active) and phosphorylated (inactive) states [139-141]. As a master regulator of cellular energy homeostasis, AMPK phosphorylates HMGCR to inhibit cholesterol synthesis, an energy intensive process. The implications of AMPK-mediated regulation of HMGCR are controversial. In mutant Drosophila lacking functional AMPK, higher activity of HMGCR and consequent higher rate of the mevalonate pathway were associated with progressive neurodegeneration [142]. On the other hand, activation of AMPK by quercetin reduced HMGCR activity, cholesterol synthesis and enhanced cognitive functions in high cholesterol fed old mice [143]. The best understood mechanism of HMGCR post transcriptional regulation is the sterol-mediated ubiquitination and proteasomal degradation. This mechanism requires binding of HMGCR to Insig-1 or Insig-2 and recruitment of Ring-finger ubiquitin ligases, Gp78, Trc8, and MARCH6 [144-146]. Insig binds to the sterol-sensing domain in HMGCR [147]. HMGCR share many sequence similarities in the sterol-sensing domain with SCAP, thus Insigs can bind with both HMGCR and SCAP [148]. The binding of Insigs has radically different consequences for SCAP and HMGCR. Upon binding Insig, HMGCR is ubiquitinated and degraded [147, 149], whereas, as indicated above SCAP is retained in the ER [89]. Both processes inhibit the mevalonate pathway. The oxysterols 25-EC (synthesized by the shunt pathway, Section 3.3.1.) and 24-HC; and the post-squalene intermediate 24, 25-dihydrolanosterol (Section 3.3.0), but not cholesterol, bind to Insigs and induce HMGCR degradation [91, 150-152]. Indeed, it is the accumulation of 24, 25-dihydrolanosterol the mechanism by which LXR$\alpha$ enhances HMGCR [102]. Adding an additional level of regulation, the non-sterol isoprenoid GGPP antagonizes LXR, blocking HMGCR degradation [153, 154]. Studies in vitro suggested that two metabolites of the non-sterol isoprenoids pathway namely farnesol (FOH) and geranylgeranyol (GGOH) enhance HMGCR degradation beyond the effect elicited by sterols. FOH and GGOH do not target the interaction between Insigs and HMGCR but seem to rely on protein prenylation [147, 155-158]. Consequently, a GGPP synthase (GGPPS) inhibitor, and a geranylgeranyl transferase I (GGTaseI) inhibitor prevented the enhancement of HMGCR degradation [155].

MK is regulated transcriptionally by SREBP-2 through an SRE in its promoter (Horton 2002). MK activity is post-translationally reduced by GGPP, FPP, GPP and dolichol phosphate via competitive inhibition at ATP binding site [159, 160]. GGPP is the strongest inhibitor of MK activity.

#### *3.2.2. Pre-squalene mevalonate pathway in AD*

Information on the status and regulation of HMGCR in AD is very limited. HMGCR is the most important enzyme of the pre-squalene mevalonate pathway. No changes in gene expression of HMGCR were found in AD brain in humans and in a mouse model of AD [161]. Genetic association of HMGCR was found in patients under the age of 75 [162], and HMGCR promoter polymorphisms alone or with polymorphisms in other proteins of cholesterol homeostasis were associated with AD risk and cognitive deterioration in some studies [163, 164], but not in all populations [165]. The AlzGene meta-analysis for HMGCR is negative [7]. Poirier's group identified HMGCR as a genetic modifier for risk, age of onset and mild cognitive impairment (MCI) conversion to AD. In their recent study they found that carriers of a specific variant of HMGCR display a protective effect that resembled in size and gender to what has been reported for APOE2 in humans [166]. Information on protein HMGCR levels and activity in the carriers' brains is expected to be available soon. Age- and sex-dependent dysregulation of HMGCR occurs in the liver [167], but to our knowledge similar mechanisms have not been reported in the brain. Studies showed high levels of the HMGCR mRNA in all areas of the brain but no obvious differences were found between AD and controls [168]; similarly levels and gene expression of HMGCR were comparable in AD and control samples in another study [169].

FPPS is the last enzyme of the pre-squalene pathway. In two small samples, polymorphisms of FPPS or their haplotypes were associated with AD [8]. But in other samples FPPS variants were not related to AD risk. The AlzGene meta- analysis for FPPS polymorphisms is negative [7].

### 3.3. Post-squalene pathway

The post-squalene mevalonate pathway is depicted in Figure 4. FPP is converted to squalene by the action of squalene synthase (farnesyl diphosphate farnesyl transferase 1) [170]. Squalene synthase is the first enzyme in the mevalonate pathway whose product, squalene, is committed to cholesterol synthesis. The lack of reports indicating genetic disorders linked to mutations in squalene synthase suggest that this enzyme may be essential in embryonic development (discussed in [114]). In fact, deletion of squalene synthase is embryonic lethal in mice [171]. Squalene synthase is inhibited by zaragozic acid.

Squalene is converted to monooxidosqualene (MOS), which can be further converted to lanosterol and dioxidosqualene (DOS). Formation of both MOS and DOS requires the action of the enzyme squalene monooxygenase (SM) (also called squalene epoxidase). Lanosterol is

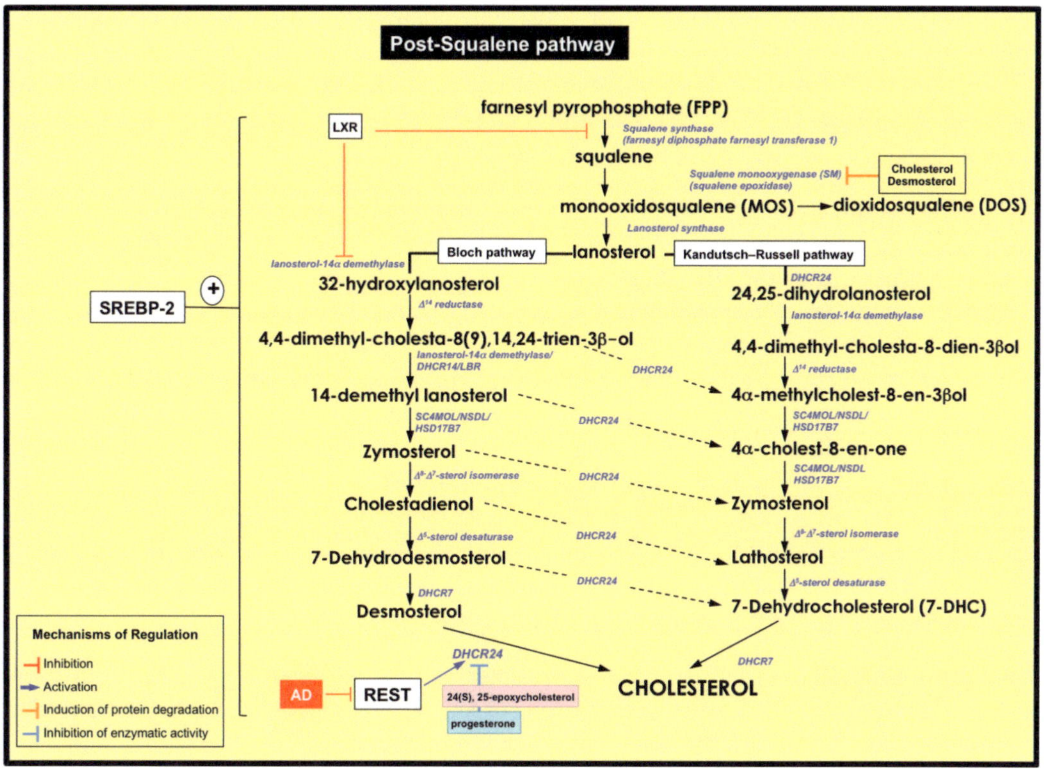


**Figure 4.** The post-squalene pathway. The final product of the post squalene pathway is cholesterol. Most enzymes of the post-squalene pathway are targets of SREBP-2. Other posttrancriptional regulatory mechanisms also exist.

the first sterol intermediate in cholesterol synthesis. Lanosterol is metabolized to cholesterol by 19 enzymatic steps. In the brain, as in the liver, there are two major pathways for the conversion of lanosterol to cholesterol. The Kandutsch–Russell pathway includes lathosterol and 7-dehydrocholesterol (7-DHC) as intermediates; while the Bloch pathway, uses desmosterol as an intermediate (reviewed in [172]. Post lanosterol precursors are present in all cells that synthesize cholesterol, although they might represent a minor sterol component due to their rapid conversion to downstream metabolites, or to their release from cells [173, 174]. A special scenario is present in embryonic mouse astrocytes, which, freshly dissociated from the striatum or after being cultured for several days, contain desmosterol as a major membrane sterol, accounting for roughly 50% of total sterols [175]. In young rodents, brain cholesterol is mainly synthesized via the desmosterol pathway, while the Kandutsch–Russell pathway is predominant in older rodents [176, 177]. Desmosterol transiently accumulates up to 30% of total sterols in the mammalian brain during development and in the perinatal period indicating the activity of the Bloch pathway [178-183]. In humans the Bloch-pathway plays a minor role in the formation of CNS cholesterol during aging [22]. Neurons and glia seem to use different pathways downstream of lanosterol. Neurons contain precursors for the Kandutsch-Russel pathway (*e.g.*, 7-DHC) whereas astrocytes contain precursors for the Bloch pathway (e.g., desmosterol) [25]. Disturbances in either of these two pathways may result in replacement of cholesterol with its precursors in the brain, which causes serious disorders of the nervous system [184, 185]. Serum lathosterol is considered an indicator of whole body cholesterol synthesis in humans [22, 186, 187]. Lanosterol and desmosterol together with lathosterol are regarded as tissue markers of local cholesterol synthesis [22].

7-DHC and desmosterol are the immediate cholesterol precursors of the Kandutsch-Russel and the Bloch pathways respectively. 7-DHC is converted to cholesterol by 7-DHC reductase (DHCR7). Mutations in the DHCR7 gene cause the human genetic disease Smith-Lemli-Opitz syndrome, characterized by a wide spectrum of developmental anomalies that may result from decreased cholesterol, increased 7-DHC, or a combination of both [184, 188, 189]. Desmosterol is reduced to cholesterol by the enzyme DHCR24, also known as seladin-1 [190]. DHCR24 catalyzes the 24,25-reduction reactions in the cholesterol biosynthesis pathway and may act on most intermediates of the Bloch pathway [23, 114, 191, 192]. Disruption of the DHCR24 gene results in accumulation of desmosterol and is characterized by multiple congenital anomalies in humans and mice [190, 193, 194]. Desmosterol is an abundant structural membrane component in astrocytes [175]. In the brain, high desmosterol levels are present during development [181, 182]. During aging, hippocampal levels of desmosterol decrease significantly in the rat [176]. Desmosterol is a natural ligand of LXR [195].

From the two reductases that participate in the later steps of cholesterol synthesis production, DHCR24 is important in AD and therefore is discussed here in more detail. DHCR24 is encoded by a single gene (Dhcr24) on chromosome 1, an evolutionarily conserved gene with homologies to a family of flavin adenine dinucleotide-dependent oxidoreductases [196]. DHCR24 is detected in many tissues, including brain, adrenal glands, pituitary, thyroid gland, ovary, testis, and prostate [197-199]. Dhcr24 was initially identified as a gene down-regulated in affected brain regions in AD [196] and consequently its product has also been called Seladin-1 from **Sel**ective **A**lzheimer's **d**isease **in**dicator 1. However, current evidence indicates that DHCR24 has functions that go beyond those expected from its enzymatic activity in the mevalonate pathway. The roles of DHCR24 in oxidative stress, hepatitis C virus infection, cardiovascular disease, prostate cancer and other conditions have been recently discussed in detail [200]. The role of DHCR24 in AD is discussed in Section 3.3.3.

#### *3.3.1. Shunt in the post-squalene pathway*

Conversion of MOS to DOS establishes an alternate pathway leading to the production of (24S, 25)-epoxycholesterol (25-EC) [201] (Figure 2). This shunt in the mevalonate pathway functions in parallel to the conversion of lanosterol to cholesterol [202]. 25-EC is the only oxysterol that does not derive from cholesterol. It is present in rodent brain [203], where it is proportionally more important than 24-HC during development and the perinatal period, but not in the adult [204]. Production of 25-EC represents a cellular defense mechanism against accumulation of cholesterol that derives from the mevalonate pathway (as opposed to exogenously-derived cholesterol) [202]. 25-EC is responsible of the fine-tuning of cholesterol synthesis, and without it, acute cholesterol synthesis is exaggerated [205]. 25-EC is synthesized in both human neurons and astrocytes, and the proportion synthesized by astrocytes is an order of magnitude higher than that of neurons [206]. Astrocytes but not neurons secrete 25-EC and neurons internalize this oxysterol. Interestingly, 25-EC reduced the expression of SREBP-2 target genes and increased expression of LXR target genes in both astrocytes and neurons [205-208]. 25-EC may represent an additional regulatory signal between astrocytes and neurons in cholesterol homeostasis [206]. 25-EC is an important negative regulator of the mevalonate pathway (Section 3.2.1).

### *3.3.2. Regulation of enzymes of post-squalene pathway*

All the enzymes of the post-squalene pathway are transcriptionally activated by SREBP-2 [67, 132, 209]. In addition, LXR$\alpha$ represses transcription of squalene synthase and lanosterol-14$\alpha$ demethylase directly [102].

Posttranslationally, cholesterol and desmosterol but none of the oxysterols enhance SM degradation [210]. MARCH6, also known as Teb4, functions as a selective ubiquitin ligase for SM ubiquitination and consequent proteasomal degradation [146, 211]. Cholesterol-induced degradation of SM is a novel feedback mechanism regulating the mevalonate pathway to prevent cholesterol accumulation without affecting isoprenoid supply.

DHCR24 is regulated by diverse mechanisms at the transcriptional and posttranslational levels. Several studies have identified the Dhcr24 gene as a target of SREBPs [67, 212-214]. In brains of statin-treated mice, there is activation of SREBP-2 and significant up-regulation of DHCR24 in cortex and hippocampus [215]. SREBP-2 binds to two (SREs) present within the Dhcr24 promoter, inducing a novel mode of transcriptional regulation for SREBP-2, characterized by homotypic cooperativity [77]. This type of regulation may warrant that a threshold of active SREBP-2 is reached before committing to the energetically expensive process of cholesterol synthesis [77, 200]. A novel mechanism of DHCR24 transcriptional activation by the transcription factor RE1-silencing transcription factor (REST), which is normally a repressor, has been recently reported [183]. Although this may be a secondary mechanism of DHCR24, the reduced levels of REST present in the brain during development may explain, at least in part, the reduced activity of DHCR24 and the consequent elevation of desmosterol [183]. Interestingly LXR has also been implicated in the regulation of DHCR24 as data from a whole genome screen for LXR binding sites showed that the Dhcr24 gene contained a functional LXR response element [216]. LXR regulation of DHCR24 seems to be tissue specific. LXR did not influence DHCR24 expression in some studies [77], and at least in studies using mice deficient in LXR$\beta$, this regulation does not seem to take place in brain [216]. DHCR24 displays epigenetic regulation by methylation and histone acetylation due to the presence of GC rich regions within the DHCR24 promoter [217]. At the post-translational level DHCR24 activity is inhibited by certain oxysterols (25EC) [218] and by progesterone possibly by direct enzyme inhibition [182]. In addition, a novel mode of DHCR24 inhibition through phosphorylation has been demonstrated, which may allow a rapid inhibition of cholesterol synthesis [219].

### *3.3.3. Post-squalene pathway in AD*

From the enzymes involved in the post-squalene section of the mevalonate pathway, DHCR24 is the most important in AD. A study comparing gene expression by using mRNA differential display identified the down-regulation of DHCR24 in large pyramidal neurons in vulnerable regions in AD but not in healthy brains [196]. This finding was confirmed by others [220], although this may not apply to all AD patients [221]. The down-regulation in DHCR24 transcription was associated with hyperphosphorylated tau but not with β-amyloid deposition [220]. Single nucleotide polymorphisms of DHCR24 have been associated with AD risk [222]. However, these associations have not been confirmed, and other polymorphisms of DHCR24 only associated with AD in men but not in women [223]. Based on the evidence that DHCR24 expression is higher in neural stem cells than in differentiated neurons [224] it was hypothesized that reduced DHCR24 expression might be due to the existence of an impaired neuronal stem cell compartment [225]. Alternatively, transcriptional regulation of DHCR24 may be altered in AD. Indeed, recent studies indicated that the transcription factor REST, identified as a DHCR24 transcriptional activator [183] is lost in mild cognitive impairment and AD [226]. In addition, we have demonstrated that Aβ causes a significant decrease of SREBP-2 activation in neurons [106]; and we found reduced SREBP-2 activation in brain cortex of the AD mouse model CRND8 [107]. These observations suggest that, as the disease progresses reduced DHCR24 levels would not be unique, and that other enzymes of the mevalonate pathway would also be affected in brain cells that accumulate Aβ. However, taking in consideration the cooperative transcriptional mechanism of regulation exerted by SREBP-2 on DHCR24 [77], it is expected that DHCR24 would be particularly sensitive to reduced SREBP-2 activation. A general reduction of the mevalonate pathway could also explain why the levels of desmosterol are decreased in AD brains [227], contrary to what would be predicted if only DHCR24 were down-regulated. If these mechanisms exist in vivo in the brain, then the decrease of DHCR24 would be a consequence, rather than a cause of AD. Contrary to the findings in humans, the levels of desmosterol were elevated in the APPSLxPS1mut mouse model of AD, which also showed a significant decrease in DHCR24 in those brain areas [161]. DHCR24 has neuroprotective effects against Aβ toxicity, ER stress and oxidative stress-induced apoptosis, inhibiting caspase 3 activity and directly scavenging reactive oxygen species [196, 228, 229]. Many other studies have reported the antioxidant properties of DHCR24 in a variety of tissues and in the context of different diseases (reviewed in [200]). Importantly, DHCR24 mediates the protective effects of estrogens in cultured human neuroblasts since estrogen and selective estrogen receptor modulators (SERMs) stimulate the expression of DHCR24 in human neuroblast long-term cell cultures [230, 231]. The neuroprotective action of DHCR24 against Aβ may be due to its ability to maintain plasma membrane cholesterol at levels that prevent the rise of intracellular calcium and the production of ROS and lipoperoxidation that contributes to Aβ toxicity [232-234]. The relevance of these mechanisms in vivo in the brain requires confirmation, especially because there is ample evidence suggesting that high plasma membrane cholesterol may be detrimental in Aβ-induced toxicity (reviewed in [11]). The reduction of cholesterol in cell membranes due to DHCR24 may impair lipid raft functions and favor Aβ accumulation by a combination of inefficient Aβ degradation (due to low plasmin activity) and increased APP amyloidogenic cleavage [235]. Thus, all these mechanisms suggest the existence of vicious feedback cycles involving Aβ and DHCR24.

The post-squalene pathway results in production of cholesterol. There is little consensus about total brain cholesterol alterations in patients with AD [236-238]. Using different methods for measuring cholesterol (discussed in [237]), some studies found no change in cholesterol content in any portion of the brain [239, 240] or the hippocampus [241] in AD brains, while other studies reported changes in cholesterol levels in specific brain areas, particularly in regions with extensive Aβ deposits and neurofibrillary tangles (NFTs). Xiong and collaborators found an increase in cholesterol in the cortex of AD brains [104], Heverin et al. described a significant increase of cholesterol concentration in the basal ganglia but not in other brain areas in a small group of AD brains [242] and Cutler at al. reported accumulation of free cholesterol in the middle frontal gyrus and frontal cortex but not the unaffected cerebellum in AD brains from individuals expressing apoE4 [243]. It was also indicated that, as the severity of the disease progressed, there was an increase in membrane- and amyloid plaque-associated cholesterol [243-245]. Cholesterol levels were lower in the temporal gyrus of autopsied brains of AD patients compared to control subjects [246].

Analysis of post squalene cholesterol precursors also provided conflicting results. Lathosterol was reported to be elevated in the basal ganglia and the pons in AD but the ratio of lathosterol to cholesterol, used as a marker for cholesterol synthesis, was not significantly different between controls and AD patients suggesting that cholesterol synthesis is normal [242]. More recently a model for cholesterol homeostasis deregulation was proposed based on the measurement of post-squalene cholesterol precursors, cholesterol and oxysterol in brains of individuals with no-cognitive impairment, MCI and AD [247]. In 'compensated' MCI and initial AD there would be a heme oxygenase-1-mediated stimulation of cholesterol synthesis and cholesterol efflux in the astroglial compartment to allow cholesterol delivery for neuronal repair. As the disease progresses, massive uptake of cholesterol derived from widespread neuronal degeneration would overwhelm glial efflux pathways resulting in increased brain cholesterol levels and feed-back suppression of de novo cholesterol synthesis. This model could explain the findings in CSF. In CSF, cholesterol levels were significantly lower in AD patients as compared to controls [248, 249], and absolute levels of lanosterol, lathosterol and desmosterol and ratios of cholesterol precursors/cholesterol were also significantly reduced strongly indicating that *de novo* cholesterol synthesis within the CNS of AD patients might be impaired [248]. In the latter study, only the ratio of desmosterol/cholesterol was not significantly different in AD patients as compared to controls, but the increased CSF ratios of desmosterol/lathosterol suggests that the activity of the Kandutsch–Russell pathway might be reduced more than the Bloch pathway. The authors proposed that reduced expression of DHCR24 also contributes to decreased levels of cholesterol in AD patients and may explain the high levels of desmosterol found in AD in some studies [220, 250]. However, in other cases brain levels of desmosterol were reduced in AD [227]. This last finding agrees with the possibility that mevalonate pathway enzymes other than DHCR24 may also be down-regulated in AD, perhaps by a mechanism that involves SREBP-2 inhibititon. A further indication that cholesterol synthesis might be inhibited in AD is the finding that neurosteroids, which result from cholesterol metabolism, are reduced in AD temporal cortex as compared to control subjects [251]. It is important to highlight that changes in levels of cholesterol intermediates in brains of mouse AD models do not parallel changes in human patients. In the APP transgenic mice carrying the Swedish mutation (APP23), no differences in the levels of lathosterol, desmosterol or cholesterol and were found when compared with wild-type animals [177]. These differences must be considered when using animal models to study the mevalonate pathway.

It is possible that a change in the distribution of cholesterol inside brain cells rather than a change in total cholesterol content may influence AD pathology [252]. We have shown that Aβ induces cholesterol sequestration within the neuronal endosomal/lysosomal system, and impairs intracellular trafficking [106]. Our findings provide an explanation to the cellular cholesterol overload reported in brains of AD patients [253]. They also agree with previous work that showed cholesterol sequestration specifically in Aβ-immunopositive neurons [104, 254, 255], and with studies in transgenic mouse models of AD where cholesterol sequestration in the brain was preceded by Aβ accumulation and/or coincided with areas of Aβ accumulation [244, 256, 257]. These studies underscored the relevance of cholesterol sequestration in AD. This is important because a causal relationship between cellular cholesterol sequestration and cell death has been found in Niemann-Pick Type C (NPC) pathology [258]. NPC is a disorder characterized by impairment of intracellular cholesterol trafficking and cholesterol sequestration in the endosomal compartment [259]. Accumulation of cholesterol within the endosomal-lysosomal system in NPC not only triggers degeneration of neurons in selected brain regions but also leads to abnormal processing of APP and Aβ generation as observed in AD pathology. The similarities between AD and NPC include the presence of immunologically similar tau-positive NFTs [254, 260], the influence of ε4 isoform of apoE in promoting disease pathology [261], and endosomal abnormalities associated with the accumulation of cleaved APP derivatives and/or Aβ peptides in vulnerable neurons [262, 263]. Importantly, strategies previously used to reduce cholesterol sequestration in NPC and strategies that reduce cholesterol levels by increasing cholesterol metabolism improved pathological symptoms in mouse models of AD [264, 265].

Preclinical and clinical studies have indicated the critical role of cholesterol in AD. This topic has been reviewed extensively and thoroughly in the past years [11, 12, 18, 236, 238, 266-268], thus it is not discussed in this chapter. The best-studied role of cholesterol is in the production of Aβ from amyloid precursor protein (APP). Overall, the evidence indicates that increase in cellular cholesterol causes an increase in Aβ production, although some studies showed the opposite [11, 12, 269]. Cholesterol regulates Aβ uptake and toxicity, but the evidence on whether cholesterol reduces or favors Aβ toxicity is controversial [11, 12]. Brain cholesterol is important in synapse development and maintenance [27, 270, 271]. Synaptic dysfunction is one of the earliest significant events in AD and synapse loss is the strongest anatomical correlate of the degree of clinical impairment [272, 273]. Significant decrease in dendritic spine density is present in the hippocampus of patients with AD and in transgenic mouse models of AD [274-278]. Alterations in cholesterol levels, even locally at synapses, may play a role in synapse dysfunction in AD [279].

### 3.4. Non-sterol isoprenoids pathway

The branch of the mevalonate pathway that leads to the production of non-sterol isoprenoids is depicted in Figure 5. The enzymes involved in these steps have been extensively reviewed [59]. The importance of this pathway is emphasized by the number of diseases

http://dx.doi.org/10.5772/59904

that are associated with its dysfunction, including AD, Parkinson's disease, cancer, and tuberculosis [129, 280-282].

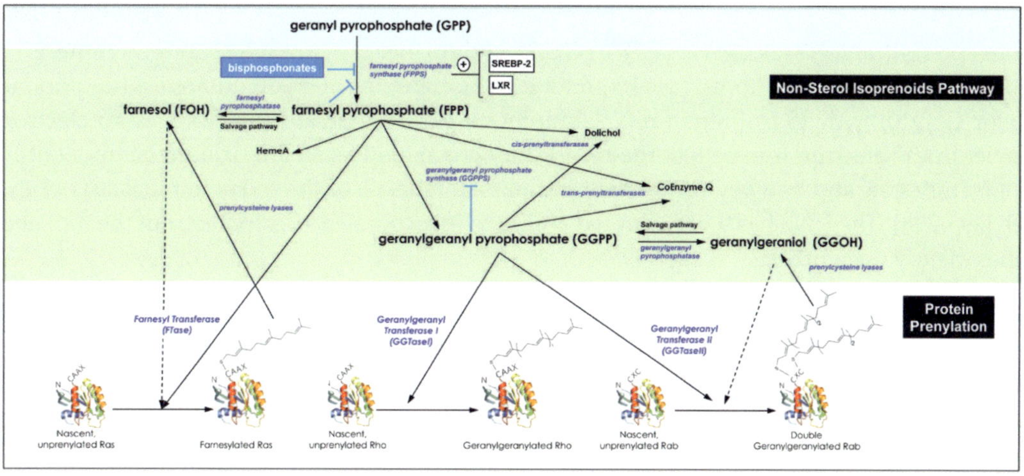


**Figure 5.** The non-sterol isoprenoid pathway.

FPP is the common substrate for synthesis of several end products and for the lipid modification of proteins. The enzymes responsible for synthesis of FPP and its non-sterol derivatives are prenyl-transferases that catalyze consecutive condensations of IPPs with primer substrates to form linear backbones for all isoprenoid compounds [130]. The enzyme GGPPS catalyzes the conversion of FPP into GGPP [283]. The main role of FPP and GGPP is in the posttranslational isoprenylation (*i.e.* farnesylation and geranylgeranylation) of proteins (Section 3.4.1.). Two different GGPPS activities have been described: a membrane-associated protein that produces GGPP for dolichol biosynthesis and a cytosolic protein that produces GGPP for protein prenylation [284]. In mouse brain cytosol, FPPS and GGPPS activities were higher than those in the corresponding fractions from the liver, perhaps reflecting a higher demand for protein prenylation in the brain [284]. FPPS and GGPPS activities were differentially distributed across various subregions of the brain. FPPS activity was present in all brain regions as expected by the several products that derive from FPP [285]. GGPPS activity was ~100 fold lower than FPPS activity, which agrees with the more limited use of GGPP, mostly for protein prenylation and as a precursor of a limited number of metabolites. GGPPS activity was lowest in the cerebellum [285].There have not been any reported cases of FPPS or GGPPS deficiency in humans [128]. FPPS is the target of nitrogen-containing bisphosphonate (N-BP) inhibitors, drugs used extensively to treat bone diseases [286]. A few bisphosphonate selective inhibitors for GGPPS have been reported but a clinically proven inhibitor of GGPPS has not yet been identified, limiting the validation of this enzyme as a therapeutic target [287].

Cis-prenyltransferases enzymes use FPP and GGPP for synthesis of dolichols [288, 289]. Dolichol phosphate is a lipid carrier embedded in the ER membrane, essential for the synthesis of N-glycans, GPI-anchors and protein C- and O-mannosylation [290, 291]. Dolichol is present, as a family with different chain lengths, in the hippocampus and spinal cord in a relatively low concentration compared to other areas of the brain [285]. Dolichol increases in brain and in peripheral organs during aging [292] and is associated with increased HMGCR activity [293]. The use of dolichol level as a marker for aging has been proposed [294].

Trans-prenyltransferases convert FPP to GGPP and further polyprenyl-PP in the synthesis of Coenzyme Q (CoQ), also known as ubiquinone. In humans, the main ubiquinone is ubiquinone 10, or CoQ10, with 10 isoprene units. Ubiquinone performs major functions as an electron carrier in the electron transfers of the respiratory chain, and as an antioxidant component in cell membranes and as a key component in the maintenance of the redox homeostasis of the cell [295-298]. The CNS has a very limited ability to incorporate ubiquinone from the diet and relies mainly on synthesis "in situ" [299].

FPP and GGPP can be converted to their correspondent alcohols farnesol (FOH) and geranylgeranyol (GGOH) by farnesyl and geranylgeranyl pyrophosphatases [300, 301]. Salvage pathways for the conversion of FOH and GGOH back to their pyrophosphate counterpart seem to exist in mammalian cells [302]. FOH and GGOH can also be formed by degradation of isoprenylated proteins in reactions catalyzed by prenylcysteine lyases, enzymes highly expressed in the brain [303]. FOH and GGOH may down-regulate HMGCR (Section 3.2.1 and Figure 3) (reviewed in [128]). The role of FOH and GGOH in protein prenylation is unclear. Some studies showed that mammalian cells utilize exogenously supplied FOH and GGOH for protein isoprenylation and, when mevalonate biosynthesis is blocked by statins, free FOH and GGOH can restore the pools of FPP and GGPP, although FOH may not be converted to GGPP [302, 304, 305]. The use of FOH and/or GGOH for protein prenylation might occur preferentially under conditions of reduced FPP and GGPP production from mevalonate [306]. Contrary to the existence of a salvage pathway that uses FOH and GGOH for protein prenylation, it was demonstrated that overexpressing phosphatases that convert FPP and GGPP to FOH and GGOH in mammalian cells, decreases rather than increases protein isoprenylation (as evaluated by a decreased of Rho protein level in cell membranes) and results in defects in cell growth and cytoskeletal organization that are associated with dysregulation of Rho family GTPases [301]. Moreover, work in cancer cells proposed that GGOH would reduce protein prenylation by down-regulating HMGCR leading to a shortage of FPP and GGPP [307]. Whether any of these mechanisms take place in the brain is uncertain. FOH is present at physiologically relevant concentrations in the brain of rodents and humans, where it may act in the regulation of brain $Ca^{2+}$ homeostasis and neurotransmitter release by inhibiting N-type $Ca^{2+}$ channels [308]. FOH has been shown to modulate the activity of the farnesoid X receptor (FXR), a member of the nuclear hormone receptor superfamily [309].

#### *3.4.1. Non-sterol isoprenoids and protein prenylation*

FPP and GGPP are substrates for protein farnesylation and geranylgeranylation (collectively called isoprenylation). In the human genome, there are approximately 300 hypothetical prenylated proteins [310]. Among them heterotrimeric G protein subunits, nuclear lamins and small GTPases have been confirmed to be prenylated [311]. Small GTPases represent the largest group of prenylated proteins. All small GTPases are able to specifically bind GDP and GTP, being inactive when bound to GDP (cytosolic location) and active when bound to GTP (membrane location). They also have an intrinsic GTPase activity to hydrolyze bound GTP to GDP and phosphate (Pi) [312]. FPP and GGPP are covalently attached via thioester linkage to C-terminal cysteine residues in the context of a prenylation motif. Farnesylation is catalyzed by farnesyl protein transferase (FTase), whereas GGTase-I and geranylgeranyl transferase type II (GGTase II) or RabGGTase catalyze the addition of GGPP to specific subsets of proteins [313-315] (Figure 5). FTase and GGTase I are responsible for posttranslational lipidation of proteins with C- terminal "CAAX" motifs, where C is cysteine, A is often an aliphatic amino acid, and X at the C-terminus determines the specificity of protein prenylation. When X is a methionine or serine, as in Ras proteins, then the protein is farnesylated by FTase. However, when X is a leucine residue, as in Rho proteins (e.g. Rac1, Cdc42, RhoA), or a phenylalanine residue, then the protein is geranylgeranylated by GGTase I [316, 317]. GGTase II catalyzes prenylation of Rab proteins, which contain at their C-termini either one or, more frequently, two cysteine residues, both of which are modified by geranylgeranyl groups [318, 319]. Protein prenyltransferase inhibitors, namely FTase inhibitors (FTIs) and GGTase inhibitors (GGTIs) have been developed and evaluated as anticancer agents.

The covalent attachment of the lipophilic isoprenyl group(s) enables prenylated proteins to anchor to cell membranes, which is an essential requirement for biological function [311]. The localization of small GTPases in distinct subcellular sites defines which signaling pathways they activate, thus defining their participation in disease. As an example, some singly prenylated Rabs are mistargeted and dysfunctional [320]. Inhibiting the membrane localization of small GTPases is a therapeutic strategy in cancer [321]. In addition, isoprenoid moieties are essential in the protein-protein interaction functions of prenylated proteins since they work as molecular handles that bind to hydrophobic grooves on the surface of soluble protein factors; these factors remove the prenylated protein from membranes in a regulated manner [322]. There is evidence that unprenylated versions of some proteins may also have physiological functional effects [323, 324] or may interfere with the activity of the isoprenylated proteins during disease [325, 326]. The requirement of prenylation for membrane association has also been recently challenged [327]. Prenylated proteins may undergo other posttranslational modifications such as palmitoylation, miristoylation and/or carboxymethylation [328].

The interest in understanding the regulation of isoprenoid production and protein prenylation in the brain has increased considerably in the past few years due to the importance of protein prenylation in several cellular processes such as cell growth, cytoskeletal organization and remodeling, and vesicle trafficking; and to the fact that some of the beneficial effects of statins in neurodegenerative diseases have been attributed to changes of protein prenylation [129, 329-334]. Non-sterol isoprenoids and protein prenyltransferases have emerged as attractive therapeutic targets for several diseases [321, 329] but we still need a deeper understanding of their roles in the brain in order to determine their value for treating neurodegeneration in general, and AD in particular.

Until recently, protein prenylation was considered to function constitutively. However, there is evidence that signaling cascades activated by druggable surface receptors affect prenylation of specific small GTPases by posttranslational modifications (e.g. phosphorylation) of unprenylated versions of the protein [326], or by regulating protein prenyltransferases directly [335]. Prenyltransferases are expressed in the brain, which contains the highest activity of GGTase I [336]. GGTase I plays important roles in synapse formation, where it is activated through acetylcholine receptor clustering at the postsynaptic membrane [335]. The effects of GGTase I at the synapse were suggested to be due to geranylgeranylation of Rho GTPases, although prenylation was not directly examined. Neuronal depolarization and BDNF activated GGTase I and this activity was required for dendritic arborization in hippocampal neurons and Purkinje cells [337-339].

There is a growing body of evidence indicating that inhibition of protein prenyltransferases and inhibition of the mevalonate pathway to an extent that reduces the levels of FPP and GGPP, alter many mechanisms critical for normal brain function. When analyzing studies in which statins are used it is important to consider that different statins differ in terms of their potency, stability and ability to cross the BBB [329, 331, 340]. Studies on the effect of statins or protein prenyl transferase inhibitors on neurite (dendrites or axons) extension and branching provided conflicting results depending on the type of neurons, the class of statin used and the duration of the treatments. Some studies showed that statins or inhibitors of protein prenyltransferases enhanced neurite outgrowth, number, length and/or branching [341-344] while we and others, discovered inhibition of neurite outgrowth, extension or branching [345-347]. Statins decreased neurite initiation but increased neurite branching in neuroblastoma cells [348]. The field of AD research will benefit from a deeper understanding of the roles of non-sterol isoprenoids and protein prenylation in axon regrowth.

Under certain experimental conditions statins affect survival of neurons and neuron-like cells, acting through the decrease of non-sterol isoprenoids and protein prenylation. Lovastatin but not pravastatin induced apoptosis of rat brain neuroblasts and caused a significant reduction of the membrane pool of Ras and RhoA proteins, suggesting an impairment of protein prenylation as the result of reduced isoprenoid production [349]. Similarly, we found no effect of pravastatin on survival of sympathetic and cortical neurons at concentrations that significantly reduced cholesterol synthesis [106, 347, 350]. Under these conditions, however, pravastatin did not affect protein prenylation [106]. Statins induced stellation, followed by apoptosis in cerebellar astrocytes and cell death of cerebellar neurons [351]. These latter effects were independent of reduced cholesterol synthesis but were prevented by GGPP. A very interesting discovery from the work of Marz and colleagues [351] was that neuronal cell death was significantly reduced in astrocyte/neuron co-cultures treated with statins. The authors speculated that astroglia cells might provide neuroprotective signals, perhaps GGPP, against the damaging effects that result from downregulation the mevalonate pathway. This idea of communication between glia and neurons through intermediates of the mevalonate pathway is further discussed in Section 4.

Non-sterol isoprenoids and protein prenylation may play a role in inflammatory events in the brain since statins were able to activate microglia in cultured rat hippocampal slices [352], and inhibitors of protein prenyltransferases and statins caused a reduction of apoE secretion by cultured microglia and organotypic hippocampal cultures [353]. Contradictory evidence was reported on the role of non-sterol isoprenoids and protein prenylation in long-term potentiation (LTP), an experimental model to study the synaptic basis of learning and memory [354]. While inhibitors of FTase and GGTase I had no effects on LTP in one study [355], FPP depletion and farnesylation inhibition were implicated in the enhancement of the LTP magnitude in hippocampal slices [356].

In the majority of the studies the conclusion that the effects of statins were due to the reduction of non-sterol isoprenoids and protein prenylation resulted from experiments in which FPP, GGPP or their correspondent alcohols, but not cholesterol were able to prevent the particular effect [343, 345, 346, 348, 352, 353, 357]. It will be important however, to confirm that protein prenylation is impaired upon statin treatment, especially when the duration of the treatment is short such as in the studies by Mans et al. [356]. Different prenylated proteins have half-lives that vary between 4hs and 24hs and will be differentially affected. The time required for depletion of the non-sterol isoprenoids pools may also be tissue-or cell-specific. Only a few studies examined the effect of statins on protein prenylation directly and found decreased prenylation of specific proteins under specific experimental conditions [341, 346].

The Rho family of GTPases has received a lot of attention as the mediators of the effects that result from reduction of non-sterol isoprenoids and/or inhibition of protein prenyl transferases [335, 337, 338, 341, 346, 352, 358]. This family represents a major branch of the Ras superfamily, and like Ras and Rabs, Rho proteins (e.g., RhoA, Rac1, Cdc42) function as GTP/GDP switches and alternate between an active GTP-bound state and an inactive GDP-bound state. Members of the Rho family are farnersylated and/or geranylgeranylated through the action of GGTase I [359]. Rho GTPases are pivotal in the integration of extracellular and intracellular signals. They are key regulators of the actin cytoskeleton which plays essential roles in orchestrating the development and remodeling of spines and synapses [360, 361]. Precise spatio-temporal regulation of Rho GTPase activity is critical for their function. Aberrant Rho GTPase signaling due to mutations or other causes can cause spine and synapse defects resulting in abnormal neuronal connectivity and deficient cognitive functioning in humans [360, 361]. Recent findings indicate that Rho GTPases are key components of neuronal cell degeneration pathways [362]. A number of studies examined the localization of Rho proteins to the membranes as an indication of their prenylation status. A caveat of this approach is that some prenylated Rho proteins interact with the guanidine dissociation inhibitor RhoGDI, which keep prenylated Rho proteins in the cytosol in an inactive state [363]. RhoGDI expression is affected during disease [363]. A decreased in RhoA or Rac association with membranes has been observed upon treatment with statins or protein prenyltransferase inhibitors [337, 338, 341, 346, 352]. A decrease in GTP-bound forms of Rho family proteins was also detected upon statin or protein prenyltransferase inhibitor treatments [338, 343] Moreover, RhoA was identified as a modulator of statins effects by using an unbiased genome-wide filter approach that examine more than 10,000 genes to identify gene expression changes that correlated with altered expression of HMGCR [364].

Non-sterol isoprenoids and protein prenylation not only determine the targeting of prenylated proteins to membranes, but also regulate the expression of a subset of prenylated proteins in a protein-specific manner [365, 366]. Depletion of mevalonate or treatment with protein prenyltransferase inhibitors resulted in up-regulation of Ras, Rac1, RhoB, Rab5 and Rab7 [365, 367-369]. The increase occurs at the levels of mRNA and protein in most cases, and both unprenylated and isoprenylated forms of the proteins accumulate [365]. Reduction of non-sterol isoprenoids decreases protein degradation, including that of already isoprenylated proteins, which suggests the existence of regulatory mechanisms to sustain levels of isoprenylated proteins under conditions that would otherwise limit protein isoprenylation [370]. FPP or GGPP prevented protein up-regulation [367, 370] by transcriptional and posttranscriptional mechanisms still unidentified but independent of protein prenylation [370]. In the case of Rab proteins it has been proposed that the membrane pool of Rabs, which decreases upon depletion of GGPP, may serve as an intracellular signal for Rab expression regulation [369].

### *3.4.2. Regulation of enzymes of non-sterol isoprenoids pathway*

FPPS is transcriptionally regulated by SREBP-2 [66, 371] and LXR [372]. A LXR response element sequence exists in the FPPS promoter overlapping with the SREBP-2 response element [372]. LXR activation of FPPS occurs under high cholesterol levels, thus SREBP-2 processing is inhibited. In this way LXR could drive the expression of FPPS in order to maintain isoprenoid supply exclusively [372]. FPPS is post-translationally regulated by a product-feedback competitive inhibition as FPP (product) competes with GPP (substrate) for the active site [373, 374].

GGPPS does not seem to be transcriptionally regulated by SREBP-2 [66, 284, 375, 376]. GGPPS activity is inhibited by GGPP [373]. The crystal structure of human GGPPS demonstrated GGPP binding to a pocket/cavity away from the chain elongation site (active site) of GGPPS, suggesting a product-feedback allosteric inhibition [377, 378]. Mammalian GGPPS can catalyze the formation of FPP as well as GGPP [379].

### *3.4.3. Coordination of the post-squalene and non-sterol isoprenoids branches of the mevalonate pathway*

Since cells have two alternative sources of cholesterol namely intracellular synthesis and uptake but only the intracellular synthesis provides non-sterol isoprenoids, the mevalonate pathway has to maintain the minimum requirement of isoprenoids at all times irrespective of cholesterol levels. Analysis of the affinity of the enzymes in the different branches of the pathway uncovers the mechanisms that mediate such regulation. The affinity of GGPPS for FPP ($K_m$ value of 0.6 μM) [284] is much higher than the affinity of squalene synthase for FPP (Km value of ~15 μM) [380]. Moreover, both coenzyme Q and dolichol synthesis are saturated at a much lower concentration of isoprene intermediates than the concentration required to saturate cholesterol synthesis [381, 382]. Thus, under limited concentrations of mevalonate and FPP, the non-sterol isoprenoid branch will be favored. Furthermore, inhibition of the mevalonate production by statins will reduce FPP supply for the production of cholesterol first. Because of the very high affinity of protein farnesyl transferase for FPP (Km below 0.1 μM) [383], farnesylation is preserved under many statin treatments [297, 384] and would be favored over geranylgeranylation.

### *3.4.4. Non-sterol isoprenoid pathway in AD*

Up-regulation of 6 out of 10 genes of isoprenoid metabolism was found in autopsied hippocampus of patients with incipient AD [105], which may represent an attempt to compensate the posttranslational inhibition of the mevalonate pathway during disease.

Dolichol is decreased in all areas of the AD brain, especially those regions affected by the disease, and dolichol-P increases in brain regions that showed morphological changes [239, 385]. In the frontal cortex and in the hippocampus the concentration of dolichol decreased by as much as 45%. The increase in dolichol-P may reflect an increased rate of glycosylation in AD brain, which may be related to the formation of amyloid plaques. Changes in dolichol and dolichol-P in AD are opposite to those present during normal aging. The amount of dolichol in different regions of the human brain, but especially in the hippocampus, increases several folds with age in humans [239, 292, 386] and rats [387, 388]. An upper limit for dolichol accumulation in tissues seems to exist since after 70 years of age there is no further increase in dolichol concentration in human brains [239]. Dolichol is present in the brain as a family with 17-21 isoprene units. This pattern of dolichol lengths is unchanged during aging; however, there are regional differences [239, 386]. Levels of dolichyl-P are already high at the time of birth and only show a moderate increase, although it varies between different brain regions [292, 386].

With respect to ubiquinone, there is a significant elevation in most regions of AD brain [239], which may reflect a futile attempt to protect the brain from oxidative stress [385]. Interestingly, the pattern of ubiquinone is also reversed in AD when compared with normal aging. Brain ubiquinone is unchanged up to the age of 55 but decreases significantly in older age groups in areas where it concentrates in human brains, mainly the nucleus caudatus, gray matter, and hippocampus [239, 386]. This decrease may indicate a reduced anti-oxidative capacity in the aging brain. Thus, when considering dolichol, dolichol-P and ubiquinone, AD cannot be regarded as a result of premature aging.

### 3.4.5. *FPP, GGPP and protein prenylation in AD*

There is limited information with respect to levels and regulation of FPP and GGPP in normal and AD brains. Recent studies showed that GGPP, FPP, and the mRNA of their respective synthases, FPPS and GGPPS, were elevated in brains of 13 male patients with AD [169], in brains of aged mice [129, 287] and in neuroblastoma SH-SY5Y cells expressing APP695 [389]. The significance of this elevation is still unknown because protein prenylation was not examined in these studies, and elevation of isoprenoids does not warrant an increase in protein prenylation. Indeed, even when GGPP levels were elevated in the aging mouse brain, the pools of Rac1, RhoA and Cdc42, associated to membranes were decreased, while Rab proteins had a mixed behavior [287]. The reduction of the subunit β of GGTase I in the aging brain may be responsible for the decreased prenylation.

The roles of non-sterol isoprenoids and protein prenylation in AD have been identified mainly by using statins and inhibitors of protein prenyltransferases. FPP, GGPP and prenylated proteins are involved in diverse processes important in AD pathology including APP metabolism, LTP and synaptic plasticity, Aβ toxicity, and oxidative stress.

The effects of statin-induced non-sterol isoprenoids depletion or inhibition of protein prenyltransferases on APP/Aβ metabolism are complex. In some cases treatment with statins or a FTase inhibitor stimulated the shedding of APP and the production of sAPPα in neuroblastoma cells overexpressing APPswe [390], while in other cases statins reduced the release of

Aβ from cells but increased the intracellular accumulation of APP and Aβ, in a process prevented by GGPP [391, 392]. The proteins affected by shortage of non-sterol isoprenoids, and responsible for the regulation APP/Aβ metabolism have been identified or proposed. The increase in APP shedding was mediated by RHO proteins [390]. Rho was also suggested to be responsible for the reduction of brain Aβ levels in the AD CRND8 mouse treated with statins, although there was no direct evidence that isoprenylation was affected [393]. The accumulation of APP and Aβ within neurons that received statins was due to decreased delivery of Rab proteins to cell membranes [392]. It is known that Rabs participate in intracellular APP trafficking and processing [394]. A study of mice treated with statins has shown significant reduction of brain levels of Aβ and the C-terminal fragments (CTFs) due to enhanced trafficking of APP-CTFs to the lysosomes for degradation [395]. The authors suggested that the process may involve a decrease in isoprenoids, and would be mediated by Rabs. However, Rab prenylation was not measured in this study and the conclusion of the involvement of isoprenoids resulted from experiments in cultured neurons in which mevalonate prevented the changes in trafficking. Unless the concentration of mevalonate is titrated to recover specifically the non-sterol isoprenoid pathway, mevalonate would also affect cholesterol levels. The regulation of APP cleavage and Aβ production by non-sterol isoprenoids and protein prenylation also involved APP secretases, although it is unclear if the decrease or the increase in isoprenoids and protein prenylation favors amyloidogenic processing of APP. Inhibition of farnesylation reduced the association of the β-secretase enzyme BACE1 with APP (although BACE itself is not farnesylated) and resulted in a dose-dependent decrease in Aβ release and production within the cell [396]. Moreover, statins caused inhibition of β-secretase dimerization into its more active form, which may be a mechanism of the reduction in Aβ production [397]. Statins also significantly decreased the association of the γ-secretase complex with lipid rafts and GGOH prevented this [398]. Contrary to this notion, in a separate study statins induced an increase of BACE levels in neurons, which was linked to the increase in Aβ production [391]. GGOH, GGPP and FPP increased Aβ production by targeting γ-secretase [399-401] but there is no consensus if this effect is dependent [401] or independent [400] of protein prenylation.

Aβ production is not significantly altered in sporadic forms of AD, which represent approximately 95% of cases [402-404]. Instead, defects in Aβ removal may be key in the development of sporadic AD [405, 406]. Statins and an FTase inhibitor promoted degradation of extracellular Aβ by microglia by stimulating the secretion of IDE (insulin degrading enzyme), an enzyme that degrades Aβ in the brain [407]. The secretion of IDE from peripheral organs into the circulation was also increased in mice treated with statins [407]. Moreover FTase but not GGTase I haplodeficiency in the APPPS1 mice increased steady-state levels of IDE [408]. The mechanisms by which farnesylation may regulate IDE secretion, are still unclear.

We have discovered that in neurons challenged with oligomeric $A\beta_{42}$, and in the cortex of the AD mouse CRND8, prenylation of Rabs and Ras proteins were reduced [106]. Since the deficit in protein prenylation induced by Aβ was prevented by GGPP we concluded that protein prenylation inhibition was due to a shortage of GGPP. More importantly GGPP was able to prevent Aβ-induced neuronal death.

Non-sterol isoprenoids have been associated with the regulation of neuroinflammation in AD. The role of inflammation in the AD brain is well known. The pro-inflammatory response mediated mainly by microglial may exacerbate and drive the pathogenic processes leading to neuronal loss. Microglia activation may occur as a response to Aβ accumulation in the brain. Statins inhibited the production of IL-1β by monocytes after stimulation with Aβ, in a process that is independent of cholesterol but prevented by GGPP [409]. The effect was mimicked by a GGTase I inhibitor and by inactivation of Rho proteins. Statins also induced cholesterol-independent inhibition of ROS production after stimulation with Aβ [409]. Statin treatment of microglia resulted in perturbation of the cytoskeleton and morphological changes due to alteration in Rho family function [410].

During the course of AD, tau is hyper-phosphorylated, detaches from the microtubules, and aggregates in the somatodendritic compartment in NFTs [411, 412]. There is very limited information about the existence of any relationship between tau pathology and isoprenoids and/or protein prenylation. Statins caused changes in tau phosphorylation that were characteristic of those observed in preclinical stages of AD [413]. These changes were mimicked by GGTase I inhibitors and compensated by GGPP suggesting that decreased prenylation of a Rho family member may be involved. The dose of statins seems to be critical in the effects on tau. In a cellular model of tauopathy, and in primary neurons, low-to-moderate doses of statins, reduced total and phosphorylated tau levels but high doses activated caspase 3 and increased levels of caspase-cleaved tau, which may facilitate tau Aβ toxicity/apoptosis [414]. A decrease in membrane localization of several small GTPases occurred concomitantly with tau reduction and GGPP reversed statin-induced decreases in tau levels. The authors focused their attention on RhoA, speculating that the statin-induced decrease in phosphorylated tau was caused by glycogen synthase kinase 3β (GSK3β) inactivation through RhoA [414].

Some recent work in genetically modified mice supported the concept that non-sterol isoprenoids and protein prenylation may have a detrimental role in AD and suggested that inhibition of protein prenylation could be a potential strategy for effectively treating AD. The increase of isoprenoids and protein prenylation has been suggested (although not tested) to contribute to tau pathology in a transgenic APP/PS1 mouse that constitutively overexpresses (P)SREBP-2 [415]. In a different mouse model the expression of protein prenyltransferases was genetically modified in order to reduce protein prenylation independent of non-sterol isoprenoids. Heterozygous deletion of FTase reduced Aβ deposition and neuroinflammation and rescued spatial learning and memory function in APPPS1 mice. Heterozygous deletion of GGTase I reduced the levels of Aβ and neuroinflammation but had no impact on learning and memory [408]. These studies in vivo are exciting but will benefit from direct measurement of brain levels of isoprenoids or protein prenylation. Based on the complex regulation of isoprenoid production, it will be important to determine if brain isoprenoid levels change in these mice since the existence of negative-feedback regulatory mechanisms downstream SREBP-2, argue that increased levels of active SREBP-2 does not warrant an increase in non-sterol isoprenoids.

A few prenylated proteins have been linked to AD. The contributions of Rho GTPases to AD are of particular interest. Rho-family GTPases are key proteins that integrate extracellular and intracellular signals. They are important regulators of the actin cytoskeleton that play essential roles in orchestrating the development and remodeling of spines and synapses [360, 361]. Precise spatio-temporal regulation of Rho GTPase activity is critical for their function. Aberrant Rho GTPase signaling due to mutations or other causes can cause spine and synapse defects resulting in abnormal neuronal connectivity and deficient cognitive functioning in humans [360, 361]. Deregulation of RhoGTPases may contribute to dendritic spine loss during AD and might be a key pathogenic event contributing to synaptic deficits in AD (reviewed in [362, 416]). RhoA protein was lower in the AD brain hippocampus, reflecting the loss of the membrane bound, presumably active, GTPase [417]. Rab proteins regulate intracellular membrane trafficking, motility and fusion [418]. In the nervous system Rabs participate in important processes such as axonal endocytosis, retrograde transport of growth signals, synaptic function, and polarized neurite growth [419]. Rab5 and Rab7 protein levels were upregulated within basal forebrain, frontal cortex, and hippocampus but not in the less vulnerable cerebellum and striatum in MCI and AD [420, 421]. Importantly, this upregulation correlated with cognitive decline and neuropathological criteria for AD. The increase of Rab7 and Rab5 in AD brains has been interpreted as overactivation of the endosomal pathway. In addition increased levels of Rab7 have been found in cerebrospinal fluid (CSF) from AD patients and may represent a novel AD CSF biomarker [422]. Evidence from our laboratory demonstrated increased levels of Rab7 in Aβ-treated neurons and in the cortex of CRND8 mice [107]. Rab-6 was increased in AD brain, and correlated with ER stress [423]. The increased level of Rab6 in AD was unable to protect against ER stress, suggesting that Rab6 is non-functional. Based on our discoveries, we anticipate that Rab6 prenylation may be decreased. Since the number of proteins that are prenylated is high and considering that a reduction of non-sterol isoprenoids or the inhibition of protein prenyltransferases will affect several prenylated proteins, the challenge in the next years will be to identify which prenylated proteins are affected in AD.

## 4. Conclusions

The analysis of the mevalonate pathway in AD reveals dysregulation. The abnormalities not only affect cholesterol but also non-sterol isoprenoids. There is a reciprocal regulation between Aβ and cholesterol at the subcellular level [11]. The evidence discussed here suggest that similar reciprocity may exist between Aβ and non-sterol isoprenoids such that isoprenylation determines the levels of intracellular Aβ [391, 392] and Aβ inhibits the mevalonate pathway causing reduction of non-sterol isoprenoid levels and protein prenylation [106]. The dysregulation of the mevalonate pathway in AD may affect neurons and glia in different ways. Our findings suggest that inhibition of the mevalonate pathway will take place specifically in cells that accumulate Aβ, most likely neurons. Depending on the size of the cell population that contains intracellular Aβ, this might or might not impact the overall content of cholesterol and isoprenoids in the brain. The decreased synthesis of cholesterol in neurons may be compensated by synthesis in astrocytes [21]. In addition, an interesting model has been proposed in which SREBPs in astrocytes would be involved in synthesis of fatty acids and perhaps other lipids for neuronal supply [424]. According to this model, glia SREBPs may work as control points of neuronal function, providing neurons with appropriate lipids when neurons cannot

http://dx.doi.org/10.5772/59904

make their own. The shuttle of non-sterol isoprenoids and 25-EC from astrocytes to neurons has been suggested [206, 351]. These possible homeostatic mechanisms should be taken in consideration when brain levels of lipids are analyzed. The increase of non-sterol isoprenoids in AD brains, if confirmed in a larger cohort, may represent an astrocytic attempt to compensate for the decrease in SREBP-dependent metabolic pathways in neurons. Compensatory attempt mechanisms in brain cholesterol homeostasis in AD have been described before. The amount of CYP46, the enzyme that converts cholesterol into 24-HC decreases in neuronal cells in AD brains, but this decrease is at least in part compensated for by an induction of the enzyme in glial cells [425]. In conclusion, our knowledge on the impairment of the mevalonate pathway in AD is still very limited. The extremely complex regulation of this pathway represents a challenge for the complete understanding of the defects present during AD. Defects at the cellular level are important but ultimately we need to comprehend how the interaction neuron-glia regulates the mevalonate pathway in the brain.

## 5. Abreviations

**24-HC**: 24(S)-hydroxycholesterol; **25-HC**: 24(S),25-epoxycholesterol; **7-DHC**: 7-dehydrocholesterol; **ABC**: adenosine triphosphate-binding cassette transporter; **ACAT**: acyl coA-cholesterol acyltransferase; **AD**: Alzheimer's disease; **AMPK**: adenosine monophosphate-activated protein kinase; **apoE4**: apolipoprotein E ε4; **Aβ**: amyloid-beta peptide; **BACE-1**: beta-site APP cleaving enzyme 1; **BBB**: blood-brain-barrier; **CNS**: central nervous system; **CoA**: coenzyme A; **CSF**: cerebrospinal fluid; **CYP46A1**: 24-hydroxylase; **DHCR24**: 24-dehydrocholesterol reductase; **DMPP**: dimethylallyl pyrophosphate; **DOS**: dioxidosqualene; **FOH**: farnesol; **FPP**: farnesyl pyrophosphate; **FPPS**: FPP synthase; **FTase**: farnesyl protein transferase; **GDP**: guanosine diphosphate; **GGOH**: geranylgeraniol; **GGPP**: geranylgeranyl pyrophosphate; **GGPPS**: GGPP synthase; **GGTase-I**: geranylgeranyl transferase type I; **GPP**: geranyl pyrophosphate; **HMG**: 3-hydroxy-3-methylglutaryl-CoA; **IDE**: insulin degrading enzyme; **Insig**: insulin-induced gene; **IPP**: isopentenylpyrophosphate; **LTP**: long-term potentiation; **LXR**: liver-X-receptor; **MCI**: mild cognitive impairment; **MK**: mevalonate kinase; **MOS**: monooxidosqualene; **NFT**: neurofibrillary tangle; **NPC**: Niemann-Pick type C; **REST**: RE1-silencing transcription factor; **SCAP**: SREBP-cleavage activating protein; **SR**EBP: sterol-regulatory element binding protein; TRP: transient receptor potential

## Author details

Amany Mohamed[1,2], Kevan Smith[1,2] and Elena Posse de Chaves[1,2*]

*Address all correspondence to: elena.chaves@ualberta.ca

1 Department of Pharmacology, University of Alberta, Edmonton, AB, Canada

2 Neuroscience and Mental Health Institute, University of Alberta, Edmonton, AB, Canada

## References


[1] O'Brien, J.S. and E.L. Sampson, *Lipid composition of the normal human brain: gray matter, white matter, and myelin.* J Lipid Res, 1965. 6(4): p. 537-44.

[2] Dietschy, J.M. and S.D. Turley, *Thematic review series: brain Lipids. Cholesterol metabolism in the central nervous system during early development and in the mature animal.* J Lipid Res, 2004. 45(8): p. 1375-97.

[3] Dietschy, J.M., *Central nervous system: cholesterol turnover, brain development and neurodegeneration.* Biol Chem, 2009. 390(4): p. 287-93.

[4] Corder, E.H., et al., *Gene dose of apolipoprotein E type 4 allele and the risk of Alzheimer's disease in late onset families.* Science, 1993. 261(5123): p. 921-3.

[5] Martins, I.J., et al., *Cholesterol metabolism and transport in the pathogenesis of Alzheimer's disease.* J Neurochem, 2009. 111(6): p. 1275-308.

[6] Carter, C.J., *Convergence of genes implicated in Alzheimer's disease on the cerebral cholesterol shuttle: APP, cholesterol, lipoproteins, and atherosclerosis.* Neurochemistry international, 2007. 50(1): p. 12-38.

[7] Wollmer, M.A., *Cholesterol-related genes in Alzheimer's disease.* Biochim Biophys Acta, 2010. 1801(8): p. 762-73.

[8] Wollmer, M.A., et al., *Association study of cholesterol-related genes in Alzheimer's disease.* Neurogenetics, 2007. 8(3): p. 179-88.

[9] Bertram, L., C.M. Lill, and R.E. Tanzi, *The genetics of Alzheimer disease: back to the future.* Neuron, 2010. 68(2): p. 270-81.

[10] Di Paolo, G. and T.W. Kim, *Linking lipids to Alzheimer's disease: cholesterol and beyond.* Nat Rev Neurosci, 2011. 12(5): p. 284-96.

[11] Posse de Chaves, E., *Reciprocal regulation of cholesterol and beta amyloid at the subcellular level in Alzheimer's disease.* Can J Physiol Pharmacol, 2012. 90(6): p. 753-64.

[12] Maulik, M., et al., *Role of cholesterol in APP metabolism and its significance in Alzheimer's disease pathogenesis.* Mol Neurobiol, 2013. 47(1): p. 37-63.

[13] Jick, H., et al., *Statins and the risk of dementia.* Lancet, 2000. 356(9242): p. 1627-31.

[14] Wolozin, B., et al., *Decreased prevalence of Alzheimer disease associated with 3-hydroxy-3-methyglutaryl coenzyme A reductase inhibitors.* Arch Neurol, 2000. 57(10): p. 1439-43.

[15] Arvanitakis, Z. and D.S. Knopman, *Clinical trial efforts in Alzheimer disease: why test statins?* Neurology, 2010. 74(12): p. 945-6.

[16] Rea, T.D., et al., *Statin use and the risk of incident dementia: the Cardiovascular Health Study.* Arch Neurol, 2005. 62(7): p. 1047-51.

[17] Kandiah, N. and H.H. Feldman, *Therapeutic potential of statins in Alzheimer's disease.* J Neurol Sci, 2009. 283(1-2): p. 230-4.

[18] Shepardson, N.E., G.M. Shankar, and D.J. Selkoe, *Cholesterol level and statin use in Alzheimer disease: I. Review of epidemiological and preclinical studies.* Archives of neurology, 2011. 68(10): p. 1239-44.

[19] Shepardson, N.E., G.M. Shankar, and D.J. Selkoe, *Cholesterol level and statin use in Alzheimer disease: II. Review of human trials and recommendations.* Arch Neurol, 2011. 68(11): p. 1385-92.

[20] Jones, L., et al., *Genetic evidence implicates the immune system and cholesterol metabolism in the aetiology of Alzheimer's disease.* PloS one, 2010. 5(11): p. e13950.

[21] Pfrieger, F.W. and N. Ungerer, *Cholesterol metabolism in neurons and astrocytes.* Progress in lipid research, 2011. 50(4): p. 357-371.

[22] Thelen, K.M., et al., *Cholesterol synthesis rate in human hippocampus declines with aging.* Neurosci Lett, 2006. 403(1-2): p. 15-9.

[23] Waterham, H.R., *Defects of cholesterol biosynthesis.* FEBS letters, 2006. 580(23): p. 5442-9.

[24] Bjorkhem, I., V. Leoni, and S. Meaney, *Genetic connections between neurological disorders and cholesterol metabolism.* Journal of lipid research, 2010. 51(9): p. 2489-503.

[25] Nieweg, K., H. Schaller, and F.W. Pfrieger, *Marked differences in cholesterol synthesis between neurons and glial cells from postnatal rats.* J Neurochem, 2009. 109(1): p. 125-34.

[26] Ullian, E.M., K.S. Christopherson, and B.A. Barres, *Role for glia in synaptogenesis.* Glia, 2004. 47(3): p. 209-16.

[27] Mauch, D.H., et al., *CNS synaptogenesis promoted by glia-derived cholesterol.* Science, 2001. 294(5545): p. 1354-7.

[28] Funfschilling, U., et al., *Survival of adult neurons lacking cholesterol synthesis in vivo.* BMC Neurosci, 2007. 8: p. 1.

[29] Valdez, C.M., et al., *Cholesterol homeostasis markers are localized to mouse hippocampal pyramidal and granule layers.* Hippocampus, 2010.

[30] Wahrle, S.E., et al., *ABCA1 is required for normal central nervous system ApoE levels and for lipidation of astrocyte-secreted apoE.* The Journal of Biological Chemistry, 2004. 279(39): p. 40987-93.

[31] Holtzman, D.M., J. Herz, and G. Bu, *Apolipoprotein E and apolipoprotein E receptors: normal biology and roles in Alzheimer disease.* Cold Spring Harb Perspect Med, 2012. 2(3): p. a006312.

[32] Pitas, R.E., et al., *Lipoproteins and their receptors in the central nervous system. Characterization of the lipoproteins in cerebrospinal fluid and identification of apolipoprotein B,E(LDL) receptors in the brain.* J Biol Chem, 1987. 262(29): p. 14352-60.

[33] LaDu, M.J., et al., *Nascent astrocyte particles differ from lipoproteins in CSF.* J Neurochem, 1998. 70(5): p. 2070-81.

[34] Bjorkhem, I. and S. Meaney, *Brain cholesterol: long secret life behind a barrier.* Arterioscler Thromb Vasc Biol, 2004. 24(5): p. 806-15.

[35] Lutjohann, D., et al., *Cholesterol homeostasis in human brain: evidence for an age-dependent flux of 24S-hydroxycholesterol from the brain into the circulation.* Proc Natl Acad Sci U S A, 1996. 93(18): p. 9799-804.

[36] Lund, E.G., J.M. Guileyardo, and D.W. Russell, *cDNA cloning of cholesterol 24-hydroxylase, a mediator of cholesterol homeostasis in the brain.* Proc Natl Acad Sci U S A, 1999. 96(13): p. 7238-43.

[37] Ramirez, D.M., S. Andersson, and D.W. Russell, *Neuronal expression and subcellular localization of cholesterol 24-hydroxylase in the mouse brain.* J Comp Neurol, 2008. 507(5): p. 1676-93.

[38] Abildayeva, K., et al., *24(S)-hydroxycholesterol participates in a liver X receptor-controlled pathway in astrocytes that regulates apolipoprotein E-mediated cholesterol efflux.* J Biol Chem, 2006. 281(18): p. 12799-808.

[39] Buhman, K.F., M. Accad, and R.V. Farese, *Mammalian acyl-CoA:cholesterol acyltransferases.* Biochim Biophys Acta, 2000. 1529(1-3): p. 142-54.

[40] Johnson, R.C. and S.N. Shah, *Cholesterol ester metabolizing enzymes in human brain: properties, subcellular distribution and relative levels in various diseased conditions.* J Neurochem, 1978. 31(4): p. 895-902.

[41] Bryleva, E.Y., et al., *ACAT1 gene ablation increases 24(S)-hydroxycholesterol content in the brain and ameliorates amyloid pathology in mice with AD.* Proc Natl Acad Sci U S A, 2010. 107(7): p. 3081-6.

[42] Huttunen, H.J. and D.M. Kovacs, *ACAT as a drug target for Alzheimer's disease.* Neurodegener Dis, 2008. 5(3-4): p. 212-4.

[43] Rubinsztein, D.C. and D.F. Easton, *Apolipoprotein E genetic variation and Alzheimer's disease. a meta-analysis.* Dement Geriatr Cogn Disord, 1999. 10(3): p. 199-209.

[44] Harold, D., et al., *Genome-wide association study identifies variants at CLU and PICALM associated with Alzheimer's disease.* Nat Genet, 2009. 41(10): p. 1088-93.

[45] Katzov, H., et al., *Genetic variants of ABCA1 modify Alzheimer disease risk and quantitative traits related to beta-amyloid metabolism.* Hum Mutat, 2004. 23(4): p. 358-67.

[46] Sundar, P.D., et al., *Gender-specific association of ATP-binding cassette transporter I (ABCA1) polymorphisms with the risk of late-onset Alzheimer's disease.* Neurobiology of Aging, 2007. 28(6): p. 856-862.

[47] Li, Y.H., et al., *Association of ABCA1 with late-onset Alzheimer's disease is not observed in a case-control study.* Neuroscience Letters, 2004. 366(3): p. 268-271.

[48] Wollmer, M.A., et al., *ABCA1 modulates CSF cholesterol levels and influences the age at onset of Alzheimer's disease.* Neurobiology of aging, 2003. 24(3): p. 421-6.

[49] Kolsch, H., et al., *Polymorphism in the cholesterol 24S-hydroxylase gene is associated with Alzheimer's disease.* Molecular Psychiatry, 2002. 7(8): p. 899-902.

[50] Desai, P., S.T. DeKosky, and M.I. Kamboh, *Genetic variation in the cholesterol 24-hydroxylase (CYP46) gene and the risk of Alzheimer's disease.* Neuroscience letters, 2002. 328(1): p. 9-12.

[51] Papassotiropoulos, A., et al., *Increased brain beta-amyloid load, phosphorylated tau, and risk of Alzheimer disease associated with an intronic CYP46 polymorphism.* Arch Neurol, 2003. 60(1): p. 29-35.

[52] Johansson, A., et al., *Variants of CYP46A1 may interact with age and APOE to influence CSF A beta 42 levels in Alzheimer's disease.* Human Genetics, 2004. 114(6): p. 581-587.

[53] Kolsch, H., et al., *Association of the C766T polymorphism of the low-density lipoprotein receptor-related protein gene with Alzheimer's disease.* Am J Med Genet B Neuropsychiatr Genet, 2003. 121B(1): p. 128-30.

[54] Causevic, M., et al., *Lack of association between the levels of the low-density lipoprotein receptor-related protein (LRP) and either Alzheimer dementia or LRP exon 3 genotype.* Journal of Neuropathology and Experimental Neurology, 2003. 62(10): p. 999-1005.

[55] Lendon, C.L., et al., *Genetic association studies between dementia of the Alzheimer's type and three receptors for apolipoprotein E in a Caucasian population.* Neuroscience Letters, 1997. 222(3): p. 187-190.

[56] Wollmer, M.A., et al., *Genetic association of acyl-coenzyme A: cholesterol acyltransferase with cerebrospinal fluid cholesterol levels, brain amyloid load, and risk for Alzheimer's disease.* Molecular psychiatry, 2003. 8(6): p. 635-8.

[57] Bloch, K., *The biological synthesis of cholesterol.* Science, 1965. 150(3692): p. 19-28.

[58] Panda, T., et al., *Kinetic Mechanisms of Cholesterol Synthesis: A Review.* Industrial & Engineering Chemistry Research, 2011. 50(23): p. 12847-12864.

[59] Miziorko, H.M., *Enzymes of the mevalonate pathway of isoprenoid biosynthesis.* Arch Biochem Biophys, 2011. 505(2): p. 131-43.

[60] Korade, Z., et al., *Expression and p75 neurotrophin receptor dependence of cholesterol synthetic enzymes in adult mouse brain.* Neurobiology of aging, 2007. 28(10): p. 1522-31.

[61] Levin, M.S., et al., *Developmental changes in the expression of genes involved in cholesterol biosynthesis and lipid transport in human and rat fetal and neonatal livers.* Biochim Biophys Acta, 1989. 1003(3): p. 293-300.

[62] Ness, G.C., *Developmental regulation of the expression of genes encoding proteins involved in cholesterol homeostasis.* Am J Med Genet, 1994. 50(4): p. 355-7.

[63] Kanungo, S., et al., *Sterol metabolism disorders and neurodevelopment-an update.* Dev Disabil Res Rev, 2013. 17(3): p. 197-210.

[64] Cedazo-Minguez, A., M.A. Ismail, and L. Mateos, *Plasma cholesterol and risk for late-onset Alzheimer's disease.* Expert review of neurotherapeutics, 2011. 11(4): p. 495-8.

[65] Rockwood, K., *Epidemiological and clinical trials evidence about a preventive role for statins in Alzheimer's disease.* Acta Neurol Scand Suppl, 2006. 185: p. 71-7.

[66] Horton, J.D., J.L. Goldstein, and M.S. Brown, *SREBPs: activators of the complete program of cholesterol and fatty acid synthesis in the liver.* The Journal of clinical investigation, 2002. 109(9): p. 1125-31.

[67] Horton, J.D., et al., *Combined analysis of oligonucleotide microarray data from transgenic and knockout mice identifies direct SREBP target genes.* Proceedings of the National Academy of Sciences of the United States of America, 2003. 100(21): p. 12027-32.

[68] Brown, M.S. and J.L. Goldstein, *The SREBP pathway: regulation of cholesterol metabolism by proteolysis of a membrane-bound transcription factor.* Cell, 1997. 89(3): p. 331-40.

[69] Rawson, R.B., *Control of lipid metabolism by regulated intramembrane proteolysis of sterol regulatory element binding proteins (SREBPs).* Biochem Soc Symp, 2003(70): p. 221-31.

[70] Horton, A.C. and M.D. Ehlers, *Dual modes of endoplasmic reticulum-to-Golgi transport in dendrites revealed by live-cell imaging.* J Neurosci, 2003. 23(15): p. 6188-99.

[71] Suzuki, R., et al., *Reduction of the cholesterol sensor SCAP in the brains of mice causes impaired synaptic transmission and altered cognitive function.* PLoS Biol, 2013. 11(4): p. e1001532.

[72] Espenshade, P.J., et al., *Autocatalytic processing of site-1 protease removes propeptide and permits cleavage of sterol regulatory element-binding proteins.* J Biol Chem, 1999. 274(32): p. 22795-804.

[73] Zelenski, N.G., et al., *Membrane topology of S2P, a protein required for intramembranous cleavage of sterol regulatory element-binding proteins.* J Biol Chem, 1999. 274(31): p. 21973-80.

[74] McPherson, R. and A. Gauthier, *Molecular regulation of SREBP function: the Insig-SCAP connection and isoform-specific modulation of lipid synthesis.* Biochem Cell Biol, 2004. 82(1): p. 201-11.

[75] Inoue, J., R. Sato, and M. Maeda, *Multiple DNA elements for sterol regulatory element-binding protein and NF-Y are responsible for sterol-regulated transcription of the genes for*

*human 3-hydroxy-3-methylglutaryl coenzyme A synthase and squalene synthase.* J Biochem, 1998. 123(6): p. 1191-8.

[76] Yieh, L., H.B. Sanchez, and T.F. Osborne, *Domains of transcription factor Sp1 required for synergistic activation with sterol regulatory element binding protein 1 of low density lipoprotein receptor promoter.* Proc Natl Acad Sci U S A, 1995. 92(13): p. 6102-6.

[77] Zerenturk, E.J., L.J. Sharpe, and A.J. Brown, *Sterols regulate 3beta-hydroxysterol Delta24-reductase (DHCR24) via dual sterol regulatory elements: cooperative induction of key enzymes in lipid synthesis by Sterol Regulatory Element Binding Proteins.* Biochim Biophys Acta, 2012. 1821(10): p. 1350-60.

[78] Horie, T., et al., *MicroRNA-33 encoded by an intron of sterol regulatory element-binding protein 2 (Srebp2) regulates HDL in vivo.* Proceedings of the National Academy of Sciences of the United States of America, 2010. 107(40): p. 17321-6.

[79] Gerin, I., et al., *Expression of miR-33 from an SREBP2 intron inhibits cholesterol export and fatty acid oxidation.* The Journal of Biological Chemistry, 2010. 285(44): p. 33652-61.

[80] Najafi-Shoushtari, S.H., et al., *MicroRNA-33 and the SREBP host genes cooperate to control cholesterol homeostasis.* Science, 2010. 328(5985): p. 1566-9.

[81] Marquart, T.J., et al., *miR-33 links SREBP-2 induction to repression of sterol transporters.* Proceedings of the National Academy of Sciences of the United States of America, 2010. 107(27): p. 12228-32.

[82] Rayner, K.J., et al., *MiR-33 contributes to the regulation of cholesterol homeostasis.* Science, 2010. 328(5985): p. 1570-3.

[83] Bommer, G.T. and O.A. MacDougald, *Regulation of lipid homeostasis by the bifunctional SREBF2-miR33a locus.* Cell metabolism, 2011. 13(3): p. 241-7.

[84] Adlakha, Y.K., et al., *Pro-apoptotic miRNA-128-2 modulates ABCA1, ABCG1 and RXRalpha expression and cholesterol homeostasis.* Cell Death Dis, 2013. 4: p. e780.

[85] Kim, J.H. and W.Y. Ong, *Localization of the transcription factor, sterol regulatory element binding protein-2 (SREBP-2) in the normal rat brain and changes after kainate-induced excitotoxic injury.* J Chem Neuroanat, 2009. 37(2): p. 71-7.

[86] Radhakrishnan, A., et al., *Switch-like control of SREBP-2 transport triggered by small changes in ER cholesterol: a delicate balance.* Cell Metab, 2008. 8(6): p. 512-21.

[87] Brown, A.J., et al., *Cholesterol addition to ER membranes alters conformation of SCAP, the SREBP escort protein that regulates cholesterol metabolism.* Mol Cell, 2002. 10(2): p. 237-45.

[88] Radhakrishnan, A., et al., *Direct binding of cholesterol to the purified membrane region of SCAP: mechanism for a sterol-sensing domain.* Mol Cell, 2004. 15(2): p. 259-68.

[89] Yang, T., et al., *Crucial step in cholesterol homeostasis: sterols promote binding of SCAP to INSIG-1, a membrane protein that facilitates retention of SREBPs in ER.* Cell, 2002. 110(4): p. 489-500.

[90] Rodriguez-Acebes, S., et al., *Desmosterol can replace cholesterol in sustaining cell proliferation and regulating the SREBP pathway in a sterol-Delta24-reductase-deficient cell line.* Biochem J, 2009. 420(2): p. 305-15.

[91] Song, B.L., N.B. Javitt, and R.A. DeBose-Boyd, *Insig-mediated degradation of HMG CoA reductase stimulated by lanosterol, an intermediate in the synthesis of cholesterol.* Cell Metab, 2005. 1(3): p. 179-89.

[92] Radhakrishnan, A., et al., *Sterol-regulated transport of SREBPs from endoplasmic reticulum to Golgi: oxysterols block transport by binding to Insig.* Proc Natl Acad Sci U S A, 2007. 104(16): p. 6511-8.

[93] Sato, R., et al., *Sterol-dependent transcriptional regulation of sterol regulatory element-binding protein-2.* J Biol Chem, 1996. 271(43): p. 26461-4.

[94] Jeon, T.I., et al., *An SREBP-responsive microRNA operon contributes to a regulatory loop for intracellular lipid homeostasis.* Cell Metab, 2013. 18(1): p. 51-61.

[95] Hu, Y.W., L. Zheng, and Q. Wang, *Regulation of cholesterol homeostasis by liver X receptors.* Clin Chim Acta, 2010. 411(9-10): p. 617-25.

[96] Beaven, S.W. and P. Tontonoz, *Nuclear receptors in lipid metabolism: targeting the heart of dyslipidemia.* Annual review of medicine, 2006. 57: p. 313-29.

[97] Jakobsson, T., et al., *Liver X receptor biology and pharmacology: new pathways, challenges and opportunities.* Trends Pharmacol Sci, 2012. 33(7): p. 394-404.

[98] Whitney, K.D., et al., *Regulation of cholesterol homeostasis by the liver X receptors in the central nervous system.* Mol Endocrinol, 2002. 16(6): p. 1378-85.

[99] Wong, J., C.M. Quinn, and A.J. Brown, *SREBP-2 positively regulates transcription of the cholesterol efflux gene, ABCA1, by generating oxysterol ligands for LXR.* Biochem J, 2006. 400(3): p. 485-91.

[100] Eckert, G.P., et al., *Regulation of central nervous system cholesterol homeostasis by the liver X receptor agonist TO-901317.* Neurosci Lett, 2007. 423(1): p. 47-52.

[101] Zelcer, N., et al., *LXR regulates cholesterol uptake through Idol-dependent ubiquitination of the LDL receptor.* Science, 2009. 325(5936): p. 100-4.

[102] Wang, Y., et al., *Regulation of cholesterologenesis by the oxysterol receptor, LXRalpha.* J Biol Chem, 2008. 283(39): p. 26332-9.

[103] Wang, L., et al., *Liver X receptors in the central nervous system: from lipid homeostasis to neuronal degeneration.* Proc Natl Acad Sci U S A, 2002. 99(21): p. 13878-83.

[104] Xiong, H., et al., *Cholesterol retention in Alzheimer's brain is responsible for high beta- and gamma-secretase activities and Abeta production.* Neurobiol Dis, 2008. 29(3): p. 422-37.

[105] Blalock, E.M., et al., *Incipient Alzheimer's disease: microarray correlation analyses reveal major transcriptional and tumor suppressor responses.* Proc Natl Acad Sci U S A, 2004. 101(7): p. 2173-8.

[106] Mohamed, A., et al., *beta-amyloid inhibits protein prenylation and induces cholesterol sequestration by impairing SREBP-2 cleavage.* J Neurosci, 2012. 32(19): p. 6490-500.

[107] Mohamed, A.a.P.d.C., EI, *Abeta Inhibits SREBP-2 Cleavage by Reducing Cellular Levels of Activated Akt* The 11th International Conference on Alzheimer's and Parkinson's Diseases, 2013- Florence, Italy, March 6-10.

[108] Pierrot, N., et al., *Amyloid precursor protein controls cholesterol turnover needed for neuronal activity.* EMBO Mol Med, 2013. 5(4): p. 608-25.

[109] Ferguson, J.J., I.F. Durr, and H. Rudney, *The Biosynthesis of Mevalonic Acid.* Proc Natl Acad Sci U S A, 1959. 45(4): p. 499-504.

[110] Rodwell, V.W., J.L. Nordstrom, and J.J. Mitschelen, *Regulation of HMG-CoA reductase.* Adv Lipid Res, 1976. 14: p. 1-74.

[111] Goldstein, J.L. and M.S. Brown, *Regulation of the mevalonate pathway.* Nature, 1990. 343(6257): p. 425-30.

[112] Simmons, C.R., et al., *Evaluation of the global association between cholesterol-associated polymorphisms and Alzheimer's disease suggests a role for rs3846662 and HMGCR splicing in disease risk.* Molecular neurodegeneration, 2011. 6: p. 62.

[113] Kovacs, W.J., et al., *Purification of brain peroxisomes and localization of 3-hydroxy-3-methylglutaryl coenzyme A reductase.* Eur J Biochem, 2001. 268(18): p. 4850-9.

[114] Horvat, S., J. McWhir, and D. Rozman, *Defects in cholesterol synthesis genes in mouse and in humans: lessons for drug development and safer treatments.* Drug Metab Rev, 2011. 43(1): p. 69-90.

[115] Tchen, T.T., *Mevalonic kinase: purification and properties.* J Biol Chem, 1958. 233(5): p. 1100-3.

[116] van der Burgh, R., et al., *Mevalonate kinase deficiency, a metabolic autoinflammatory disease.* Clin Immunol, 2013. 147(3): p. 197-206.

[117] Tada, M. and F. Lynen, *[On the biosynthesis of terpenes. XIV. On the determination of phosphomevalonic acid kinase and pyrophosphomevalonic acid decarboxylase in cell extracts].* J Biochem, 1961. 49: p. 758-64.

[118] Agranoff, B.W., et al., *Biosynthesis of terpenes. VII. Isopentenyl pyrophosphate isomerase.* J Biol Chem, 1960. 235: p. 326-32.

[119] Moosmann, B. and C. Behl, *Selenoproteins, cholesterol-lowering drugs, and the consequences: revisiting of the mevalonate pathway.* Trends Cardiovasc Med, 2004. 14(7): p. 273-81.

[120] Warner, G.J., et al., *Inhibition of selenoprotein synthesis by selenocysteine tRNA[Ser]Sec lacking isopentenyladenosine.* J Biol Chem, 2000. 275(36): p. 28110-9.

[121] Bellinger, F.P., et al., *Regulation and function of selenoproteins in human disease.* Biochem J, 2009. 422(1): p. 11-22.

[122] Zhang, S., C. Rocourt, and W.H. Cheng, *Selenoproteins and the aging brain.* Mech Ageing Dev, 2010. 131(4): p. 253-60.

[123] Wirth, E.K., et al., *Neuronal selenoprotein expression is required for interneuron development and prevents seizures and neurodegeneration.* FASEB J, 2010. 24(3): p. 844-52.

[124] Seeher, S., et al., *Impaired selenoprotein expression in brain triggers striatal neuronal loss leading to co-ordination defects in mice.* Biochem J, 2014. 462(1): p. 67-75.

[125] Moosmann, B. and C. Behl, *Selenoprotein synthesis and side-effects of statins.* Lancet, 2004. 363(9412): p. 892-4.

[126] Bang, S., et al., *Isopentenyl pyrophosphate is a novel antinociceptive substance that inhibits TRPV3 and TRPA1 ion channels.* Pain, 2011. 152(5): p. 1156-64.

[127] Bang, S., et al., *Nociceptive and pro-inflammatory effects of dimethylallyl pyrophosphate via TRPV4 activation.* Br J Pharmacol, 2012. 166(4): p. 1433-43.

[128] Holstein, S.A. and R.J. Hohl, *Isoprenoids: remarkable diversity of form and function.* Lipids, 2004. 39(4): p. 293-309.

[129] Hooff, G.P., et al., *Isoprenoids, small GTPases and Alzheimer's disease.* Biochim Biophys Acta, 2010. 1801(8): p. 896-905.

[130] Wang, K.C. and S. Ohnuma, *Isoprenyl diphosphate synthases.* Biochim Biophys Acta, 2000. 1529(1-3): p. 33-48.

[131] Vallett, S.M., et al., *A direct role for sterol regulatory element binding protein in activation of 3-hydroxy-3-methylglutaryl coenzyme A reductase gene.* J Biol Chem, 1996. 271(21): p. 12247-53.

[132] Sharpe, L.J. and A.J. Brown, *Controlling Cholesterol Synthesis beyond 3-Hydroxy-3-methylglutaryl-CoA Reductase (HMGCR).* J Biol Chem, 2013. 288(26): p. 18707-15.

[133] Medina, M.W., et al., *Coordinately regulated alternative splicing of genes involved in cholesterol biosynthesis and uptake.* PLoS One, 2011. 6(4): p. e19420.

[134] Nakanishi, M., J.L. Goldstein, and M.S. Brown, *Multivalent control of 3-hydroxy-3-methylglutaryl coenzyme A reductase. Mevalonate-derived product inhibits translation of mRNA and accelerates degradation of enzyme.* J Biol Chem, 1988. 263(18): p. 8929-37.

[135] Peffley, D. and M. Sinensky, *Regulation of 3-hydroxy-3-methylglutaryl coenzyme A reductase synthesis by a non-sterol mevalonate-derived product in Mev-1 cells. Apparent translational control.* J Biol Chem, 1985. 260(18): p. 9949-52.

[136] Straka, M.S. and S.R. Panini, *Post-transcriptional regulation of 3-hydroxy-3-methylglutaryl coenzyme A reductase by mevalonate.* Arch Biochem Biophys, 1995. 317(1): p. 235-43.

[137] Peffley, D.M. and A.K. Gayen, *Plant-derived monoterpenes suppress hamster kidney cell 3-hydroxy-3-methylglutaryl coenzyme a reductase synthesis at the post-transcriptional level.* J Nutr, 2003. 133(1): p. 38-44.

[138] Peffley, D.M. and A.K. Gayen, *Mevalonate regulates polysome distribution and blocks translation-dependent suppression of 3-hydroxy-3-methylglutaryl coenzyme A reductase mRNA: relationship to translational control.* Somat Cell Mol Genet, 1995. 21(3): p. 189-204.

[139] Ching, Y.P., S.P. Davies, and D.G. Hardie, *Analysis of the specificity of the AMP-activated protein kinase by site-directed mutagenesis of bacterially expressed 3-hydroxy 3-methylglutaryl-CoA reductase, using a single primer variant of the unique-site-elimination method.* Eur J Biochem, 1996. 237(3): p. 800-8.

[140] Clarke, P.R. and D.G. Hardie, *Regulation of HMG-CoA reductase: identification of the site phosphorylated by the AMP-activated protein kinase in vitro and in intact rat liver.* EMBO J, 1990. 9(8): p. 2439-46.

[141] Gaussin, V., et al., *Distinct type-2A protein phosphatases activate HMGCoA reductase and acetyl-CoA carboxylase in liver.* FEBS Lett, 1997. 413(1): p. 115-8.

[142] Cook, M., et al., *Increased RhoA prenylation in the loechrig (loe) mutant leads to progressive neurodegeneration*. PLoS One, 2012. 7(9): p. e44440.

[143] Lu, J., et al., *Quercetin activates AMP-activated protein kinase by reducing PP2C expression protecting old mouse brain against high cholesterol-induced neurotoxicity.* The Journal of pathology, 2010. 222(2): p. 199-212.

[144] Song, B.L., N. Sever, and R.A. DeBose-Boyd, *Gp78, a membrane-anchored ubiquitin ligase, associates with Insig-1 and couples sterol-regulated ubiquitination to degradation of HMG CoA reductase.* Mol Cell, 2005. 19(6): p. 829-40.

[145] Jo, Y., et al., *Sterol-induced degradation of HMG CoA reductase depends on interplay of two Insigs and two ubiquitin ligases, gp78 and Trc8.* Proc Natl Acad Sci U S A, 2011. 108(51): p. 20503-8.

[146] Zelcer, N., et al., *The E3 ubiquitin ligase MARCH6 degrades squalene monooxygenase and affects 3-hydroxy-3-methyl-glutaryl coenzyme A reductase and the cholesterol synthesis pathway.* Mol Cell Biol, 2014. 34(7): p. 1262-70.

[147] Sever, N., et al., *Insig-dependent ubiquitination and degradation of mammalian 3-hydroxy-3-methylglutaryl-CoA reductase stimulated by sterols and geranylgeraniol.* The Journal of Biological Chemistry, 2003. 278(52): p. 52479-90.

[148] Hua, X., et al., *Sterol resistance in CHO cells traced to point mutation in SREBP cleavage-activating protein.* Cell, 1996. 87(3): p. 415-26.

[149] Sever, N., et al., *Accelerated degradation of HMG CoA reductase mediated by binding of insig-1 to its sterol-sensing domain.* Molecular cell, 2003. 11(1): p. 25-33.

[150] Song, B.L. and R.A. DeBose-Boyd, *Ubiquitination of 3-hydroxy-3-methylglutaryl-CoA reductase in permeabilized cells mediated by cytosolic E1 and a putative membrane-bound ubiquitin ligase.* J Biol Chem, 2004. 279(27): p. 28798-806.

[151] DeBose-Boyd, R.A., *Feedback regulation of cholesterol synthesis: sterol-accelerated ubiquitination and degradation of HMG CoA reductase.* Cell research, 2008. 18(6): p. 609-21.

[152] Lange, Y., et al., *Effectors of rapid homeostatic responses of endoplasmic reticulum cholesterol and 3-hydroxy-3-methylglutaryl-CoA reductase.* J Biol Chem, 2008. 283(3): p. 1445-55.

[153] Forman, B.M., et al., *The orphan nuclear receptor LXRalpha is positively and negatively regulated by distinct products of mevalonate metabolism.* Proc Natl Acad Sci U S A, 1997. 94(20): p. 10588-93.

[154] Gan, X., et al., *Dual mechanisms of ABCA1 regulation by geranylgeranyl pyrophosphate.* J Biol Chem, 2001. 276(52): p. 48702-8.

[155] Leichner, G.S., et al., *Metabolically Regulated Endoplasmic Reticulum-associated Degradation of 3-Hydroxy-3-methylglutaryl-CoA Reductase: EVIDENCE FOR REQUIREMENT OF A GERANYLGERANYLATED PROTEIN.* The Journal of Biological Chemistry, 2011. 286(37): p. 32150-61.

[156] Meigs, T.E., D.S. Roseman, and R.D. Simoni, *Regulation of 3-hydroxy-3-methylglutaryl-coenzyme A reductase degradation by the nonsterol mevalonate metabolite farnesol in vivo.* J Biol Chem, 1996. 271(14): p. 7916-22.

[157] Meigs, T.E. and R.D. Simoni, *Farnesol as a regulator of HMG-CoA reductase degradation: characterization and role of farnesyl pyrophosphatase.* Arch Biochem Biophys, 1997. 345(1): p. 1-9.

[158] Correll, C.C., L. Ng, and P.A. Edwards, *Identification of farnesol as the non-sterol derivative of mevalonic acid required for the accelerated degradation of 3-hydroxy-3-methylglutaryl-coenzyme A reductase.* J Biol Chem, 1994. 269(26): p. 17390-3.

[159] Dorsey, J.K. and J.W. Porter, *The inhibition of mevalonic kinase by geranyl and farnesyl pyrophosphates.* J Biol Chem, 1968. 243(18): p. 4667-70.

[160] Hinson, D.D., et al., *Post-translational regulation of mevalonate kinase by intermediates of the cholesterol and nonsterol isoprene biosynthetic pathways.* J Lipid Res, 1997. 38(11): p. 2216-23.

[161] Vanmierlo, T., et al., *Alterations in brain cholesterol metabolism in the APPSLxPS1mut mouse, a model for Alzheimer's disease.* J Alzheimers Dis, 2010. 19(1): p. 117-27.

[162] Licastro, F., et al., *Genetic risk profiles for Alzheimer's disease: integration of APOE genotype and variants that up-regulate inflammation.* Neurobiol Aging, 2007. 28(11): p. 1637-43.

[163] Porcellini, E., et al., *The hydroxy-methyl-glutaryl CoA reductase promoter polymorphism is associated with Alzheimer's risk and cognitive deterioration.* Neuroscience Letters, 2007. 416(1): p. 66-70.

[164] Rodriguez-Rodriguez, E., et al., *Interaction between HMGCR and ABCA1 cholesterol-related genes modulates Alzheimer's disease risk.* Brain Res, 2009. 1280: p. 166-71.

[165] Keller, L., et al., *A functional polymorphism in the HMGCR promoter affects transcriptional activity but not the risk for Alzheimer disease in Swedish populations.* Brain Res, 2010. 1344: p. 185-91.

[166] Leduc, V., et al., *HMGCR is a genetic modifier for risk, age of onset and MCI conversion to Alzheimer's disease in a three cohorts study.* Mol Psychiatry, 2014.

[167] Trapani, L. and V. Pallottini, *Age-Related Hypercholesterolemia and HMG-CoA Reductase Dysregulation: Sex Does Matter (A Gender Perspective).* Curr Gerontol Geriatr Res, 2010: p. 420139.

[168] Yasojima, K., E.G. McGeer, and P.L. McGeer, *3-hydroxy-3-methylglutaryl-coenzyme A reductase mRNA in Alzheimer and control brain.* Neuroreport, 2001. 12(13): p. 2935-8.

[169] Eckert, G.P., et al., *Regulation of the brain isoprenoids farnesyl- and geranylgeranylpyrophosphate is altered in male Alzheimer patients.* Neurobiol Dis, 2009. 35(2): p. 251-7.

[170] Do, R., et al., *Squalene synthase: a critical enzyme in the cholesterol biosynthesis pathway.* Clin Genet, 2009. 75(1): p. 19-29.

[171] Tozawa, R., et al., *Embryonic lethality and defective neural tube closure in mice lacking squalene synthase.* J Biol Chem, 1999. 274(43): p. 30843-8.

[172] Lutjohann, D., *Cholesterol metabolism in the brain: importance of 24S-hydroxylation.* Acta Neurol Scand Suppl, 2006. 185: p. 33-42.

[173] Lusa, S., S. Heino, and E. Ikonen, *Differential mobilization of newly synthesized cholesterol and biosynthetic sterol precursors from cells.* J Biol Chem, 2003. 278(22): p. 19844-51.

[174] Johnson, W.J., et al., *Efflux of Newly Synthesized Cholesterol and Biosynthetic Sterol Intermediates from Cells: Dependence on Acceptor Type and on Enrichment of Cells with Cholesterol.* Journal of Biological Chemistry, 1995. 270(42): p. 25037-25046.

[175] Mutka, A.L., et al., *Secretion of sterols and the NPC2 protein from primary astrocytes.* J Biol Chem, 2004. 279(47): p. 48654-62.

[176] Smiljanic, K., et al., *Aging Induces Tissue-Specific Changes in Cholesterol Metabolism in Rat Brain and Liver.* Lipids, 2013.

[177] Lutjohann, D., *Profile of cholesterol-related sterols in aged amyloid precursor protein transgenic mouse brain.* The Journal of Lipid Research, 2002. 43(7): p. 1078-1085.

[178] Tint, G.S., et al., *The use of the Dhcr7 knockout mouse to accurately determine the origin of fetal sterols.* J Lipid Res, 2006. 47(7): p. 1535-41.

[179] Hinse, C.H. and S.N. Shah, *The desmosterol reductase activity of rat brain during development.* J Neurochem, 1971. 18(10): p. 1989-98.

[180] Kritchevsky, D. and W.L. Holmes, *Occurrence of desmosterol in developing rat brain.* Biochem Biophys Res Commun, 1962. 7: p. 128-31.

[181] Fumagalli, R. and R. Paoletti, *The identification and significance of desmosterol in the developing human and animal brain.* Life Sci, 1963. 5: p. 291-5.

[182] Jansen, M., et al., *What dictates the accumulation of desmosterol in the developing brain?* FASEB J, 2013. 27(3): p. 865-70.

[183] Tint, G.S., et al., *Desmosterol in brain is elevated because DHCR24 needs REST for Robust Expression but REST is poorly expressed.* Dev Neurosci, 2014. 36(2): p. 132-42.

[184] Tint, G.S., et al., *The Smith-Lemli-Opitz syndrome: a potentially fatal birth defect caused by a block in the last enzymatic step in cholesterol biosynthesis.* Subcell Biochem, 1997. 28: p. 117-44.

[185] Jira, P., *Cholesterol metabolism deficiency.* Handb Clin Neurol, 2013. 113: p. 1845-50.

[186] Kempen, H.J.M., et al., *Serum Lathosterol Concentration Is an Indicator of Whole-Body Cholesterol-Synthesis in Humans.* Journal of Lipid Research, 1988. 29(9): p. 1149-1155.

[187] Bjorkhem, I., et al., *Correlation between Serum Levels of Some Cholesterol Precursors and Activity of Hmg-Coa Reductase in Human-Liver.* Journal of Lipid Research, 1987. 28(10): p. 1137-1143.

[188] Irons, M., et al., *Defective cholesterol biosynthesis in Smith-Lemli-Opitz syndrome.* Lancet, 1993. 341(8857): p. 1414.

[189] Nowaczyk, M.J. and M.B. Irons, *Smith-Lemli-Opitz syndrome: phenotype, natural history, and epidemiology.* Am J Med Genet C Semin Med Genet, 2012. 160C(4): p. 250-62.

[190] Waterham, H.R., et al., *Mutations in the 3beta-hydroxysterol Delta24-reductase gene cause desmosterolosis, an autosomal recessive disorder of cholesterol biosynthesis.* Am J Hum Genet, 2001. 69(4): p. 685-94.

[191] Belic, A., et al., *An algorithm for rapid computational construction of metabolic networks: a cholesterol biosynthesis example.* Comput Biol Med, 2013. 43(5): p. 471-80.

[192] Bae, S.H. and Y.K. Paik, *Cholesterol biosynthesis from lanosterol: development of a novel assay method and characterization of rat liver microsomal lanosterol delta 24-reductase.* Biochem J, 1997. 326 (Pt 2): p. 609-16.

[193] Wechsler, A., et al., *Generation of viable cholesterol-free mice.* Science, 2003. 302(5653): p. 2087.

[194] FitzPatrick, D.R., et al., *Clinical phenotype of desmosterolosis.* Am J Med Genet, 1998. 75(2): p. 145-52.

[195] Yang, C.D., et al., *Sterol intermediates from cholesterol biosynthetic pathway as liver X receptor ligands.* Journal of Biological Chemistry, 2006. 281(38): p. 27816-27826.

[196] Greeve, I., et al., *The human DIMINUTO/DWARF1 homolog seladin-1 confers resistance to Alzheimer's disease-associated neurodegeneration and oxidative stress.* The Journal of neuroscience : the official journal of the Society for Neuroscience, 2000. 20(19): p. 7345-52.

[197] Luciani, P., et al., *Expression of the antiapoptotic gene seladin-1 and octreotide-induced apoptosis in growth hormone-secreting and nonfunctioning pituitary adenomas.* J Clin Endocrinol Metab, 2005. 90(11): p. 6156-61.

[198] Fuller, P.J., et al., *Seladin-1/DHCR24 expression in normal ovary, ovarian epithelial and granulosa tumours.* Clin Endocrinol (Oxf), 2005. 63(1): p. 111-5.

[199] Biancolella, M., et al., *Effects of dutasteride on the expression of genes related to androgen metabolism and related pathway in human prostate cancer cell lines.* Invest New Drugs, 2007. 25(5): p. 491-7.

[200] Zerenturk, E.J., et al., *Desmosterol and DHCR24: unexpected new directions for a terminal step in cholesterol synthesis.* Prog Lipid Res, 2013. 52(4): p. 666-80.

[201] Nelson, J.A., S.R. Steckbeck, and T.A. Spencer, *Biosynthesis of 24,25-epoxycholesterol from squalene 2,3;22,23-dioxide.* J Biol Chem, 1981. 256(3): p. 1067-8.

[202] Wong, J., C.M. Quinn, and A.J. Brown, *Synthesis of the oxysterol, 24(S), 25-epoxycholesterol, parallels cholesterol production and may protect against cellular accumulation of newly-synthesized cholesterol.* Lipids Health Dis, 2007. 6: p. 10.

[203] Wang, Y., et al., *24S,25-Epoxycholesterol in mouse and rat brain.* Biochem Biophys Res Commun, 2014. 449(2): p. 229-234.

[204] Griffiths, W.J. and Y. Wang, *Analysis of oxysterol metabolomes.* Biochim Biophys Acta, 2011. 1811(11): p. 784-99.

[205] Wong, J., et al., *Endogenous 24(S),25-epoxycholesterol fine-tunes acute control of cellular cholesterol homeostasis.* J Biol Chem, 2008. 283(2): p. 700-7.

[206] Wong, J., et al., *Primary human astrocytes produce 24(S),25-epoxycholesterol with implications for brain cholesterol homeostasis.* J Neurochem, 2007. 103(5): p. 1764-73.

[207] Janowski, B.A., et al., *Structural requirements of ligands for the oxysterol liver X receptors LXRalpha and LXRbeta.* Proc Natl Acad Sci U S A, 1999. 96(1): p. 266-71.

[208] Beyea, M.M., et al., *Selective up-regulation of LXR-regulated genes ABCA1, ABCG1, and APOE in macrophages through increased endogenous synthesis of 24(S),25-epoxycholesterol.* J Biol Chem, 2007. 282(8): p. 5207-16.

[209] Horton, J.D., *Sterol regulatory element-binding proteins: transcriptional activators of lipid synthesis.* Biochem Soc Trans, 2002. 30(Pt 6): p. 1091-5.

[210] Gill, S., et al., *Cholesterol-dependent degradation of squalene monooxygenase, a control point in cholesterol synthesis beyond HMG-CoA reductase.* Cell Metab, 2011. 13(3): p. 260-73.

[211] Foresti, O., et al., *Sterol homeostasis requires regulated degradation of squalene monooxygenase by the ubiquitin ligase Doa10/Teb4.* Elife, 2013. 2: p. e00953.

[212] Daimiel, L.A., et al., *Promoter analysis of the DHCR24 (3beta-hydroxysterol Delta(24)-reductase) gene: characterization of SREBP (sterol-regulatory-element-binding protein)-mediated activation.* Biosci Rep, 2013. 33(1): p. 57-69.

[213] Demoulin, J.B., et al., *Platelet-derived growth factor stimulates membrane lipid synthesis through activation of phosphatidylinositol 3-kinase and sterol regulatory element-binding proteins.* J Biol Chem, 2004. 279(34): p. 35392-402.

[214] Reed, B.D., et al., *Genome-wide occupancy of SREBP1 and its partners NFY and SP1 reveals novel functional roles and combinatorial regulation of distinct classes of genes.* PLoS Genet, 2008. 4(7): p. e1000133.

[215] Ramos, M.C., et al., *Simvastatin modulates the Alzheimer's disease-related gene seladin-1.* J Alzheimers Dis, 2012. 28(2): p. 297-301.

[216] Wang, Y., et al., *The selective Alzheimer's disease indicator-1 gene (Seladin-1/DHCR24) is a liver X receptor target gene.* Molecular pharmacology, 2008. 74(6): p. 1716-21.

[217] Drzewinska, J., A. Walczak-Drzewiecka, and M. Ratajewski, *Identification and analysis of the promoter region of the human DHCR24 gene: involvement of DNA methylation and histone acetylation.* Mol Biol Rep, 2011. 38(2): p. 1091-101.

[218] Zerenturk, E.J., et al., *The endogenous regulator 24(S),25-epoxycholesterol inhibits cholesterol synthesis at DHCR24 (Seladin-1).* Biochim Biophys Acta, 2012. 1821(9): p. 1269-77.

[219] Luu, W., et al., *Signaling regulates activity of DHCR24, the final enzyme in cholesterol synthesis.* J Lipid Res, 2014. 55(3): p. 410-20.

[220] Iivonen, S., et al., *Seladin-1 transcription is linked to neuronal degeneration in Alzheimer's disease.* Neuroscience, 2002. 113(2): p. 301-10.

[221] Sharpe, L.J., et al., *Is seladin-1 really a selective Alzheimer's disease indicator?* J Alzheimers Dis, 2012. 30(1): p. 35-9.

[222] Lamsa, R., et al., *The association study between DHCR24 polymorphisms and Alzheimer's disease.* Am J Med Genet B Neuropsychiatr Genet, 2007. 144B(7): p. 906-10.

[223] Feher, A., et al., *Gender dependent effect of DHCR24 polymorphism on the risk for Alzheimer's disease.* Neurosci Lett, 2012. 526(1): p. 20-3.

[224] Benvenuti, S., et al., *Neuronal differentiation of human mesenchymal stem cells: changes in the expression of the Alzheimer's disease-related gene seladin-1.* Exp Cell Res, 2006. 312(13): p. 2592-604.

[225] Peri, A., et al., *New insights on the neuroprotective role of sterols and sex steroids: the seladin-1/DHCR24 paradigm.* Front Neuroendocrinol, 2009. 30(2): p. 119-29.

[226] Lu, T., et al., *REST and stress resistance in ageing and Alzheimer's disease.* Nature, 2014. 507(7493): p. 448-54.

[227] Wisniewski, T., K. Newman, and N.B. Javitt, *Alzheimer's disease: brain desmosterol levels.* J Alzheimers Dis, 2013. 33(3): p. 881-8.

[228] Peri, A. and M. Serio, *Neuroprotective effects of the Alzheimer's disease-related gene seladin-1.* J Mol Endocrinol, 2008. 41(5): p. 251-61.

[229] Lu, X., et al., *3 beta-hydroxysteroid-Delta 24 reductase (DHCR24) protects neuronal cells from apoptotic cell death induced by endoplasmic reticulum (ER) stress.* PLoS One, 2014. 9(1): p. e86753.

[230] Luciani, P., et al., *Seladin-1 is a fundamental mediator of the neuroprotective effects of estrogen in human neuroblast long-term cell cultures.* Endocrinology, 2008. 149(9): p. 4256-66.

[231] Benvenuti, S., et al., *Estrogen and selective estrogen receptor modulators exert neuroprotective effects and stimulate the expression of selective Alzheimer's disease indicator-1, a recently discovered antiapoptotic gene, in human neuroblast long-term cell cultures.* J Clin Endocrinol Metab, 2005. 90(3): p. 1775-82.

[232] Peri, A., et al., *Membrane cholesterol as a mediator of the neuroprotective effects of estrogens.* Neuroscience, 2011. 191: p. 107-17.

[233] Cecchi, C., et al., *Seladin-1/DHCR24 protects neuroblastoma cells against Abeta toxicity by increasing membrane cholesterol content.* Journal of cellular and molecular medicine, 2008. 12(5B): p. 1990-2002.

[234] Pensalfini, A., et al., *Membrane cholesterol enrichment prevents Abeta-induced oxidative stress in Alzheimer's fibroblasts.* Neurobiol Aging, 2011. 32(2): p. 210-22.

[235] Crameri, A., et al., *The role of seladin-1/DHCR24 in cholesterol biosynthesis, APP processing and Abeta generation in vivo.* EMBO J, 2006. 25(2): p. 432-43.

[236] Martin, M., C.G. Dotti, and M.D. Ledesma, *Brain cholesterol in normal and pathological aging.* Biochim Biophys Acta, 2010. 1801(8): p. 934-944.

[237] Cossec, J.C., et al., *Cholesterol changes in Alzheimer's disease: Methods of analysis and impact on the formation of enlarged endosomes.* Biochim Biophys Acta, 2010.

[238] Wood, W.G., et al., *Cholesterol as a causative factor in Alzheimer's disease: a debatable hypothesis.* J Neurochem, 2014. 129(4): p. 559-72.

[239] Edlund, C., et al., *Ubiquinone, dolichol, and cholesterol metabolism in aging and Alzheimer's disease.* Biochemistry and cell biology = Biochimie et biologie cellulaire, 1992. 70(6): p. 422-8.

[240] Snipes, G.J. and U. Suter, *Cholesterol and myelin.* Subcell Biochem, 1997. 28: p. 173-204.

[241] Eckert, G.P., et al., *Cholesterol modulates the membrane-disordering effects of beta-amyloid peptides in the hippocampus: specific changes in Alzheimer's disease.* Dement Geriatr Cogn Disord, 2000. 11(4): p. 181-6.

[242] Heverin, M., et al., *Changes in the levels of cerebral and extracerebral sterols in the brain of patients with Alzheimer's disease.* J Lipid Res, 2004. 45(1): p. 186-93.

[243] Cutler, R.G., et al., *Involvement of oxidative stress-induced abnormalities in ceramide and cholesterol metabolism in brain aging and Alzheimer's disease.* Proc Natl Acad Sci U S A, 2004. 101(7): p. 2070-5.

[244] Mori, T., et al., *Cholesterol accumulates in senile plaques of Alzheimer disease patients and in transgenic APP(SW) mice.* J Neuropathol Exp Neurol, 2001. 60(8): p. 778-85.

[245] Panchal, M., et al., *Enrichment of cholesterol in microdissected Alzheimer's disease senile plaques as assessed by mass spectrometry.* J Lipid Res, 2010. 51(3): p. 598-605.

[246] Mason, R.P., et al., *Evidence for changes in the Alzheimer's disease brain cortical membrane structure mediated by cholesterol.* Neurobiol Aging, 1992. 13(3): p. 413-9.

[247] Hascalovici, J.R., et al., *Brain sterol dysregulation in sporadic AD and MCI: relationship to heme oxygenase-1.* J Neurochem, 2009. 110(4): p. 1241-53.

[248] Kolsch, H., et al., *Alterations of cholesterol precursor levels in Alzheimer's disease.* Biochim Biophys Acta, 2010. 1801(8): p. 945-50.

[249] Mulder, M., et al., *Reduced levels of cholesterol, phospholipids, and fatty acids in cerebrospinal fluid of Alzheimer disease patients are not related to apolipoprotein E4.* Alzheimer Dis Assoc Disord, 1998. 12(3): p. 198-203.

[250] Wender, M., Z. Adamczewska-Goncerzewicz, and J. Szczech, *Free sterols in senile human brain.* Folia Neuropathol, 1994. 32(2): p. 75-9.

[251] Naylor, J.C., et al., *Allopregnanolone levels are reduced in temporal cortex in patients with Alzheimer's disease compared to cognitively intact control subjects.* Biochim Biophys Acta, 2010. 1801(8): p. 951-9.

[252] Burns, M. and K. Duff, *Cholesterol in Alzheimer's disease and tauopathy.* Annals of the New York Academy of Sciences, 2002. 977: p. 367-75.

[253] Lazar, A.N., et al., *Time-of-flight secondary ion mass spectrometry (TOF-SIMS) imaging reveals cholesterol overload in the cerebral cortex of Alzheimer disease patients.* Acta Neuropathol, 2013. 125(1): p. 133-44.

[254] Ohm, T.G., et al., *Cholesterol and tau protein--findings in Alzheimer's and Niemann Pick C's disease.* Pharmacopsychiatry, 2003. 36 Suppl 2: p. S120-6.

[255] Gomez-Ramos, P. and M. Asuncion Moran, *Ultrastructural localization of intraneuronal Abeta-peptide in Alzheimer disease brains.* J Alzheimers Dis, 2007. 11(1): p. 53-9.

[256] Fernandez, A., et al., *Mitochondrial cholesterol loading exacerbates amyloid beta peptide-induced inflammation and neurotoxicity.* J Neurosci, 2009. 29(20): p. 6394-405.

[257] Sole-Domenech, S., et al., *Localization of cholesterol, amyloid and glia in Alzheimer's disease transgenic mouse brain tissue using time-of-flight secondary ion mass spectrometry (ToF-SIMS) and immunofluorescence imaging.* Acta Neuropathol, 2013. 125(1): p. 145-57.

[258] Aqul, A., et al., *Unesterified cholesterol accumulation in late endosomes/lysosomes causes neurodegeneration and is prevented by driving cholesterol export from this compartment.* J Neurosci, 2011. 31(25): p. 9404-13.

[259] Yamazaki, T., et al., *Accumulation and aggregation of amyloid beta-protein in late endosomes of Niemann-pick type C cells.* J Biol Chem, 2001. 276(6): p. 4454-60.

[260] Auer, I.A., et al., *Paired helical filament tau (PHFtau) in Niemann-Pick type C disease is similar to PHFtau in Alzheimer's disease.* Acta Neuropathol (Berl), 1995. 90(6): p. 547-51.

[261] Saito, Y., et al., *Niemann-Pick type C disease: accelerated neurofibrillary tangle formation and amyloid beta deposition associated with apolipoprotein E epsilon 4 homozygosity.* Ann Neurol, 2002. 52(3): p. 351-5.

[262] Nixon, R.A., *Niemann-Pick Type C disease and Alzheimer's disease: the APP-endosome connection fattens up.* Am J Pathol, 2004. 164(3): p. 757-61.

[263] Jin, L.W., et al., *Intracellular accumulation of amyloidogenic fragments of amyloid-beta precursor protein in neurons with Niemann-Pick type C defects is associated with endosomal abnormalities.* Am J Pathol, 2004. 164(3): p. 975-85.

[264] Yao, J., et al., *Neuroprotection by cyclodextrin in cell and mouse models of Alzheimer disease.* J Exp Med, 2012. 209(13): p. 2501-13.

[265] Hudry, E., et al., *Adeno-associated virus gene therapy with cholesterol 24-hydroxylase reduces the amyloid pathology before or after the onset of amyloid plaques in mouse models of Alzheimer's disease.* Molecular therapy : the journal of the American Society of Gene Therapy, 2010. 18(1): p. 44-53.

[266] Bu, G., *Apolipoprotein E and its receptors in Alzheimer's disease: pathways, pathogenesis and therapy.* Nat Rev Neurosci, 2009. 10(5): p. 333-44.

[267] Verghese, P.B., J.M. Castellano, and D.M. Holtzman, *Apolipoprotein E in Alzheimer's disease and other neurological disorders*. Lancet Neurol, 2011. 10(3): p. 241-52.

[268] Grimm, M.O., et al., *The impact of cholesterol, DHA, and sphingolipids on Alzheimer's disease.* Biomed Res Int, 2013. 2013: p. 814390.

[269] Fonseca, A.C., et al., *Cholesterol and statins in Alzheimer's disease: current controversies.* Exp Neurol, 2010. 223(2): p. 282-93.

[270] Pfrieger, F.W., *Role of cholesterol in synapse formation and function.* Biochim Biophys Acta, 2003. 1610(2): p. 271-80.

[271] Dotti, C.G., J.A. Esteban, and M.D. Ledesma, *Lipid dynamics at dendritic spines.* Front Neuroanat, 2014. 8: p. 76.

[272] Selkoe, D.J., *Alzheimer's disease is a synaptic failure.* Science, 2002. 298(5594): p. 789-91.

[273] Tanzi, R.E., *The synaptic Abeta hypothesis of Alzheimer disease.* Nat Neurosci, 2005. 8(8): p. 977-9.

[274] Ferrer, I. and F. Gullotta, *Down's syndrome and Alzheimer's disease: dendritic spine counts in the hippocampus.* Acta Neuropathol, 1990. 79(6): p. 680-5.

[275] Moolman, D.L., et al., *Dendrite and dendritic spine alterations in Alzheimer models.* J Neurocytol, 2004. 33(3): p. 377-87.

[276] Spires, T.L., et al., *Dendritic spine abnormalities in amyloid precursor protein transgenic mice demonstrated by gene transfer and intravital multiphoton microscopy.* J Neurosci, 2005. 25(31): p. 7278-87.

[277] Jacobsen, J.S., et al., *Early-onset behavioral and synaptic deficits in a mouse model of Alzheimer's disease.* Proc Natl Acad Sci U S A, 2006. 103(13): p. 5161-6.

[278] Knafo, S., et al., *Widespread changes in dendritic spines in a model of Alzheimer's disease.* Cereb Cortex, 2009. 19(3): p. 586-92.

[279] Koudinov, A.R. and N.V. Koudinova, *Cholesterol homeostasis failure as a unifying cause of synaptic degeneration.* J Neurol Sci, 2005. 229-230: p. 233-40.

[280] Rajanikant, G.K., et al., *The therapeutic potential of statins in neurological disorders.* Curr Med Chem, 2007. 14(1): p. 103-12.

[281] Obiol-Pardo, C., J. Rubio-Martinez, and S. Imperial, *The Methylerythritol Phosphate (MEP) Pathway for Isoprenoid Biosynthesis as a Target for the Development of New Drugs Against Tuberculosis.* Current Medicinal Chemistry, 2011. 18(9): p. 1325-1338.

[282] Wiemer, A.J., R.J. Hohl, and D.F. Wiemer, *The Intermediate Enzymes of Isoprenoid Metabolism as Anticancer Targets.* Anti-Cancer Agents in Medicinal Chemistry, 2009. 9(5): p. 526-542.

[283] Kandutsch, A.A., et al., *Purification of Geranylgeranyl Pyrophosphate Synthetase from Micrococcus Lysodeikticus.* J Biol Chem, 1964. 239: p. 2507-15.

[284] Ericsson, J., et al., *Distribution of prenyltransferases in rat tissues. Evidence for a cytosolic all-trans-geranylgeranyl diphosphate synthase.* J Biol Chem, 1993. 268(2): p. 832-8.

[285] Runquist, M., et al., *Distribution of branch point prenyltransferases in regions of bovine brain.* J Neurochem, 1995. 65(5): p. 2299-306.

[286] Park, J., et al., *Human isoprenoid synthase enzymes as therapeutic targets.* Front Chem, 2014. 2: p. 50.

[287] Afshordel, S., et al., *Impaired geranylgeranyltransferase-I regulation reduces membrane-associated Rho protein levels in aged mouse brain.* J Neurochem, 2014. 129(4): p. 732-42.

[288] Schenk, B., F. Fernandez, and C.J. Waechter, *The ins(ide) and out(side) of dolichyl phosphate biosynthesis and recycling in the endoplasmic reticulum.* Glycobiology, 2001. 11(5): p. 61R-70R.

[289] Crick, D.C., J.S. Rush, and C.J. Waechter, *Characterization and localization of a long-chain isoprenyltransferase activity in porcine brain: proposed role in the biosynthesis of dolichyl phosphate.* J Neurochem, 1991. 57(4): p. 1354-62.

[290] Takeda, J. and T. Kinoshita, *GPI-anchor biosynthesis.* Trends Biochem Sci, 1995. 20(9): p. 367-71.

[291] Kornfeld, R. and S. Kornfeld, *Assembly of asparagine-linked oligosaccharides.* Annu Rev Biochem, 1985. 54: p. 631-64.

[292] Andersson, M., et al., *Age-dependent changes in the levels of dolichol and dolichyl phosphates in human brain.* Acta Chem Scand B, 1987. 41(2): p. 144-6.

[293] Pallottini, V., et al., *Age-related changes of isoprenoid biosynthesis in rat liver and brain.* Biogerontology, 2003. 4(6): p. 371-8.

[294] Parentini, I., et al., *Accumulation of dolichol in older tissues satisfies the proposed criteria to be qualified a biomarker of aging.* J Gerontol A Biol Sci Med Sci, 2005. 60(1): p. 39-43.

[295] Dallner, G. and P.J. Sindelar, *Regulation of ubiquinone metabolism.* Free Radic Biol Med, 2000. 29(3-4): p. 285-94.

[296] Teclebrhan, H., et al., *Biosynthesis of the side chain of ubiquinone:trans-prenyltransferase in rat liver microsomes.* J Biol Chem, 1993. 268(31): p. 23081-6.

[297] Rauthan, M. and M. Pilon, *The mevalonate pathway in C. elegans.* Lipids Health Dis, 2011. 10: p. 243.

[298] Lopez-Lluch, G., et al., *Is coenzyme Q a key factor in aging?* Mech Ageing Dev, 2010. 131(4): p. 225-35.

[299] Bentinger, M., et al., *Distribution and breakdown of labeled coenzyme Q10 in rat.* Free Radic Biol Med, 2003. 34(5): p. 563-75.

[300] Bansal, V.S. and S. Vaidya, *Characterization of two distinct allyl pyrophosphatase activities from rat liver microsomes.* Arch Biochem Biophys, 1994. 315(2): p. 393-9.

[301] Miriyala, S., et al., *Functional characterization of the atypical integral membrane lipid phosphatase PDP1/PPAPDC2 identifies a pathway for interconversion of isoprenols and isoprenoid phosphates in mammalian cells.* J Biol Chem, 2010. 285(18): p. 13918-29.

[302] Crick, D.C., D.A. Andres, and C.J. Waechter, *Novel salvage pathway utilizing farnesol and geranylgeraniol for protein isoprenylation.* Biochem Biophys Res Commun, 1997. 237(3): p. 483-7.

[303] Beigneux, A., et al., *Prenylcysteine lyase deficiency in mice results in the accumulation of farnesylcysteine and geranylgeranylcysteine in brain and liver.* J Biol Chem, 2002. 277(41): p. 38358-63.

[304] Onono, F., et al., *Efficient use of exogenous isoprenols for protein isoprenylation by MDA-MB-231 cells is regulated independently of the mevalonate pathway.* J Biol Chem, 2013. 288(38): p. 27444-55.

[305] Crick, D.C., C.J. Waechter, and D.A. Andres, *Utilization of geranylgeraniol for protein isoprenylation in C6 glial cells.* Biochem Biophys Res Commun, 1994. 205(1): p. 955-61.

[306] Ownby, S.E. and R.J. Hohl, *Isoprenoid alcohols restore protein isoprenylation in a time-dependent manner independent of protein synthesis.* Lipids, 2003. 38(7): p. 751-9.

[307] Fernandes, N.V., et al., *Geranylgeraniol suppresses the viability of human DU145 prostate carcinoma cells and the level of HMG CoA reductase.* Exp Biol Med (Maywood), 2013. 238(11): p. 1265-74.

[308] Roullet, J.B., et al., *Modulation of neuronal voltage-gated calcium channels by farnesol.* J Biol Chem, 1999. 274(36): p. 25439-46.

[309] Forman, B.M., et al., *Identification of a nuclear receptor that is activated by farnesol metabolites.* Cell, 1995. 81(5): p. 687-93.

[310] Sebti, S.M., *Protein farnesylation: implications for normal physiology, malignant transformation, and cancer therapy.* Cancer Cell, 2005. 7(4): p. 297-300.

[311] McTaggart, S.J., *Isoprenylated proteins.* Cell Mol Life Sci, 2006. 63(3): p. 255-67.

[312] Bento, C.F., et al., *The role of membrane-trafficking small GTPases in the regulation of autophagy.* J Cell Sci, 2013. 126(Pt 5): p. 1059-69.

[313] Wiemer, A.J., D.F. Wiemer, and R.J. Hohl, *Geranylgeranyl diphosphate synthase: an emerging therapeutic target.* Clin Pharmacol Ther, 2011. 90(6): p. 804-12.

[314] Lane, K.T. and L.S. Beese, *Thematic review series: lipid posttranslational modifications. Structural biology of protein farnesyltransferase and geranylgeranyltransferase type I.* J Lipid Res, 2006. 47(4): p. 681-99.

[315] Leung, K.F., R. Baron, and M.C. Seabra, *Thematic review series: lipid posttranslational modifications. geranylgeranylation of Rab GTPases.* J Lipid Res, 2006. 47(3): p. 467-75.

[316] Desnoyers, L., J.S. Anant, and M.C. Seabra, *Geranylgeranylation of Rab proteins.* Biochem Soc Trans, 1996. 24(3): p. 699-703.

[317] Wu, S.K., et al., *Structural insights into the function of the Rab GDI superfamily.* Trends Biochem Sci, 1996. 21(12): p. 472-6.

[318] Seabra, M.C., et al., *Rab geranylgeranyl transferase. A multisubunit enzyme that prenylates GTP-binding proteins terminating in Cys-X-Cys or Cys-Cys.* J Biol Chem, 1992. 267(20): p. 14497-503.

[319] Farnsworth, C.C., et al., *Rab geranylgeranyl transferase catalyzes the geranylgeranylation of adjacent cysteines in the small GTPases Rab1A, Rab3A, and Rab5A.* Proc Natl Acad Sci U S A, 1994. 91(25): p. 11963-7.

[320] Gomes, A.Q., et al., *Membrane targeting of Rab GTPases is influenced by the prenylation motif.* Mol Biol Cell, 2003. 14(5): p. 1882-99.

[321] Holstein, S.A. and R.J. Hohl, *Is there a future for prenyltransferase inhibitors in cancer therapy?* Curr Opin Pharmacol, 2012. 12(6): p. 704-9.

[322] Gelb, M.H., et al., *Therapeutic intervention based on protein prenylation and associated modifications.* Nat Chem Biol, 2006. 2(10): p. 518-28.

[323] Lebowitz, P.F., W. Du, and G.C. Prendergast, *Prenylation of RhoB is required for its cell transforming function but not its ability to activate serum response element-dependent transcription.* J Biol Chem, 1997. 272(26): p. 16093-5.

[324] Allal, C., et al., *RhoA prenylation is required for promotion of cell growth and transformation and cytoskeleton organization but not for induction of serum response element transcription.* J Biol Chem, 2000. 275(40): p. 31001-8.

[325] Miyake, M., et al., *Unfarnesylated transforming Ras mutant inhibits the Ras-signaling pathway by forming a stable Ras.Raf complex in the cytosol.* FEBS Lett, 1996. 378(1): p. 15-8.

[326] Ntantie, E., et al., *An Adenosine-Mediated Signaling Pathway Suppresses Prenylation of the GTPase Rap1B and Promotes Cell Scattering.* Science Signaling, 2013. 6(277): p. ra39-ra39.

[327] Khan, O.M., et al., *Geranylgeranyltransferase type I (GGTase-I) deficiency hyperactivates macrophages and induces erosive arthritis in mice.* J Clin Invest, 2011. 121(2): p. 628-39.

[328] Konstantinopoulos, P.A., M.V. Karamouzis, and A.G. Papavassiliou, *Post-translational modifications and regulation of the RAS superfamily of GTPases as anticancer targets.* Nat Rev Drug Discov, 2007. 6(7): p. 541-55.

[329] Li, L., et al., *Isoprenoids and Related Pharmacological Interventions: Potential Application in Alzheimer's Disease.* Mol Neurobiol, 2012.

[330] Cole, S.L. and R. Vassar, *Isoprenoids and Alzheimer's disease: a complex relationship.* Neurobiol Dis, 2006. 22(2): p. 209-22.

[331] Butterfield, D.A., E. Barone, and C. Mancuso, *Cholesterol-independent neuroprotective and neurotoxic activities of statins: perspectives for statin use in Alzheimer disease and other age-related neurodegenerative disorders.* Pharmacological research : the official journal of the Italian Pharmacological Society, 2011. 64(3): p. 180-6.

[332] van der Most, P.J., et al., *Statins: mechanisms of neuroprotection.* Prog Neurobiol, 2009. 88(1): p. 64-75.

[333] Wood, W.G., et al., *Statins and neuroprotection: a prescription to move the field forward.* Ann N Y Acad Sci, 2010. 1199: p. 69-76.

[334] Liao, J.K., *Isoprenoids as mediators of the biological effects of statins.* J Clin Invest, 2002. 110(3): p. 285-8.

[335] Luo, Z.G., et al., *Implication of geranylgeranyltransferase I in synapse formation.* Neuron, 2003. 40(4): p. 703-17.

[336] Joly, A., G. Popjak, and P.A. Edwards, *In vitro identification of a soluble protein:geranylgeranyl transferase from rat tissues.* J Biol Chem, 1991. 266(21): p. 13495-8.

[337] Zhou, X.P., et al., *TrkB-mediated activation of geranylgeranyltransferase I promotes dendritic morphogenesis.* Proc Natl Acad Sci U S A, 2008. 105(44): p. 17181-6.

[338] Li, Z., et al., *Geranylgeranyltransferase I mediates BDNF-induced synaptogenesis.* J Neurochem, 2013. 125(5): p. 698-712.

[339] Wu, K.Y., X.P. Zhou, and Z.G. Luo, *Geranylgeranyltransferase I is essential for dendritic development of cerebellar Purkinje cells.* Mol Brain, 2010. 3: p. 18.

[340] Wood, W.G., W.E. Mupsilonller, and G.P. Eckert, *Statins and Neuroprotection: Basic Pharmacology Needed.* Mol Neurobiol, 2014.

[341] Pooler, A.M., S.C. Xi, and R.J. Wurtman, *The 3-hydroxy-3-methylglutaryl co-enzyme A reductase inhibitor pravastatin enhances neurite outgrowth in hippocampal neurons.* Journal of neurochemistry, 2006. 97(3): p. 716-23.

[342] Maltese, W.A. and K.M. Sheridan, *Differentiation of neuroblastoma cells induced by an inhibitor of mevalonate synthesis: relation of neurite outgrowth and acetylcholinesterase activity to changes in cell proliferation and blocked isoprenoid synthesis.* J Cell Physiol, 1985. 125(3): p. 540-58.

[343] Fernandez-Hernando, C., Y. Suarez, and M.A. Lasuncion, *Lovastatin-induced PC-12 cell differentiation is associated with RhoA/RhoA kinase pathway inactivation.* Molecular and cellular neurosciences, 2005. 29(4): p. 591-602.

[344] Holmberg, E., et al., *Simvastatin promotes neurite outgrowth in the presence of inhibitory molecules found in central nervous system injury.* J Neurotrauma, 2006. 23(9): p. 1366-78.

[345] Schulz, J.G., et al., *HMG-CoA reductase inhibition causes neurite loss by interfering with geranylgeranylpyrophosphate synthesis.* Journal of neurochemistry, 2004. 89(1): p. 24-32.

[346] Kim, W.Y., et al., *Statins decrease dendritic arborization in rat sympathetic neurons by blocking RhoA activation.* J Neurochem, 2009. 108(4): p. 1057-71.

[347] de Chaves, E.I., et al., *Role of lipoproteins in the delivery of lipids to axons during axonal regeneration.* J Biol Chem, 1997. 272(49): p. 30766-73.

[348] Samuel, F., et al., *Inhibiting geranylgeranylation increases neurite branching and differentially activates cofilin in cell bodies and growth cones.* Mol Neurobiol, 2014. 50(1): p. 49-59.

[349] Garcia-Roman, N., et al., *Lovastatin induces apoptosis of spontaneously immortalized rat brain neuroblasts: involvement of nonsterol isoprenoid biosynthesis inhibition.* Molecular and cellular neurosciences, 2001. 17(2): p. 329-41.

[350] Saavedra, L., et al., *Internalization of beta-amyloid peptide by primary neurons in the absence of apolipoprotein E.* J Biol Chem, 2007. 282(49): p. 35722-32.

[351] Marz, P., U. Otten, and A.R. Miserez, *Statins induce differentiation and cell death in neurons and astroglia.* Glia, 2007. 55(1): p. 1-12.

[352] Bi, X.N., et al., *Inhibition of geranylgeranylation mediates the effects of 3-hydroxy-3-methylglutaryl (HMG)-CoA reductase inhibitors on microglia.* Journal of Biological Chemistry, 2004. 279(46): p. 48238-48245.

[353] Naidu, A., et al., *Secretion of apolipoprotein E by brain glia requires protein prenylation and is suppressed by statins.* Brain Res, 2002. 958(1): p. 100-11.

[354] Bliss, T.V. and G.L. Collingridge, *A synaptic model of memory: long-term potentiation in the hippocampus.* Nature, 1993. 361(6407): p. 31-9.

[355] Kotti, T., et al., *Biphasic requirement for geranylgeraniol in hippocampal long-term potentiation.* Proceedings of the National Academy of Sciences of the United States of America, 2008. 105(32): p. 11394-9.

[356] Mans, R.A., L.L. McMahon, and L. Li, *Simvastatin-mediated enhancement of long-term potentiation is driven by farnesyl-pyrophosphate depletion and inhibition of farnesylation.* Neuroscience, 2012. 202: p. 1-9.

[357] Posada-Duque, R.A., et al., *Atorvastatin requires geranylgeranyl transferase-I and Rac1 activation to exert neuronal protection and induce plasticity.* Neurochem Int, 2013. 62(4): p. 433-445.

[358] Samuel, F. and D.L. Hynds, *RHO GTPase signaling for axon extension: is prenylation important?* Molecular neurobiology, 2010. 42(2): p. 133-42.

[359] Roberts, P.J., et al., *Rho Family GTPase modification and dependence on CAAX motif-signaled posttranslational modification.* J Biol Chem, 2008. 283(37): p. 25150-63.

[360] Ramakers, G.J., *Rho proteins, mental retardation and the cellular basis of cognition.* Trends Neurosci, 2002. 25(4): p. 191-9.

[361] Tolias, K.F., J.G. Duman, and K. Um, *Control of synapse development and plasticity by Rho GTPase regulatory proteins.* Prog Neurobiol, 2011. 94(2): p. 133-48.

[362] DeGeer, J. and N. Lamarche-Vane, *Rho GTPases in neurodegeneration diseases.* Exp Cell Res, 2013. 319(15): p. 2384-94.

[363] Garcia-Mata, R., E. Boulter, and K. Burridge, *The 'invisible hand': regulation of RHO GTPases by RHOGDIs.* Nature reviews. Molecular cell biology, 2011. 12(8): p. 493-504.

[364] Medina, M.W., et al., *RHOA is a modulator of the cholesterol-lowering effects of statin.* PLoS Genet, 2012. 8(11): p. e1003058.

[365] Holstein, S.A., C.L. Wohlford-Lenane, and R.J. Hohl, *Consequences of mevalonate depletion. Differential transcriptional, translational, and post-translational up-regulation of Ras, Rap1a, RhoA, AND RhoB.* J Biol Chem, 2002. 277(12): p. 10678-82.

[366] Dimster-Denk, D., W.R. Schafer, and J. Rine, *Control of RAS mRNA level by the mevalonate pathway.* Mol Biol Cell, 1995. 6(1): p. 59-70.

[367] Stubbs, E.B., Jr. and C.L. Von Zee, *Prenylation of Rho G-proteins: a novel mechanism regulating gene expression and protein stability in human trabecular meshwork cells.* Mol Neurobiol, 2012. 46(1): p. 28-40.

[368] Laezza, C., et al., *Control of Rab5 and Rab7 expression by the isoprenoid pathway.* Biochem Biophys Res Commun, 1998. 248(3): p. 469-72.

[369] Bifulco, M., *Role of the isoprenoid pathway in ras transforming activity, cytoskeleton organization, cell proliferation and apoptosis.* Life Sci, 2005. 77(14): p. 1740-9.

[370] Holstein, S.A., C.L. Wohlford-Lenane, and R.J. Hohl, *Isoprenoids influence expression of Ras and Ras-related proteins.* Biochemistry, 2002. 41(46): p. 13698-704.

[371] Ericsson, J., et al., *Sterol regulatory element binding protein binds to a cis element in the promoter of the farnesyl diphosphate synthase gene.* Proceedings of the National Academy of Sciences of the United States of America, 1996. 93(2): p. 945-950.

[372] Fukuchi, J., et al., *Transcriptional regulation of farnesyl pyrophosphate synthase by liver X receptors.* Steroids, 2003. 68(7-8): p. 685-691.

[373] Lutz, R.J., T.M. McLain, and M. Sinensky, *Feedback inhibition of polyisoprenyl pyrophosphate synthesis from mevalonate in vitro. Implications for protein prenylation.* J Biol Chem, 1992. 267(12): p. 7983-6.

[374] Laskovics, F.M., J.M. Krafcik, and C.D. Poulter, *Prenyltransferase. Kinetic studies of the 1'-4 coupling reaction with avian liver enzyme.* J Biol Chem, 1979. 254(19): p. 9458-63.

[375] Ericsson, J., et al., *Human geranylgeranyl diphosphate synthase: isolation of the cDNA, chromosomal mapping and tissue expression.* J Lipid Res, 1998. 39(9): p. 1731-9.

[376] Shimano, H., *Sterol regulatory element-binding proteins (SREBPs): transcriptional regulators of lipid synthetic genes.* Progress in lipid research, 2001. 40(6): p. 439-52.

[377] Kavanagh, K.L., et al., *The crystal structure of human geranylgeranyl pyrophosphate synthase reveals a novel hexameric arrangement and inhibitory product binding.* J Biol Chem, 2006. 281(31): p. 22004-12.

[378] Wiemer, A.J., et al., *Digeranyl bisphosphonate inhibits geranylgeranyl pyrophosphate synthase.* Biochem Biophys Res Commun, 2007. 353(4): p. 921-5.

[379] Vicent, D., E. Maratos-Flier, and C.R. Kahn, *The branch point enzyme of the mevalonate pathway for protein prenylation is overexpressed in the ob/ob mouse and induced by adipogenesis.* Mol Cell Biol, 2000. 20(6): p. 2158-66.

[380] Biller, S.A., et al., *Isoprenoid (Phosphinylmethyl)Phosphonates as Inhibitors of Squalene Synthetase.* Journal of Medicinal Chemistry, 1988. 31(10): p. 1869-1871.

[381] James, M.J. and A.A. Kandutsch, *Regulation of hepatic dolichol synthesis by beta-hydroxy-beta-methylglutaryl coenzyme A reductase.* J Biol Chem, 1980. 255(18): p. 8618-22.

[382] Gold, P.H. and R.E. Olson, *Studies on coenzyme Q. The biosynthesis of coenzyme Q9 in rat tissue slices.* J Biol Chem, 1966. 241(15): p. 3507-16.

[383] Sinensky, M., et al., *Differential inhibitory effects of lovastatin on protein isoprenylation and sterol synthesis.* J Biol Chem, 1990. 265(32): p. 19937-41.

[384] Winter-Vann, A.M. and P.J. Casey, *Opinion - Post-prenylation-processing enzymes as new targets in oncogenesis.* Nature Reviews Cancer, 2005. 5(5): p. 405-412.

[385] Edlund, C., M. Soderberg, and K. Kristensson, *Isoprenoids in aging and neurodegeneration.* Neurochem Int, 1994. 25(1): p. 35-8.

[386] Soderberg, M., et al., *Lipid compositions of different regions of the human brain during aging.* J Neurochem, 1990. 54(2): p. 415-23.

[387] Andersson, M., et al., *Age-dependent modifications in the metabolism of mevalonate pathway lipids in rat brain.* Mech Ageing Dev, 1995. 85(1): p. 1-14.

[388] Zhang, Y., et al., *The lipid compositions of different regions of rat brain during development and aging.* Neurobiol Aging, 1996. 17(6): p. 869-75.

[389] Hooff, G.P., et al., *Modulation of cholesterol, farnesylpyrophosphate, and geranylgeranyl-pyrophosphate in neuroblastoma SH-SY5Y-APP695 cells: impact on amyloid beta-protein production.* Molecular neurobiology, 2010. 41(2-3): p. 341-50.

[390] Pedrini, S., et al., *Modulation of statin-activated shedding of Alzheimer APP ectodomain by ROCK.* PLoS Med, 2005. 2(1): p. e18.

[391] Cole, S.L., et al., *Statins cause intracellular accumulation of amyloid precursor protein, beta-secretase-cleaved fragments, and amyloid beta-peptide via an isoprenoid-dependent mechanism.* J Biol Chem, 2005. 280(19): p. 18755-70.

[392] Ostrowski, S.M., et al., *Statins Reduce Amyloid-beta Production through Inhibition of Protein Isoprenylation.* J Biol Chem, 2007. 282(37): p. 26832-44.

[393] Chauhan, N.B., G.J. Siegel, and D.L. Feinstein, *Effects of lovastatin and pravastatin on amyloid processing and inflammatory response in TgCRND8 brain.* Neurochem Res, 2004. 29(10): p. 1897-911.

[394] Jiang, S., et al., *Trafficking regulation of proteins in Alzheimer's disease.* Mol Neurodegener, 2014. 9: p. 6.

[395] Shinohara, M., et al., *Reduction of brain beta-amyloid (Abeta) by fluvastatin, a hydroxymethylglutaryl-CoA reductase inhibitor, through increase in degradation of amyloid precursor protein C-terminal fragments (APP-CTFs) and Abeta clearance.* J Biol Chem, 2010. 285(29): p. 22091-102.

[396] Parsons, R.B. and B.M. Austen, *Protein lipidation of BACE.* Biochem Soc Trans, 2005. 33(Pt 5): p. 1091-3.

[397] Parsons, R.B., et al., *Statins inhibit the dimerization of beta-secretase via both isoprenoid- and cholesterol-mediated mechanisms.* Biochem J, 2006. 399(2): p. 205-14.

[398] Urano, Y., et al., *Association of active gamma-secretase complex with lipid rafts.* J Lipid Res, 2005. 46(5): p. 904-12.

[399] Zhou, Y., et al., *Geranylgeranyl pyrophosphate stimulates gamma-secretase to increase the generation of Abeta and APP-CTFgamma.* FASEB J, 2008. 22(1): p. 47-54.

[400] Kukar, T., et al., *Diverse compounds mimic Alzheimer disease-causing mutations by augmenting Abeta42 production.* Nature medicine, 2005. 11(5): p. 545-50.

[401] Zhou, Y., et al., *Nonsteroidal anti-inflammatory drugs can lower amyloidogenic Abeta42 by inhibiting Rho.* Science, 2003. 302(5648): p. 1215-7.

[402] Selkoe, D.J. and D. Schenk, *Alzheimer's disease: molecular understanding predicts amyloid-based therapeutics.* Annu Rev Pharmacol Toxicol, 2003. 43: p. 545-84.

[403] Clippingdale, A.B., J.D. Wade, and C.J. Barrow, *The amyloid-beta peptide and its role in Alzheimer's disease.* J Pept Sci, 2001. 7(5): p. 227-49.

[404] Nathalie, P. and O. Jean-Noel, *Processing of amyloid precursor protein and amyloid peptide neurotoxicity.* Curr Alzheimer Res, 2008. 5(2): p. 92-9.

[405] Saido, T.C. and N. Iwata, *Metabolism of amyloid beta peptide and pathogenesis of Alzheimer's disease. Towards presymptomatic diagnosis, prevention and therapy.* Neuroscience research, 2006. 54(4): p. 235-53.

[406] Mawuenyega, K.G., et al., *Decreased clearance of CNS beta-amyloid in Alzheimer's disease.* Science, 2010. 330(6012): p. 1774.

[407] Tamboli, I.Y., et al., *Statins promote the degradation of extracellular amyloid {beta}-peptide by microglia via stimulation of exosome-associated insulin-degrading enzyme (IDE) secretion.* J Biol Chem, 2010. 285(48): p. 37405-14.

[408] Cheng, S., et al., *Farnesyltransferase haplodeficiency reduces neuropathology and rescues cognitive function in a mouse model of Alzheimer disease.* J Biol Chem, 2013. 288(50): p. 35952-60.

[409] Cordle, A. and G. Landreth, *3-Hydroxy-3-methylglutaryl-coenzyme A reductase inhibitors attenuate beta-amyloid-induced microglial inflammatory responses.* The Journal of neuroscience : the official journal of the Society for Neuroscience, 2005. 25(2): p. 299-307.

[410] Cordle, A., et al., *Mechanisms of statin-mediated inhibition of small G-protein function.* The Journal of Biological Chemistry, 2005. 280(40): p. 34202-9.

[411] Kidd, M., *Paired helical filaments in electron microscopy of Alzheimer's disease.* Nature, 1963. 197: p. 192-3.

[412] Iqbal, K., et al., *Tau in Alzheimer disease and related tauopathies.* Curr Alzheimer Res, 2010. 7(8): p. 656-64.

[413] Meske, V., et al., *Blockade of HMG-CoA reductase activity causes changes in microtubule-stabilizing protein tau via suppression of geranylgeranylpyrophosphate formation: implications for Alzheimer's disease.* Eur J Neurosci, 2003. 17(1): p. 93-102.

[414] Hamano, T., et al., *Pitavastatin decreases tau levels via the inactivation of Rho/ROCK.* Neurobiol Aging, 2011.

[415] Barbero-Camps, E., et al., *APP/PS1 mice overexpressing SREBP-2 exhibit combined Abeta accumulation and tau pathology underlying Alzheimer's disease.* Hum Mol Genet, 2013. 22(17): p. 3460-76.

[416] Bolognin, S., et al., *The Potential Role of Rho GTPases in Alzheimer's Disease Pathogenesis.* Mol Neurobiol, 2014.

[417] Huesa, G., et al., *Altered distribution of RhoA in Alzheimer's disease and AbetaPP overexpressing mice.* J Alzheimers Dis, 2010. 19(1): p. 37-56.

[418] Takai, Y., T. Sasaki, and T. Matozaki, *Small GTP-binding proteins.* Physiol Rev, 2001. 81(1): p. 153-208.

[419] Ng, E.L. and B.L. Tang, *Rab GTPases and their roles in brain neurons and glia.* Brain Res Rev, 2008. 58(1): p. 236-46.

[420] Ginsberg, S.D., et al., *Regional selectivity of rab5 and rab7 protein upregulation in mild cognitive impairment and Alzheimer's disease.* Journal of Alzheimer's disease : JAD, 2010. 22(2): p. 631-9.

[421] Ginsberg, S.D., et al., *Upregulation of* select rab GTPases in cholinergic basal forebrain neurons in mild cognitive impairment and Alzheimer's disease. Journal of chemical neuroanatomy, 2011.

[422] Armstrong, A., et al., Lysosomal Network Proteins as Potential Novel CSF Biomarkers for Alzheimer's Disease. Neuromolecular Med, 2014. 16(1): p. 150-60.

[423] Scheper, W., et al., Rab6 is increased in Alzheimer's disease brain and correlates with endoplasmic reticulum stress. Neuropathol Appl Neurobiol, 2007. 33(5): p. 523-32.

[424] Camargo, N., A.B. Smit, and M.H. Verheijen, SREBPs: SREBP function in glia-neuron interactions. FEBS J, 2009. 276(3): p. 628-36.

[425] Bogdanovic, N., et al., On the turnover of brain cholesterol in patients with Alzheimer's disease. Abnormal induction of the cholesterol-catabolic enzyme CYP46 in glial cells. Neurosci Lett, 2001. 314(1-2): p. 45-8.

Section 3

# Biomarkers

Chapter 8

# Recent Progress in the Identification of Non-Invasive Biomarkers to Support the Diagnosis of Alzheimer's Disease in Clinical Practice and to Assist Human Clinical Trials

Francois Bernier, Pavan Kumar, Yoshiaki Sato and Yoshiya Oda

Additional information is available at the end of the chapter

http://dx.doi.org/10.5772/60008

## 1. Introduction

Alzheimer's disease (AD) is a neurodegenerative disorder that manifests itself by progressive dementia accompanied by memory deterioration usually in elderlies and is becoming the public health crisis of the 21st century. Currently, there are an estimated 35 Million patients affected by the disease, and this number is expected to burgeon to 115 million by the year 2050 (WHO, 2012). In the United States alone, one patient is diagnosed with AD every 67 seconds according to the Alzheimer's Association website.

This situation is very alarming since Alzheimer's disease has been a graveyard for drug developers with an astonishing 99.6% of trials of potential Alzheimer's treatments aimed at preventing, curing or improving the symptoms of the disease failing or being discontinued from 2002 to 2014 [1]. Although there are FDA approved drugs available including acetylcholine esterase inhibitors (donepezil, rivastigmine, galantamine) and the NMDA receptor antagonist memantine that have been useful in temporarily alleviating short-term memory problems or improving daily functions, they are ineffective in stopping disease progression.

AD is characterized by the presence of amyloid plaques in brain and it is hypothesized that the increase levels of toxic Amyloid beta oligomers and protofibrils leads to Tau neurofibrillary tangles formation, loss of synaptic connections and selective neuronal cell death in the brain (Figure 1) and this sequence of events is referred as the amyloid cascade hypothesis [2]. The amyloid plaques are mostly composed of amyloid-beta peptides (Abeta 40-42) thought to be toxic once they self-aggregate and subsequently bind to a cell surface to disrupt neuronal signaling and cell viability [3]. It is initially thought that downstream to this event is the formation of neurofibrillary tangles composed of hyperphosphorylated Tau protein. Such hyperphosphorylation is an indicator of neuronal cell death in numerous neurodegenerative disorders or brain injuries [4, 5] indicating that both abnormal processes can take place independently [6]. Two key enzymes necessary for the cleavage of the Amyloid Precursor Protein (APP) to generate Amyloid-beta peptides are the gamma and beta-secretase. According to the amyloid cascade, it is thought that developing Inhibitors of those enzymes would prevent amyloid formation and stop disease progression. Several companies have therefore been testing such inhibitors in human trials. Unfortunately, this has proven to be harder than anticipated. While Bace1 inhibitors trials outcomes are not yet known at the time of this writing, gamma-secretase inhibitors had disappointing results in late-stage trials where worsening of cognition was observed [7]. The reason for this is not totally clear, but the fact that gamma-secretase is responsible for the cleavage of multiple substrates including NOTCH protein may have been a contributing factor.

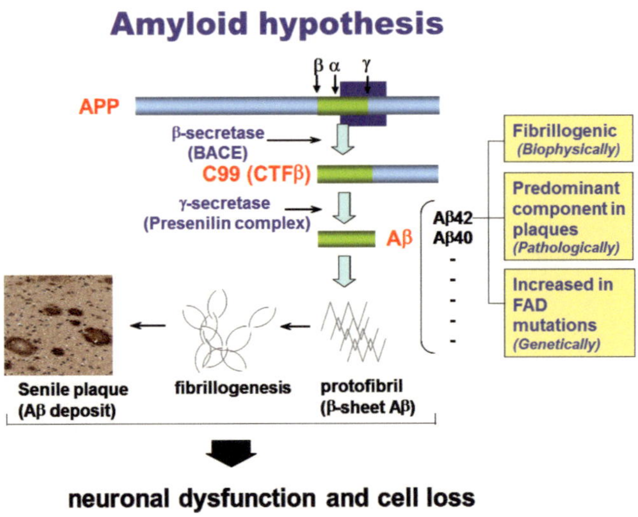


**Figure 1.** Transmembrane APP protein can be cleaved by three proteases; Beta, Alpha, and Gamma-secretase. Cleavage by B-secretase and G-secretase produces Abeta peptides (mainly 40 and 42). Aggregation of Abeta peptides into toxic oligomers and protofibrils to brain cells is a critical event prior to Abeta plaques formation and disruption of neuronal function and cellular loss.

Other clinical approaches around the amyloid cascade are focusing on passive immunization using administered human monoclonal antibodies against the amyloid-beta peptides, oligomers, protofibrils or plaques [8-10]. Several advanced phase 2 and 3 trials are still ongoing (Table 1) but at least one phase 3 trial outcome, although it did not meet its endpoints has revealed that patients with the mild form of the disease seemed to respond better to treatment [11, 12].

Based on this data, it appears that it might be too late to stop disease progression in patient with mild-to-moderate to severe AD patients with anti-amyloid therapies, so companies are now focusing their efforts on testing those drugs, including beta-secretase inhibitors, in early Mild Cognitive Impairment patients (MCI) which are known to convert to AD more rapidly, especially if patients test positive for amyloid deposition using Positron Emission Tomography scans (PET) [13, 14]. It also comes as no surprise that companies developing these new therapies are now adding being positive on amyloid PET scan as entry criteria in recent clinical trials [15] (table1). Unfortunately, the cost of amyloid PET imaging is very expensive, and PET centers are not currently available worldwide [16-18]. Even if Amyloid-PET is proven to be useful to identify a target patient population, it is important to also develop a non-invasive biomarker that could either be singly used to identify amyloid positive patients or used as a first-line test before Amyloid PET imaging confirmation.

| Drug | Trial phase | Patient population | Enriched Study population | Amyloid PET | CSF Abeta | CSF Tau | FDG-PET | VMRI |
|---|---|---|---|---|---|---|---|---|
| | | | Anti-amyloid passive immunotherapies | | | | | |
| Solanezumab | Phase 3 | mild AD | yes (Amyloid PET) | yes | yes | yes | no | yes |
| Gantenerumab | Phase 2/3 | autosomal-dominant AD | yes (Amyloid PET) | yes | yes | yes | yes | yes |
| Crenezumab | Phase 2 | mild-moderate AD | no | yes | yes | yes | yes | no |
| | | autosomal-dominant AD | yes (genetics) | yes | no | no | yes | yes |
| Ban2401 | Phase 2 | early AD | yes (Amyloid PET) | yes | yes | yes | no | yes |
| BIIB037 | Phase 1 | prodromal/mild AD | yes (Amyloid PET) | yes | no | no | no | no |
| LY3002813 | Phase 1 | mild-moderate AD | yes (Amyloid PET) | no | no | no | no | no |
| MEDI1814 | Phase 1 | mild-moderate AD | no | no | yes | no | no | no |
| | | | Bace inhibitors | | | | | |
| MK-8931 | Phase 2/3 | mild-moderate AD | no | yes | no | no | no | yes |
| | Phase 3 | prodromal AD | yes (Amyloid PET) | yes | no | no | no | yes |
| E2609 | Phase 2 | prodromal AD/mild AD | yes (Amyloid PET) | yes | yes | yes | no | no |
| JNJ-54861911 | Phase 1 | prodromal AD | yes (Amyloid PET) | yes | yes | no | no | no |
| AZD3293 | Phase 1 | mild/moderate AD | no | no | yes | no | no | no |

Source: Clinicaltrial.Gov and various press releases.

**Table 1.** Please add caption

In this book chapter, we will review the recent progress in the development of non-invasive AD biomarkers that could be used for such purpose by various research groups with a focus on AD biomarkers our group recently identified in patients' plasma.

## 2. The diagnosis of Alzheimer' Disease and the need for non-invasive markers

The disease is difficult to diagnose correctly even with the availability of cognitive tests and sophisticated Imaging technologies that include MRI, FDG-PET and Amyloid PET imaging. Currently, a diagnosis of probable AD is made using NINCDS-ADRDA criteria but this is usually possible when the condition has developed and progressed to a point where neuronal cell death and/or irreparable damages have already occurred [19]. While the accuracy of this test was thought to be around 80-90% when it was developed in the early 80's, it's accuracy, especially to diagnose patients at the early stage of the disease, is much lower which further complicates AD biomarker discovery.

The inability to correctly diagnose AD has also probably negatively affected the development of novel therapies aiming at stopping the amyloid cascade via gamma-secretase inhibitors as well passive immunization therapies using antibodies against abeta peptides or abeta plaques [7, 11]. The possible inclusion of patients suffering from non-AD dementia in those trials may have been a contributing factor to those failures.

As a result, research efforts have intensified exponentially in the recent years to identify and develop biomarkers that could be used for diagnosing AD early to support clinical practice and clinical drug development [20].

Much of these efforts have initially focus on looking at pathological changes of amyloid beta peptides, Abeta 40/42 in CSF as well as P-Tau and T-Tau and has eventually led to the development of a model that define Alzheimer's disease progression [6, 21, 22]. In that original model, gradual reduction in Abeta 42 is observed in CSF, presumably due to the aggregation of the peptide in brain and formation of plaques which is followed by gradual elevation of P-TAU and TAU in CSF, indicators of neuronal cell death or injury[23, 24]. The model was initially received with great interest because it described the temporal evolution of AD biomarkers in relation to each other and the onset and progression of clinical symptoms. However, emerging evidence appeared that challenges this model's assumptions. Refinements to the model now include indexing of individuals by the time rather than clinical symptom severity.; incorporation of inter-individual cognitive impairment variability in relation to AD pathophysiology progression; modifications to when some biomarkers changes sequentially appear; and acknowledgement that the two major proteinopathies in AD, amyloid beta (Abeta) and tau, might be initiated separately from one another in sporadic AD[6].

Although useful to assist clinical diagnosis of AD with enough sensitivity and specificity [23, 25], stiff barriers exist that prevent the comprehensive utilization of those markers by physicians and especially primary care doctors. Lumbar puncture, for example, that is required to collect CSF is still a delicate medical intervention in several developed countries and is also accompanied by increased frequency of headaches [26].The nature of the Amyloid peptides itself is also complicating the picture. Recent data have indeed shown that the Abeta 42 peptides are prone to stick to collection tubes and their detected concentration is affected by various parameters such as storage temperature, volume and thawing [27-29], probably explaining the frequent lack of correlation between labs using the same immunoassay kits.

Separately to CSF analysis, the research field has also developed a series of imaging approaches to assist clinical diagnosis such as Volumetric Magnetic Resonance Imaging (MRI) (to measure brain areas volume), FDG-PET and Amyloid PET imaging. Those are useful but currently provide only prognostic value to predict the likelihood to convert from MCI to AD [30, 31]. Amyloid PET tracers such as Pittsburgh Compound B and two new tracers, florbetapir-18 and flutemetamol-18, are approved as an *in vitro* diagnostic (IVD) but only to rule out possible AD pathology since a significant % of patients that test positive might never develop the disease [32]. Moreover, Positron Emission Tomography (PET) is very costly, and the scarcity of centers capable to handle this technology is still an issue in many countries. In UK, for example, only ~30 centers can perform this test, and the numbers are even lower in countries such as China [33]. These agents, although not reimbursed in US and other countries, are now proving useful to assist the development of novel drugs aiming to test the amyloid cascade hypothesis and are being used as enrollment criteria by several companies developing beta-secretase inhibitors as well as passive immunotherapies using anti-amyloid antibodies (Table 1). If these new therapies succeed, the availability of Amyloid-PET imaging as Companion Diagnostic (CDx) will still present the issues mentioned here as well as create additional economic burden on many healthcare systems. It is therefore accepted that having a first-line non-invasive diagnostic blood test comparable to Amyloid PET imaging would be precious in the clinical setting and could be used in tandem to diagnose patients correctly.

## 3. Recent progress in AD biomarker discoveries

### 3.1. Amyloid beta peptides and TAU in blood

Given the apparent association between Abeta accumulation and increase of P-TAU and Tau in brain and CSF of AD patients, several studies have looked at the change of Abeta 40/42 ratio in serum and plasma as non-invasive AD marker. At least 14 studies including our own that examined the change in such ratio in AD have been conducted [34] but have produced mixed results. It is not clear why such discrepancy is observed, but several factors not only related to patient's selection but also to assays themselves and how samples were stored and handled are possible explanations. It should be noted that even the Alzheimer's Disease Neuroimaging Initiative study (ADNI) data could not link Abeta40/42 plasma ratios to clinical state [35].What further complicate the use of plasma Abeta as an AD marker is the fact that it is produced not only centrally but also in the periphery and the nature itself of the peptide which tend to stick to walls and aggregate on itself affect the epitopes available during ELISA assays [34, 36].

Recently, researchers have also looked at Abeta 1-17 as a possible diagnostic marker of AD. One report showed that free-to-cell bound ratio of Abeta 1-17 could discriminate Control, MCI and AD patients with high sensitivity and specificity [37]. Additionally, plasma BACE1 enzyme, one key enzyme essential for the generation of Abeta peptides as well as soluble APP beta (sAPPbeta) have been found to be elevated in one study in AD patients plasma [38]. Despite the challenge of reliably measure Abeta 1-42 in plasma, a group demonstrated that APP669-711 appeared to be an indicator of pathological change of Abeta1-42. Ratio of APP669-711 to Abeta1-42 (APP669-711/Abeta1-42) measured by MALDI-TOF mass spectra showed a very good correlation with PIB+ signal in brain, suggesting that this plasma biomarker could be developed as a surrogate marker of cerebral amyloid deposition[39].

As for Tau and P-Tau detection in blood, demonstrating association with AD has been very challenging [40], especially for P-TAU due to the presence of circulating phosphatases in blood [24, 41] and the fact that TAU/P-TAU is elevated in multiple types of dementia including brain injuries [42]. A recent paper reporting the increase of an enzyme-generated fragment of TAU in serum that is inversely associated with cognitive function [43] seems promising. Another recently developed assay using antibodies reacting to all TAU isoforms could show with greater sensitivity than usual EIA methods the elevation of total Tau in serum of patients suffering from severe brain ischemia [44].Another group described the finding of oligomeric form of TAU in AD patients platelets [45] providing 76% sensitivity and 80% specificity. Time will tell if these TAU assays will be useful as a screening tool to support AD diagnosis.

### 3.2. Amyloid beta oligomers in blood

Amyloid beta (Aβ), especially Aβ42 oligomers play a significant role in early Alzheimer's disease (AD) pathogenesis [46, 47].In fact, AD-associated inflammation has been thought to be a secondary response to the pathological lesions triggered by Aβ oligomers in the early stage of pathogenesis. Although several studies, including our own (unpublished) have shown an elevation of such oligomers in CSF [48-52], few studies have looked at the correlation between blood oligomers concentration. In one study, levels of plasma Aβ monomers, Aβ oligomers, and soluble tumor necrosis factor $\alpha$ receptors (sTNFRs) were evaluated by ELISA in 120 controls, 32 amnestic mild cognitive impairment (aMCI) patients, and 90 mild AD patients [53]. The study found that levels of Aβ oligomers were significantly increased by ~two fold in mild AD patients compared to levels in aMCI and healthy controls. Interestingly, plasma levels of sTNFR in aMCI and mild AD patients was elevated significantly compared to controls, and both sTNFR1 and sTNFR2 levels were associated with levels of Aβ oligomers in both aMCI and mild AD individuals. Interestingly, changes in Aβ oligomer concentrations and sTNFR levels correctly differentiated mild ADfrom healthy control subjects.

In a separate study [50], another group have demonstrated that their ELISA system using BAN50 can detect signals in 60% of serum samples and 80% of CSF samples obtained from non-demented subjects.

| individual peptide/ protein (plasma,serum) | comments | reference |
|---|---|---|
| Abeta 40/42 ratio | mixed results by various group | (34) |
| Abeta 1-17 | free to bound cell ratio discriminate Control, MCI and AD | (37) |
| BACE1 enzyme, sAPPbeta | elevated in plasma | (38) |
| APP669-711/Abeta1-42 | significant correlation with brain amyloid deposition (PIB+) | (39) |
| TAU fragment | level in serum inversely correlates with cognition deline | (42) |
| multiple TAU isoforms combination | elevated in patients suffering from brain ischemia | (43) |
| Oligomeric TAU | increase levels identified in platelets | (44) |
| Abeta oligomers (serum) | higher in MCI and AD subjects, not detected in all samples | (49, 52) |
| sTNFr | higher in MCI and AD subjects | (52) |
| **proteins panels (plasma)** | | |
| 30 serum proteins combination | set of several inflammatory and vascular related markers | (54, 55) |
| | combined with clinical data | |
| 18 signalling plasma proteins combination | can differentiate AD and C, predict MCI conversion to AD | (56,57) |
| | (1 study could not reproduce this finding) | |
| Cortisol/VWF/oxidized LDL antibodies | can distinguish AD and C with 80% accuracy | (58) |
| **Lipids (plasma)** | | |
| 10 lipids combination | predicted phenoconversion from MCI to AD within 2-3 y | (61) |
| Ceramide/sphygomyelin | elevation correlates with MMSE score | (62) |
| Desmosterol/Cholesterol | decreased in MCI and AD, decrease % change in longitudinal cohorts | (66,73) |
| | correlates with rate of cognitive decline | |
| **Genes, mRNAs. miRNAs** | | |
| 96 genes signature (blood) | algorythm correctly predicts AD and discriminate Parkinson's Disease (CE mark test)) | (75) |
| 136 genes signature (blood) | algorythm identify AD patients over Controls (CE mark test) | (76) |
| 48 genes signature (blood) | identify AD patients over Controls with even more accuracy when combined with MRI | (77) |
| TOMM40 | expression in blood potentially useful to monitor AD progression/severity | (79) |
| 98-5p,885-5p,483-3p,343-3p,191-5p,7d-5p | Asian population (Serum) | (131) |
| Let-7g-5p,142-3p,15b-5p,301s-3p,545-3p,191-5p,7d-5p | Caucasian population (Plasma) | (120) |
| 7f,1285,107,103a-3p,26b-5p,26a-5p,532-5p,151a-3p,161,7d,112,5010-3p | Caucasian population (Whole blood cells) | (135) |
| miR-132,128,874,134,323-3p,382 | Caucasian population (Plasma) (MCI correlation) | (109) |
| 9,29a,29b,34a,125b,146a | Asian population (Plasma,CSF) | (158) |
| **Others** | | |
| Two retinal amyloid depositions scans | detected after oral ingestion of curcumin tracer prior to eye scan using laser | AAIC 2014 |
| | found good correlation with PIB amyloid positivity and/AV-45 | O2-05-05 |
| | ointment containing tracer applied to eye before laser scan | O3-12-01 |
| Impairment of smell detection ability | association with brain region atrophy and prediction of conversion from MCI to AD | AAIC 2014 |

**Table 2.** Summary of non-invasive AD biomarker candidates

Although the levels of serum Abeta oligomers were reported to be unexpectedly high, the authors made the suggestion that the assay could be detecting non-pathological Abeta complexes associated with serum carrier proteins. Nonetheless, they did show a significant positive correlation with the levels obtained from matched CSF samples, suggesting that this assay system might be useful to support AD diagnosis.

## 4. Emerging blood-based AD biomarkers: Reproducibility of findings difficult

Novel non-invasive AD biomarkers found in blood are emerging as being a composition of different proteins, metabolites or gene transcripts in blood cells or single analytes. In total, there are as many as 21 literature studies in recent years looking at blood-based proteins association with AD. While the studies varied in size, they all looked at more than 100 proteins and the total number of patients examined ranged from 14 to 961, the 2 largest cohorts being ADNI (566) and AIBL (961). Kiddle et al. have recently published a report where they tried to replicate the findings of those 21 studies that linked a total of 163 proteins to AD using Somalogic's SOMAscan proteomics technology. 94 of those 163 candidate AD biomarkers were assessed in a relatively large cohorts of 677 subjects [54]. Only 9 candidate protein biomarkers were actually found to be related to at least 1 AD-related phenotypes: Pancreatic prohormone, Granulocyte colony-stimulating factor, Clusterin, Complement C3, Complement C6, Insulin-like growth factor-binding protein 2, Alpha-1-antitrypsin, inter-alpha-trypsin inhibitor heavy chain H4 and C-C motif chemokine 18. The outcome of this extensive replication study illustrates well the difficulty the field has been facing when trying to confirm previous findings in different patient cohorts.

## 5. Protein panel assays in development

Various protein panel assays have been developed by several groups with the use of algorithms to predict AD correctly. This approach is based on the assumption that combining markers together will increase the power of the test to identify patients correctly. One assay, in particular, is looking at 30 serum proteins and has 80% sensitivity and 91% specificity for diagnosing AD [55].The set of proteins is composed of several inflammatory and vascular related markers and the assay, combined with clinical data, showed a correlation with neuropsychological test performance [56].

Another group identified a panel of 18 signaling plasma proteins that can differentiate AD and control with ~90% sensitivity and identify MCI patients likely to convert to AD within 2 years with 81% sensitivity [57]. However, these results could not be reproduced independently [58].Combination of 3 blood markers (cortisol, von Willebrand factor and oxidized LDL antibodies) was able to diagnose AD with 80% accuracy [59].Quantitative mass-spectrometry-based selective reaction monitoring (SRM) is also supporting the development of AD diagnostic tests [60] by using isotopic tandem mass tag (TMT) technology to evaluate specific peptides derived from selected AD-related proteins. This approach, although very sound, is more difficult that one would think. In fact, when we tried in-house a similar technique called MRM (multiple reaction monitoring), we could not replicate several AD biomarker protein candidates discovered by other groups. Intriguingly, several peptides from the same protein showed changes in opposite directions (unpublished).

## 6. Plasma lipids as non-invasive AD biomarkers

The disturbance of several lipid pathways in the brain, in particular in cholesterol biosynthesis has been associated with several brain disorders including AD [61].So it comes as a little surprise that this category of molecule changes in blood to be another rich source of potential AD biomarkers. In a recent study, 525 community-dwelling healthy participants, aged 70 and older were enrolled as part of 5 year's observation study. Over the course of the study, 74 patients developed either MCI or mild AD. Using a lipidomic approach, the authors identified and validated a set of 10 lipids from peripheral blood that predicted phenoconversion to either MCI or AD within 2-3 year period with over 90% accuracy [62]. To our knowledge, this study is the first report of blood-based marker panel that can detect preclinical AD with such accuracy although validation using other cohorts will be required before considering clinical use. As the authors pointed out, alteration of lipids found in the cell membrane may be sensitive markers of neurodegeneration in pre-clinical AD. Another study using shotgun lipidomics, compared AD with controls individuals and found a change of ceramide/sphingomyelin ratio in AD [63] and its elevation to correlate with Mini-Mental-State-Examination scores (MMSE). This small study (26 AD and 26 controls) needs to be replicated though. Interestingly, a separate group found that an increase in this ratio was associated with slower disease progression [64]. Analysis of a longitudinal cohort of AD and control samples showed that AD patients had diminished baseline levels of either phospholipids, phosphatidylcholines, sphingomyelin and sterols as opposed to controls although they could not confirm the lipid profile to be good prognostic panel for estimating the progression to AD [65].

Our group initially discovered plasma desmosterol, the precursor of cholesterol, a metabolite that was recently identified as an LXR and RORgamma agonist[66, 67], as a candidate AD plasma marker [68]. Desmosterol is an essential sterol with hormone-like activity and account for as much as 30% of all brain sterols during most species brain development [69, 70].Multiple activities of desmosterol have also been reported, and it is understood that disturbances of the cholesterol metabolism may contribute to neurodegeneration [71, 72].

In our first study, decreased levels of desmosterol were observed ($p$ value$< 0.05$, fold change$=$ 0.36) in AD plasma samples versus controls plasma as well as in CSF [68]. Other groups also reported a decrease of desmosterol in brain as well as CSF [73] in an independent study but not in plasma. The discrepancy was understood in-house after we determined that this was due to an incomplete separation of cholesterol-desmosterol peaks during Gas Chromatography (AAIC 2012 abstract). Interestingly, we also observed a decrease of desmosterol also in

MCI and in particular, more pronounced in plasma of female AD patients plasma. This change of desmosterol in contrast was not affected by ApoE4 genotype. This finding was further validated and presented recently (AAIC 2013 abstract) using two large cohorts: a commercially available Caucasian sample set and a large Asian cohort. The Caucasian sample set consisted of a total of 109 patients (Control, MCI, and AD) and the large Asian cohort (n=401, 200 C and 201 AD) were both analyzed using LCMS. Our original data showing the association between decreased desmosterol/cholesterol ratio in AD and MCI was replicated in these cohorts. Data analysis showed that desmosterol level in plasma was found to be significantly different from AD and control groups with p-values 2.3E-14 and comparable AUC of ROC curve as initially found. High correlation between plasma desmosterol level and MMSE score was observed for these two large cohorts. As for novel AD candidate markers, we believe specificity should be investigated in other dementia types in order to understand the clinical usefulness of the marker and this work is currently on-going. In addition, the longitudinal analysis revealed that plasma Desmosterol/Cholesterol ratio (DES/CHO) in AD patients shows a significant decrease at follow-up intervals. The decline in plasma DES/CHO is larger in the AD group with rapid progression than in that with slow progression and the changes in plasma DES/CHO significantly correlated with changes in MMSE score.

Altogether, this data means that plasma DES/CHO decrease in AD patients may serve as a longitudinal surrogate marker associated with cognitive decline. This data, as well as an additional longitudinal cohort data analysis, is now in press at the time of this writing[74].

Very interestingly, a minor allele of an intronic SNP within DHCR24 gene (the gene coding for the protein responsible to convert desmosterol into cholesterol) was identified in a recent ADNI study and was associated with a lower average PiB PET uptake, a first generation imaging amyloid PET agent that is used to understand amyloid deposit load in AD brain [75].It is tempting to speculate that lower desmosterol levels in the brain (reflected as well in plasma and CSF) could be directly linked to higher amyloid deposition.

In order to further understand the utility of desmosterol as an AD biomarker, we collected patients plasma samples obtained through one of our ongoing AD clinical phase 2 trial, that were either positive or negative on Amyloid Pet scans (Flurbetamol) and data analysis is now ongoing. Possible outcome of this study could help patient stratification in further trials and lead to the development of a first line test prior to conducting more expensive PET imaging scans for patients enrolment in future trials or to the development of a stand-alone *in vitro* diagnostics.

## 7. Genes, mRNA, and miRNAs

Because gene transcription and translation ultimately determine the production of proteins that regulate cells and tissue functions, several groups have been looking at molecular changes in AD vs Controls in blood components and circulating peripheral cells to identify biomarkers. Among these, one group looked at the expression of 96 different genes in blood. A whole genome analysis was conducted using oligonucleotide microarray and blood from a large clinical cohort consisting of AD patients and control healthy subjects. a. Gene analysis comparing the gene expression of 94 AD patients and 94 cognitive healthy controls was conducted, and a disease classifier algorithm developed [76].

Validation was conducted on an independent cohort consisting of 63 subjects that included 50% AD patients,40% aged-matched controls and 10% young healthy controls. The results showed the test to have an accuracy of 87% to predict AD pathology. Additionally, the algorithm also discriminated AD from Parkinson's disease in 24/27 patients (accuracy 89%).

Another group developed an alternate gene AD signature consisting of 136 different genes using 177 blood samples (90 AD patients and 87 controls) [77]. Signature validation was then later performed on a blinded independent cohort of 209 individuals (111 AD and 98 controls). Many of the genes included in the signature are found to be elevated during inflammation processes and apoptosis and have been associated with the amyloid cascade and tau pathology. In a follow-up validation study consisting of 164 patients.. This test performed relatively well and was able to identify AD patients (81.3% sensitivity) correctly and to exclude AD pathology (67.1% specificity). Both of these tests have won approval in Europe (CE Mark) as AD biomarker and are available to physicians but they still haven't been validated in large clinical cohorts such as the Alzheimer's Disease Neuroimaging Initiative (ADNI ½).

At least two other studies showed this transcriptome approach potential. In one study [78], a gene expression signature was discovered in a 156 patients cohorts consisting of AD and controls. The validation study confirmed the performance of the gene signature in a separate cohort composed of 26 AD, 26 healthy age-matched control and 118 mild MCI individuals classified as probable early AD subjects. The 48 genes signature accurately identified 70% of AD patients and when combined with MRI defined criteria, the accuracy went up to 85%.,. However, the authors indicated that these results have to be validated in other diseases or dementias.

The same group also looked at changes in gene expression in leukocytes and found alterations in blood seen mild cognitive impairment (MCI) and AD subjects indicating a peripheral response to pathology may occur very early [79].Noticeably, evidences for mitochondrial dysfunction indicated by a reduce expression of several respiratory complex I-V genes were observed, confirming changes previously seen in AD brain.

One novel single gene marker identified that is associated with AD is TOMM40 (translocase of outer mitochondrial membrane 40 homolog). The protein encoded by TOMM40 seems to transport proteins functionally to mitochondria. Risk Mutation in this gene has been found in several GWAS studies, and one group showed that its expression in blood may serve as an AD marker of disease severity and progression [80].

## 8. miRNAs

Beside the existing proteomic, metabolomics and nucleic acid based markers, small RNAs (including miRNAs) are an upcoming class of circulating biomarkers that have resulted in many new findings. miRNAs belong to the class of non-coding regulatory RNA molecules of ~22nt length that regulate gene expression post-transcriptionally by binding (in most cases) to the 3′ un-translated region (UTRs) of their targets [81-83]. It is estimated that ~5% genes in the human genome encode for miRNAs and a single miRNA can regulate multiple targets (sometimes in excess of 200) based primarily on the complementarity of the seed region (nt 2-8 of the miRNA) to target mRNA molecules [84]. MicroRNAs play regulatory roles in vital biological processes, including cell proliferation and growth, tissue differentiation, development, and cell death[85]. Interestingly, it has recently been demonstrated, that not only are miRNAs active in their cell of origin, but they can be exported/secreted out, and cause down-regulation of target mRNAs in an alternate target cell [86]. It is this unique property of miRNAs of being present in intact and functional condition in circulating biofluids including CSF, plasma, serum, urine, tears and saliva, which makes them promising biomarker candidates. They are found enclosed in membrane-bound structures (exosomes, microvesicles etc.) [87, 88], and in some cases in "free" form, protected by RNA binding proteins like NPM1, HDL [86, 89] or Argonaute2 [90, 91]. Circulating miRNA signatures have been shown to identify different tumor types [92, 93] indicate staging and progression of the disease [94] and serve as prognostic markers [95, 96]. Recently, five miRNA based diagnostic tests have been made available for clinicians to prescribe (through Rosetta Genomics and Asuragen Inc). Although the first generation of tests requires tumor biopsies, there is now significant work in progress to eliminate the need for getting biopsies, and to be able to get answers from blood, urine or other readily available circulating fluids.

Although the potential of miRNAs as diagnostic markers has been consistently demonstrated in Oncology; recent publications in other areas like neurodegenerative disorders point to their expanding role [99]. In AD, for example, miRNA profiling experiments (in brain tissue) have resulted in the identification of many disease-specific miRNAs that have been confirmed independently in two or more studies [97]. For example, hsa-miR-106, hsa-miR-153 and hsa-miR-101 have been shown to modulate APP [98-101], while BACE1 has been shown to be targeted by hsa-miRNA-29 and hsa-miR-107, linking miRNAs to regulation of amyloid production in AD brains [102]. Based on similar studies, researchers have focused on these disease-specific miRNAs to determine if differential levels are found in more-easily accessible biofluids like blood or CSF. Hsa-miR-29a/b including others was a disease-specific miRNA whose down-regulated levels in the serum of AD patients mimicked the expected down-regulation in the brain tissue [103]. This is a more disease-focused approach, where only those miRNAs that have a known link to the illness is profiled for. However, the nature of circulating fluids, which allows all organs, tissues to be potential sources of biomarkers makes a simple correlation with only diseased focus biomarkers (miRNAs, in this case) hard. There is also now a confirmed presence of a selective gating mechanism that determines a particular profile of miRNAs to be exported out (in exosomes or protein bound). This was recently demonstrated in studies that showed that secreted miRNA profiles (from culture) were not in correlation with intra-cellular profiles. This could explain why higher level of a miRNA in an affected organ is not automatically associated with an increase in its plasma level [104, 105]. Another approach, still under the umbrella of disease-relevant miRNAs looks not at the disease etiology, but broadens the net and looks for all miRNAs known to be expressed in the tissue/

organ of interest. Hence for AD for examples, miRNAs known to be enriched in neurons and synapse destruction were focused on [109-111]. As a result, miR-132 and the miR-134 family of miRNAs were discovered which showed potential for differentiation between MCI and AD, and, in fact, could also predict 1-5 years in advance of a clinical diagnosis. Potential biomarkers like these could be instrumental in identifying the population which would respond best to therapy in the future, or at least identify the correct pool of patients who are MCI for example, but would advance to AD in the absence of any treatment. On the Neurodegeneration side, some focused miRNA analysis has uncovered candidates like miR-146a and miR-155 that were found in higher levels in brain tissue extra-cellular fluid (ECF) in AD patients [112]. Along with the recent report on let-7b that is being investigated as a TLR-7 ligand [113], these recent findings point towards the potential role of inflammation, which ultimately could lead to neurodegenerative disorders.

Without limiting the miRNA profiles to either disease etiology or organ/tissue of focus, unbiased-global profiling is another approach to biomarker research. This is now especially more feasible, considering the significant technological advancements that have allowed researchers to look at thousands of biomarkers using as little as 100 ul of blood, for example. Another reason, why an unbiased approach might be appealing to certain researchers is the potential of finding novel pathways that have so far not been implicated in the disease of interest, and this is especially true for complex, heterogeneous disorders like AD, where there is still a lot of work on going in trying to understand all the biology of the disease. Of course, on the flip-side, it is often difficult to explain the biological significance and connection of the novel biomarker for the illness. The problem is more severe for miRNAs, because it is not a simple miRNA-mRNA relationship, but rather a single miRNA, and hundreds of potential mRNA targets [114-116], which makes it even harder to predict connections to disease. To put this conundrum of multiple miRNA targets into a biological context, this publication proposed [117] that usually biologically meaningful targets of miRNAs were found to be enriched in specific pathways, or a network. The first un-biased miRNA study in blood (PBMCs) was done in 2007 [106] followed by a much-cited study by Cogswell et al.[107] that identified miRNAs differentially expressed in brain and CFS of AD/matched controls. In addition to some related pathways being implicated in neuronal differentiation and actin remodeling (through targets of miR-9 and 132), novel target pathways like brain insulin signaling and oxidative stress were identified. However, the surprise finding was the lack of correlation between CSF and brain profiles, which again hinted at a particular secretion mechanism that regulated the transfer of miRNAs from the cell. In addition, differentially expressed CSF miRNAa like miR-146b (thought to be involved in immune function) were found to be decreased in AD patients, suggesting an activated immune status, potentially offering insights into the role of inflammation in the disease.

Consistent with the global profiling approach, our group had published a novel AD signature that had >95% accuracy in determining AD status from matched controls [108]. It consisted of reduced levels of 7 miRNAs (hsa-let-7d-5p, hsa-let-7g-5p, hsa-miR-15b-5p, hsa-miR-142-3p, hsa-miR-191-5p, hsa-miR-301a-3p and hsa-miR-545-3p) which was further confirmed in an independent sample-set of 20 AD and 17 NC samples, To put a biological context to the hundreds of potential miRNA target molecules, we enriched for mRNA molecules that were targeted by multiple miRNAs (at least 2) Some neurological canonical pathways identified included axonal guidance signaling, ephrin receptor signaling [109], actin cytoskeleton signaling[110], clathrin-mediated endocytosis signaling [111] and RhoA signaling [112]. These pathways, although diverse, show potential biological relationships with disease etiology [125]. Using an unbiased analysis approach, we removed the filter of neurological pathways in IPA, and got a list of pathways enriched for signature miRNA targets., A type II Diabetes Mellitus signaling canonical pathway was identified. This was interesting because there was also evidence from multiple GWAS studies indicating that SNPs in ApoE [113] Clu [114] and ABCA7 genes [115] were linked to AD biology. This was in addition to another report that linked lipid metabolism to both amyloid and tau pathology [61]. However, due to unclear outcomes after statin treatment in AD clinical trials, the role of lipid metabolism in AD pathogenesis remains to be elucidated [116]. In another global-approach driven study in serum, miRNAs were profiled from 50 AD and 50 matched control samples using next-generation sequencing [117] This was followed by a validation study using qRT-PCR in an independent cohort of 158 AD and 155 control populations. Amongst other signature miRNAs identified, miR-191-5p and let-7d-5p were identified to be down-regulated in AD patients. This was encouraging because it validated part of our miRNA signature in blood (serum) using a different profiling technology (NGS) as opposed to a hybridization-based technology (nCounter: Nanostring) used by our group. This suggested that the signature had biological relevance and was not likely a profiling or normalization artifact, which often results in little validation rates of miRNA signatures.

Having previously established that the signature miRNAs could reliably differentiate AD from a matched control population NC, we investigated if lower levels of these miRNAs could be observed at earlier stages of dementia. To address this, a new set of samples containing 27 AD, 30 MCI, and 59 NC samples was obtained. All 7signature miRNAs were confirmed to be differentially expressed between the new cohort of 27 AD and 59 NC samples (internal data, not published). In addition, these miRNAs could reliably differentiate between MCI and NC samples. Meanwhile, no significant difference was observed between MCI and AD samples. To eliminate a potential normalization bias because of our choice of normalization strategy (geometric mean of ath-159a and hsa-miR-106), the data was normalized in two additional ways. The geometric mean of hsa-miR-16-5p and ath-miR-159a was used for normalization, given previous use of hsa-miR-16 as the miRNA of choice for normalization for plasma-based miRNA profiles [118, 119]. In addition, spike-in ath-159a was used in isolation to account for the possibility that normalization with endogenous control miRNAs might prevent detection of valid and meaningful biological variation. We observed no significant change in fold-changes or p –values for AD/NC and MCI/NC confirming that the signature was robust and not sensitive to different normalization strategies. Inter-site reproducibility was also investigated and an aliquot of total RNA was tested at another site by a different operator following the described protocol. Excellent correlations were observed for all 7-miRNA signatures, demonstrating the robustness of the entire assay workflow.

It was encouraging, that the same signature set of miRNAs that could differentiate AD from NC individuals was also downregulated in MCI patients. This suggested that these signature miRNAs were potentially related to early events in the disease and could be valuable for the early identification of AD/MCI patients for potential stratification in clinical studies. However, care should be exercised in how one interpret these findings. Patients that have been diagnosed as MCI are a heterogeneous population, which can have very diverse outcomes as a result of their MCI diagnosis. Some patients continue in the MCI phase or advance to more severe MCI states while, for others, conditions might deteriorate towards dementia. While some MCI patients go on to develop dementia linked to Frontal Temporal Lobe Dementia (FTLD) or Dementia with Lewy Bodies (DLB), a majority of patients develop dementia driven by pathophysiological processes attributed to Alzheimer's with a conversion rate of ~15-20% per year [120] So it is important to follow up with more studies to understand the course of progression for the MCI population tested, and evaluate if we can predict conversion of MCI to AD (for example) using this signature set of miRNAs. In addition to the specificity of any diagnostic signature for Alzheimer's disease, determining how early in disease etiology the biomarker in question changes is also critical. Archived samples are going back years before the actual diagnosis of MCI or AD would need to be accessed and processed to understand the timing of the biomarker aberration. For a biomarker signature to be valuable for a longitudinal evaluation, it is helpful to comprehend the variation and stability of the proposed biomarker across time. We observed an average coefficient of variation between 15 and 25% for 6 out of 7 miRNAs for eight healthy individuals across samples taken from multiple 6-month visits spread over 3-4 years (unpublished). This set of data indicates that the signature miRNAs are indeed stable across time in individuals, and are therefore promising candidates to evaluate in longitudinal samples from individual patients to understand at what point, these biomarkers start to change (in Alzheimer's progression, for example).

In another global, unbiased study, researchers looked at whole blood cells from Alzheimer's and age-matched control samples to discover diagnostic miRNA signatures. They utilized a next-generation-sequencing platform for profiling the miRNAs in a discovery cohort of 48 AD and 22 unaffected control samples, while the validation was done using qRT-PCR in a larger cohort of over 200 patients comprising not only of AD patients but also patients suffering from other CNS illnesses. They achieved a 12-miRNA signature, which had an accuracy of 93% to differentiate AD from matched control samples [121] The accuracy was significantly lower (74-78%) to distinguish AD from other CNS disorders. In another study, researchers looked at profiling serum samples from 22 AD and control samples, which comprised of 18 non-inflammatory neurological disease controls (NINDCs) and eight inflammatory neurological disease controls (INDCs). Although they used an unbiased approach and did not restrict the number of miRNAs to disease-associated candidates, they only profiled the most abundantly expressed miRNAs (a panel of 192 miRNAs), and then followed up with qRT-PCR validation. MicroRNA-125b and miR-26b were found to be down-regulated in AD, and confirmed in CSF from the same patient population [122] Accuracy was determined to be 82% for differentiating between AD and NINDC cohorts. Although they had an FTD cohort (Frontotemporal Lobe Dementia), the number of patients was too small [10] to make significant conclusions about the specificity of the signature.

While there is a lot of activities, excitement, and hope for a non-invasive, specific, cost effective and quantitative biomarker for early detection of Alzheimer's, there has also been a concerning lack of concordance reported amongst individual studies trying to reproduce previous signatures for Alzheimer's (Fig. 2). This is true for miRNA signatures for other diseases as well. A number of unique, independent signatures, especially for Oncology have been reported previously [123] but most of them remained un-validated or never progressed to the clinic stage. There are several reasons for this. Throughout the process of miRNA profiling and subsequent validation, there are steps in which individual biases get introduced, which are unique to each profiling method. The choice of starting material, be it plasma, serum, whole blood cells, PBMC's, or even exosomes from the blood impact signature profiles. The extraction method is another source of variation, as evidenced by the recent retraction[124], where it was reported that Trizol based preparations were susceptible to non-uniform extraction biases depending on initial concentration of certain miRNAs (with particular GC content profiles) in the sample. Gender, ethnicity, age [125] are some other factors that are known to affect miRNA profiles. Hence if one study utilized a defined cohort of patients that were Caucasian in ethnicity, while another group tried to replicate the signature in a cohort that was mixed with Hispanic or African American patient samples, concordance between the two studies could be compromised There has also been considerable concern about presence of blood-cell derived miRNAs that are found in the plasma fraction, occurring because of hemolysis of blood cells during plasma preparation [126, 127]. Hence, subtle differences in plasma preparation methods could impact plasma signatures significantly. Platelet contamination during plasma preparation is another source of potential discordance [128]. Even in our study, we have observed center to center variation and now more work needs to be done in identifying the source of variation, be it plasma handling leading to platelet contamination from some centers, or the effect of platelet activation leading to microparticle shedding, which also could impact the miRNA signature performance.

Post sample preparation, the choice of profiling platform utilized for discovery and validation has a significant effect on miRNA levels. A study compared biases in miRNA profiling across hybridization-based array platforms and a Next Generation Sequencing (NGS) platform [129] AU-rich miRNAs were detected with higher sensitivity using NGS based platforms; while GC-rich miRNAs were preferably detected using Hybridization based array platforms. Within a NGS platform itself, biases for certain miRNAs exist, that are driven by sequence (3`nt) and secondary structure at the ligation site [130] of individual miRNAs and adapters, affecting ligase enzyme efficiency during the library construction step. What further compounds the issue is that typically after discovery using a high-throughput platform, miRNA signatures are usually validated using qPCR based methods, which adds their bias to the analysis. Stem loop RT-PCR primers, that are often the "gold standard" for miRNA detection only bind to the 3′ 8-10 nt of the miRNA in question, and hence are susceptible to stable secondary structures at the 3′ end of miRNAs that inhibit efficient primer initiation in the typical temperature range of reverse transcription (37° to 42°C). Alternatively, with the LNA (modified primers using Locked Nucleic Acid modifications to increase the Tm of smaller sized primers to accommodate size limitations of miRNAs method, polyadenylation is used to elongate the short miRNA sequence, followed by RT-qPCR detection. Due to substrate preferences and secondary structures at the 3′ end of the miRNA, certain miRNAs are better substrates than others for this first step, causing a bias. A recent analysis published in Nature captured the variability in miRNA profiling platforms [131]. They evaluated up to 12 profiling platforms using standardized sample sets. The platforms were PCR, hybridization or sequencing based. As expected, the PCR-based platforms resulted in higher sensitivity, although sometimes at a cost of accuracy and specificity. Metrics tested included reproducibility, dynamic range performance, accuracy, accuracy at lower RNA input, sensitivity, sensitivity at a lower RNA input specificity and cross assay reactivity. The lower volume metrics were designed to address applications like detection of circulating miRNAs from body fluids, where the concentrations of miRNAs are typically very small. Although differences were expected between platforms, what was surprising was the extent of discordance observed between platforms. The average validation rate between any two platforms was as low as 54%. This labors the point, that it is paramount to profile and validate using two different platforms to confirm potential signature miRNAs in order to eliminate platform artifacts. Moreover, lastly, the multiple normalization strategies that are used for circulating miRNA analysis further reduce concordance between independent studies. Because of a lack of a well-established and accepted normalization miRNA candidate (a GAPDH equivalent for miRNAs), there have been a variety of strategies utilized and have been previously reviewed [132, 133]. Each approach makes certain assumptions, and it is important to consider those when comparing different miRNA profiling studies. Given these above mentioned sources of variation, it is not surprising that multiple studies which started in 2007, where miRNAs were profiled using microarray technologies (that modified mRNA based strategies to work with the much shorter miRNAs) to today, where you have the next generation of technologies that have been built keeping miRNAs in mind, the miRNA profiles are significantly different. Furthermore, there have been constant additions/subtractions and even sequence edits to the miRBASE registry over the years, which have an impact on profiling platforms, since they have to modify probes in order to accommodate these changes. With the recent discovery and advancement in technologies to look at exosomes, another dimension of complexity has been added, where one can distinguish exosome encapsulated fractions and truly cell-free fractions, further reducing concordance between studies. Hence it is important to maintain very standard protocols, and then follow through with them till the end of the study, including multiple validations with many independent cohorts of samples taken from different centers, ethnicities and ages.

The last 3-4 years have seen the beginning of the utilization of circulating miRNAs in the neurodegenerative disorders domain, and it is still a maturing field. The potential of miRNAs to provide a cost effective, non-invasive, accurate and sensitive diagnostic assay resulting in a positive impact on patient health is undeniable, but care needs to be exercised in interpretation of these signatures in the absence of thorough validation. Furthermore, significant work detailing how these novel biomarkers tie into disease etiology is a must to increase confidence and understand the reason behind biomarker modulation due to illness or subsequent treatment.

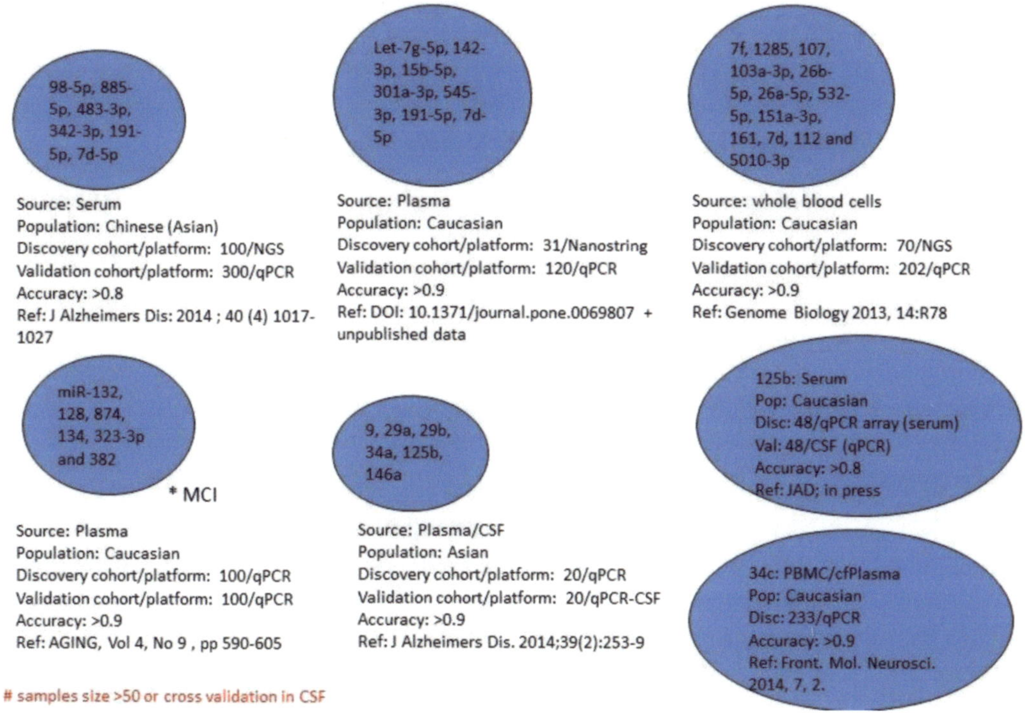


**Figure 2.** Snapshot of current circulating miRNA signatures# for Alzheimer's Disease

## 9. New non-invasive biomarkers on the horizon

Despite the promising collection of novel blood-based biomarkers as we just described, there is still a possibility to unravel additional novel non-invasive biomarkers for AD and MCI in other accessible body matrices. The human retina shares many features with the brain, including embryological origin, anatomical (ex. Microvasculature bed) and important physiological characteristics such as blood-tissue barrier [134] So researchers have looked at the possibility that the retina may offer an easily accessible and non-invasive way of examining human brain pathology. As it turned out, it is becoming evident that amyloid is also accumulating in the eyes and that this landmark event could be detected by relatively straightforward eye examinations according to data derived from multiple research trials data presented during the summer of 2014 at the Alzheimer's Association International Conference held in Copenhagen.. Data from independent studies showed that the level of beta-amyloid detected in the eye was significantly correlated with the level of beta-amyloid deposition in the brain and allowed researchers to accurately identify patients with Alzheimer's in the studies.

In the first study looking at healthy patients from the Australian Imaging, Biomarker and Lifestyle Flagship Stud Preliminary data from the first 40 participants showed that amyloid levels detected in the retina using an orally administered curcumin supplement were significantly correlated with brain amyloid levels, as shown by PiB PET imaging. In addition, Retinal Amyloid Imaging (RAI) differentiated participants with AD from those without AD with 100% sensitivity and 80.6% specificity. Furthermore, longitudinal data showed a 3.5% elevation on average in retinal amyloid signal during a 3.5-month period, suggesting that the technique may be used as a means of monitoring response to therapy.

The second separate phase 2 studies included 20 individuals with probable mild to moderate AD and 20 healthy, age-matched control participants. In this study, participants had a small proprietary molecule applied to the eye in the form of a sterile ophthalmic ointment. The compound was left to diffuse into the eye overnight and the next day the eye was scanned with the laser and results computed. As in the first study, all 40 participants also underwent PET amyloid brain imaging but this time with Amyvid PET agent. The test was capable to distinguish individuals with Alzheimer's from healthy control participants with 85% sensitivity and 95% specificity significantly and as in the first study, amyloid levels in the lens significantly correlated with PET imaging results.

Given the rapidity and simplicity of the diagnostic test (5 minutes) it is easy to understand how revolutionary this would be for the medical field as it could be used by general practitioners and specialists at point-of-care in hospitals and offices. Time will tell if it could also be used to monitor disease progression and monitor efficacy of new anti-Alzheimer's drug in development (Alzheimer's Association International Conference (AAIC) 2014. Abstracts O2-05-05 and O3-13-01).

## 10. Impairment of odor detection as early AD diagnostic

It is becoming evident that as AD sets in, impairment of the olfaction system in its ability to correctly distinguish odors appears to be an early phenomenon that could predict cognitive impairment at an early stage (AAIC 2014, in Copenhagen). In two studies, the decreased ability to identify various defined odors was significantly associated with loss of neuronal cells function and progression to Alzheimer's disease as measured by a variety of cognitive tests.

Imaging data from one study revealed that a smaller hippocampus and a thinner entorhinal cortex accompanied by higher levels of brain amyloid were linked to worsening of smell identification abilities and memory after adjusting for parameters that includes age, gender, and an estimate of cognitive reserve(AAIC 2014).

A separate study conducted at Columbia University Medical Center looked at odor Identification deficits association with Transition from Mild Cognitive Impairment to Alzheimer's. Researchers investigated a multi-ethnic sample of 1037 non-demented elderly people in New York City, (average age of 80.7) and assessed their olfaction abilities in a variety of ways at three time periods. 109 people developed dementia (101=Alzheimer's and eight non-AD dementia) a significant incapacity to correctly identify odors was found to be associated with the early development of dementia in those patients.

Although further large-scale studies will be required to confirm these results it is encouraging for the medical practice field that such relatively inexpensive test may be used one day to detect early stage of AD and those at risk of cognitive decline.

## 11. Urine

There are very few reports describing the discovery of any AD-related urine biomarker, and the few that are reported and published have met the AD research field with controversy. One of them is called NTP (Neural Thread Protein), a membrane-associated phosphoprotein that made the headlines in 2007 when a company called Nymox Corporation got an EIA kit CE approved in Europe for the diagnosis of AD using urine samples. Although Nymox claimed the utility of the test, one blinded study conducted in the Czech Republic by a reference lab using the Nymox test found that when compared to the diagnosis established by NINCDS-ADRDA for AD, the test appeared to have low sensitivity and specificity. Very recently, two studies evaluating the levels of NTP in urine were published [135, 136]. In the first study, levels of NTP in AD, PD, and Healthy participants were evaluated (AD (49, PD (20), HC (22) using Nymox AlzhemAlert test. AD patients had significantly higher levels of NTP than HC and that those of PD. Although the authors concluded that urine NTP could be used as a promising biomarker of AD, it should be noted that there was an age difference among participants that could potentially affect this interpretation. Average age for each group was as follows: AD (72.2+/-7.5), PD (66.4 +/- 8.8), Control (64.1+/-6.8).

In a second separate recent study [137], NTP levels were compared in relation to age in HC volunteers divided into 5 groups (20-29, 30-39,40-49,50-59 and >=60) using a different test called 7c Gold..It is not clear as to why the levels detected in this study are in ng/ml range as opposed to the ug/ml range for the Nymox Kit since both studies were conducted on Asian patients. The authors concluded though that urine levels of NTP increase with age significantly which might explain the controversy around NTP as an AD biomarker.

## 12. Conclusion

### 12.1. Hurdles to blood-based AD biomarker development

Replicating candidate blood biomarker findings has been the biggest challenge of the research field [138]. Several pre-analytical components factors are likely to make discoveries very challenging: choice of anticoagulant (EDTA, Heparin), addition of protease inhibitors, needle size, order of blood draw, processing time, storage condition, freeze/thaw cycles and centrifugation procedures are just a few parameters that can affect drastically the detection of several analytes [128, 138]. Longitudinal analysis from the same patient is essential to find early markers, but the success of this approach highly depends on analyte stability during >10 years storage. Blood is also a constantly changing matrix where components levels are affected by multiple factors such as diet, lifestyle, circadian changes and other co-morbidities, especially in an elderly population such as Alzheimer's Disease patients which quite frequently suffers from other diseases where inflammation is implicated such as diabetes, rheumatoid arthritis and cardiovascular diseases [139].Further complicating discoveries is the fact that several patients have mixed dementias such as Vascular Dementia, Fronto Temporal Lobe Dementia (FTLD) and Dementia with Lewy-body (DLB) making it difficult to identify a particular marker. Importantly, the integrity of the blood-brain barrier and its impact on AD-related biomarkers might differ from patient to patient based on genetics and other factors [140].Another less discussed parameter that we found that is crucial for the discovery of true AD blood biomarkers is the definition of healthy controls. We realized talking to clinical physicians in Japan, US, and EU that in many instances, healthy elderly control samples are obtained from caregivers or spouses living with the patients. This is a particular concern since epidemiological studies have demonstrated that living with an AD patient increases the risk to develop the disease by six-fold [141]. The reason is not exactly known but contributing factors such as exposure to pollutants (air, water, contaminants in food, etc) and pathogens [142, 143] by the patient and the spouse for several years living in the same environment may play a role. We also heard through interviews with clinicians that several healthy control samples are obtained from patients who went to a clinic after complaining of some abnormalities that were later ruled out as not being related to dementia. The inclusion of such patient samples in the control group category may also contribute to the difficulty of identifying a true AD biomarker.

While co-morbidities cannot be avoided when comparing AD and control groups, it is important to the research field to agree on standard practices to ensure reproducibility of data and that careful selection of healthy controls be conducted before doing any comparisons. At least, initiatives like the Blood-Based Biomarker Interest Group and the release of FDA guidelines for the analytical validation of assays that meet GCP/GLP will hopefully lead to the adoption of robust standards for the research field that applies to the analysis of proteins, metabolites, lipids and miRNAs in serum and plasma to control for precision, analytical accuracy and dilution linearity.

One more important point for the successful development and adoption of blood-based AD biomarkers is to understand the relationship with the disease as AD is essentially a brain disorder with little manifestation of illness in the peripheral system. Such understanding of the biomarker, its function, and its contribution to the illness state is essential to promote the confirmation by peers. Moreover, such clarification could lead to the discovery of even better biomarkers that could be used to detect the disease at an even earlier state or lead to the identification of novel drug targets. Such functional identification as much as the validation is critical to promote the verification of novel candidate biomarker in exploratory studies that are part of sponsored clinical trials.

In conclusion, blood tests or other non-invasive tests as biomarkers for AD are appealing as they could be applied to many uses such as patient screening, disease prognosis, diagnosis and aid to support clinical trial development. The development of such markers will be greatly facilitated once we fully understand what is causing sporadic AD in the first place and after more comprehensive studies will be able to look at correlation between endophenotypic changes in the brain using imaging technologies and the candidate biomarkers.

## Author details

Francois Bernier[1], Pavan Kumar[2], Yoshiaki Sato[1] and Yoshiya Oda[1,2*]

*Address all correspondence to: yoshiya_oda@eisai.com

1 Eisai Co., Ltd., Tokodai, Tsukuba, Ibaraki, Japan

2 Eisai IncAndover, MA, USA

## References

[1] Cummings JL, Morstorf T, Zhong K. Alzheimer's disease drug-development pipeline: few candidates, frequent failures. Alzheimers Res Ther. 2014;6(4):37.

[2] Hardy JA, Higgins GA. Alzheimer's disease: the amyloid cascade hypothesis. Science. 1992 Apr 10;256(5054):184-5.

[3] Rushworth JV, Griffiths HH, Watt NT, Hooper NM. Prion protein-mediated toxicity of amyloid-beta oligomers requires lipid rafts and the transmembrane LRP1. J Biol Chem. 2013 Mar 29;288(13):8935-51.

[4] Abisambra JF, Scheff S. Brain injury in the context of tauopathies. J Alzheimers Dis. 2014;40(3):495-518.

[5] Krstic D, Knuesel I. Deciphering the mechanism underlying late-onset Alzheimer disease. Nat Rev Neurol. 2013 Jan;9(1):25-34.

[6] Jack CR, Jr., Knopman DS, Jagust WJ, Petersen RC, Weiner MW, Aisen PS, et al. Tracking pathophysiological processes in Alzheimer's disease: an updated hypothetical model of dynamic biomarkers. Lancet Neurol. 2013 Feb;12(2):207-16.

[7] Henley DB, Sundell KL, Sethuraman G, Dowsett SA, May PC. Safety profile of semagacestat, a gamma-secretase inhibitor: IDENTITY trial findings. Curr Med Res Opin. 2014 Jul 14:1-12.

[8] Lannfelt L, Relkin NR, Siemers ER. Amyloid-ss-directed immunotherapy for Alzheimer's disease. J Intern Med. 2014 Mar;275(3):284-95.

[9] Counts SE, Lahiri DK. Editorial: Overview of Immunotherapy in Alzheimer's Disease (AD) and Mechanisms of IVIG Neuroprotection in Preclinical Models of AD. Curr Alzheimer Res. 2014;11(7):623-5.

[10] Wisniewski T, Goni F. Immunotherapy for Alzheimer's disease. Biochem Pharmacol. 2014 Apr 15;88(4):499-507.

[11] Salloway S, Sperling R, Fox NC, Blennow K, Klunk W, Raskind M, et al. Two phase 3 trials of bapineuzumab in mild-to-moderate Alzheimer's disease. N Engl J Med. 2014 Jan 23;370(4):322-33.

[12] Doody RS, Thomas RG, Farlow M, Iwatsubo T, Vellas B, Joffe S, et al. Phase 3 trials of solanezumab for mild-to-moderate Alzheimer's disease. N Engl J Med. 2014 Jan 23;370(4):311-21.

[13] Grimmer T, Wutz C, Drzezga A, Forster S, Forstl H, Ortner M, et al. The usefulness of amyloid imaging in predicting the clinical outcome after two years in subjects with mild cognitive impairment. Curr Alzheimer Res. 2013 Jan;10(1):82-5.

[14] Okello A, Koivunen J, Edison P, Archer HA, Turkheimer FE, Nagren K, et al. Conversion of amyloid positive and negative MCI to AD over 3 years: an 11C-PIB PET study. Neurology. 2009 Sep 8;73(10):754-60.

[15] Weiner MW. Commentary on "Biomarkers in Alzheimer's disease drug development." The view from Alzheimer's Disease Neuroimaging Initiative. Alzheimers Dement. 2011 May;7(3):e45-7.

[16] Mitka M. PET imaging for Alzheimer disease: are its benefits worth the cost? JAMA. 2013 Mar 20;309(11):1099-100.

[17] Lorenzi M, Donohue M, Paternico D, Scarpazza C, Ostrowitzki S, Blin O, et al. Enrichment through biomarkers in clinical trials of Alzheimer's drugs in patients with mild cognitive impairment. Neurobiol Aging. 2010 Aug;31(8):1443-51, 51 e1.

[18] High-tech scan reveals protein in the brain linked to Alzheimer's disease. A special form of PET scanning offers a more certain diagnosis for some, but at a steep out-of-pocket cost. Harv Mens Health Watch. 2014 Feb;18(7):6.

[19] McKhann G, Drachman D, Folstein M, Katzman R, Price D, Stadlan EM. Clinical diagnosis of Alzheimer's disease: report of the NINCDS-ADRDA Work Group under the auspices of Department of Health and Human Services Task Force on Alzheimer's Disease. Neurology. 1984 Jul;34(7):939-44.

[20] Tanne JH. US scientists discuss early detection and treatment of Alzheimer's disease. BMJ. 2012;344:e1068.

[21] Jack CR, Jr., Knopman DS, Jagust WJ, Shaw LM, Aisen PS, Weiner MW, et al. Hypothetical model of dynamic biomarkers of the Alzheimer's pathological cascade. Lancet Neurol. 2010 Jan;9(1):119-28.

[22] Fjell AM, Walhovd KB. Neuroimaging results impose new views on Alzheimer's disease--the role of amyloid revised. Mol Neurobiol. 2012 Feb;45(1):153-72.

[23] Blennow K. Biomarkers in Alzheimer's disease drug development. Nat Med. 2010 Nov;16(11):1218-22.

[24] Cummings JL. Biomarkers in Alzheimer's disease drug development. Alzheimers Dement. 2011 May;7(3):e13-44.

[25] Hampel H, Blennow K, Shaw LM, Hoessler YC, Zetterberg H, Trojanowski JQ. Total and phosphorylated tau protein as biological markers of Alzheimer's disease. Exp Gerontol. 2010 Jan;45(1):30-40.

[26] de Almeida SM, Shumaker SD, LeBlanc SK, Delaney P, Marquie-Beck J, Ueland S, et al. Incidence of post-dural puncture headache in research volunteers. Headache. 2011 Nov-Dec;51(10):1503-10.

[27] Schoonenboom NS, Mulder C, Vanderstichele H, Van Elk EJ, Kok A, Van Kamp GJ, et al. Effects of processing and storage conditions on amyloid beta (1-42) and tau concentrations in cerebrospinal fluid: implications for use in clinical practice. Clin Chem. 2005 Jan;51(1):189-95.

[28] Kaiser E, Schonknecht P, Thomann PA, Hunt A, Schroder J. Influence of delayed CSF storage on concentrations of phospho-tau protein (181), total tau protein and beta-amyloid (1-42). Neurosci Lett. 2007 May 1;417(2):193-5.

[29] Simonsen AH, Bahl JM, Danborg PB, Lindstrom V, Larsen SO, Grubb A, et al. Pre-analytical factors influencing the stability of cerebrospinal fluid proteins. J Neurosci Methods. 2013 May 15;215(2):234-40.

[30] Morris JC, Blennow K, Froelich L, Nordberg A, Soininen H, Waldemar G, et al. Harmonized diagnostic criteria for Alzheimer's disease: recommendations. J Intern Med. 2014 Mar;275(3):204-13.

[31] Forsberg A, Engler H, Almkvist O, Blomquist G, Hagman G, Wall A, et al. PET imaging of amyloid deposition in patients with mild cognitive impairment. Neurobiol Aging. 2008 Oct;29(10):1456-65.

[32] Yang L, Rieves D, Ganley C. Brain amyloid imaging--FDA approval of florbetapir F18 injection. N Engl J Med. 2012 Sep 6;367(10):885-7.

[33] CMS issues new instructions on PET coverage. J Nucl Med. 2014 Apr;55(4):9N-10N.

[34] Koyama A, Okereke OI, Yang T, Blacker D, Selkoe DJ, Grodstein F. Plasma amyloid-beta as a predictor of dementia and cognitive decline: a systematic review and meta-analysis. Arch Neurol. 2012 Jul;69(7):824-31.

[35] Toledo JB, Shaw LM, Trojanowski JQ. Plasma amyloid beta measurements - a desired but elusive Alzheimer's disease biomarker. Alzheimers Res Ther. 2013;5(2):8.

[36] Mehta PD, Pirttila T, Mehta SP, Sersen EA, Aisen PS, Wisniewski HM. Plasma and cerebrospinal fluid levels of amyloid beta proteins 1-40 and 1-42 in Alzheimer disease. Arch Neurol. 2000 Jan;57(1):100-5.

[37] Perez-Grijalba V, Pesini P, Allue JA, Sarasa L, Montanes M, Lacosta AM, et al. Abeta1-17 is a Major Amyloid-beta Fragment Isoform in Cerebrospinal Fluid and Blood with Possible Diagnostic Value in Alzheimer's Disease. J Alzheimers Dis. 2014 Jul 24.

[38] Wu G, Sankaranarayanan S, Wong J, Tugusheva K, Michener MS, Shi X, et al. Characterization of plasma beta-secretase (BACE1) activity and soluble amyloid precursor proteins as potential biomarkers for Alzheimer's disease. J Neurosci Res. 2012 Dec; 90(12):2247-58.

[39] Kaneko N, Nakamura A, Washimi Y, Kato T, Sakurai T, Arahata Y, et al. Novel plasma biomarker surrogating cerebral amyloid deposition. Proc Jpn Acad Ser B Phys Biol Sci. 2014;90(9):353-64.

[40] Noguchi-Shinohara M, Hamaguchi T, Nozaki I, Sakai K, Yamada M. Serum tau protein as a marker for the diagnosis of Creutzfeldt-Jakob disease. J Neurol. 2011 Aug; 258(8):1464-8.

[41] Blennow K, Hampel H, Weiner M, Zetterberg H. Cerebrospinal fluid and plasma biomarkers in Alzheimer disease. Nat Rev Neurol. 2010 Mar;6(3):131-44.

[42] Neselius S, Zetterberg H, Blennow K, Marcusson J, Brisby H. Increased CSF levels of phosphorylated neurofilament heavy protein following bout in amateur boxers. PLoS One. 2013;8(11):e81249.

[43] Neselius S, Zetterberg H, Blennow K, Randall J, Wilson D, Marcusson J, et al. Olympic boxing is associated with elevated levels of the neuronal protein tau in plasma. Brain Inj. 2013;27(4):425-33.

[44] Randall J, Mortberg E, Provuncher GK, Fournier DR, Duffy DC, Rubertsson S, et al. Tau proteins in serum predict neurological outcome after hypoxic brain injury from cardiac arrest: results of a pilot study. Resuscitation. 2013 Mar;84(3):351-6.

[45] Neumann K, Farias G, Slachevsky A, Perez P, Maccioni RB. Human platelets tau: a potential peripheral marker for Alzheimer's disease. J Alzheimers Dis. 2011;25(1): 103-9.

[46] Upadhaya AR, Lungrin I, Yamaguchi H, Fandrich M, Thal DR. High-molecular weight Abeta oligomers and protofibrils are the predominant Abeta species in the native soluble protein fraction of the AD brain. J Cell Mol Med. 2012 Feb;16(2):287-95.

[47] Yoshiike Y, Chui DH, Akagi T, Tanaka N, Takashima A. Specific compositions of amyloid-beta peptides as the determinant of toxic beta-aggregation. J Biol Chem. 2003 Jun 27;278(26):23648-55.

[48] Savage MJ, Kalinina J, Wolfe A, Tugusheva K, Korn R, Cash-Mason T, et al. A sensitive abeta oligomer assay discriminates Alzheimer's and aged control cerebrospinal fluid. J Neurosci. 2014 Feb 19;34(8):2884-97.

[49] Herskovits AZ, Locascio JJ, Peskind ER, Li G, Hyman BT. A Luminex assay detects amyloid beta oligomers in Alzheimer's disease cerebrospinal fluid. PLoS One. 2013;8(7):e67898.

[50] Kasai T, Tokuda T, Taylor M, Kondo M, Mann DM, Foulds PG, et al. Correlation of Abeta oligomer levels in matched cerebrospinal fluid and serum samples. Neurosci Lett. 2013 Sep 13;551:17-22.

[51] Funke SA. Detection of Soluble Amyloid-beta Oligomers and Insoluble High-Molecular-Weight Particles in CSF: Development of Methods with Potential for Diagnosis and Therapy Monitoring of Alzheimer's Disease. Int J Alzheimers Dis. 2011;2011:151645.

[52] Yang T, Hong S, O'Malley T, Sperling RA, Walsh DM, Selkoe DJ. New ELISAs with high specificity for soluble oligomers of amyloid beta-protein detect natural Abeta oligomers in human brain but not CSF. Alzheimers Dement. 2013 Mar;9(2):99-112.

[53] Zhang J, Peng M, Jia J. Plasma Amyloid-beta Oligomers and Soluble Tumor Necrosis Factor Receptors as Potential Biomarkers of AD. Curr Alzheimer Res. 2014 Mar 16.

[54] Kiddle SJ, Sattlecker M, Proitsi P, Simmons A, Westman E, Bazenet C, et al. Candidate blood proteome markers of Alzheimer's disease onset and progression: a systematic review and replication study. J Alzheimers Dis. 2014;38(3):515-31.

[55] O'Bryant SE, Xiao G, Barber R, Reisch J, Doody R, Fairchild T, et al. A serum protein-based algorithm for the detection of Alzheimer disease. Arch Neurol. 2010 Sep;67(9): 1077-81.

[56] O'Bryant SE, Xiao G, Barber R, Reisch J, Hall J, Cullum CM, et al. A blood-based algorithm for the detection of Alzheimer's disease. Dement Geriatr Cogn Disord. 2011;32(1):55-62.

[57] Ray S, Britschgi M, Herbert C, Takeda-Uchimura Y, Boxer A, Blennow K, et al. Classification and prediction of clinical Alzheimer's diagnosis based on plasma signaling proteins. Nat Med. 2007 Nov;13(11):1359-62.

[58] Soares HD, Chen Y, Sabbagh M, Roher A, Schrijvers E, Breteler M. Identifying early markers of Alzheimer's disease using quantitative multiplex proteomic immunoassay panels. Ann N Y Acad Sci. 2009 Oct;1180:56-67.

[59] Laske C, Leyhe T, Stransky E, Hoffmann N, Fallgatter AJ, Dietzsch J. Identification of a blood-based biomarker panel for classification of Alzheimer's disease. Int J Neuropsychopharmacol. 2011 Oct;14(9):1147-55.

[60] O'Brien D LS, Kuhn K, Shulz-Knappe P, Ward M,Byers H, Pike I, editor. Tandem mass tags and MRM mass spectrometry for the evaluation of biomarkers implicated in Alzheimer's disease. MP309 Proceedings of the 56th American Society of MAss Spectrometry conference Denver, CO; 2008.

[61] Di Paolo G, Kim TW. Linking lipids to Alzheimer's disease: cholesterol and beyond. Nat Rev Neurosci. 2011 May;12(5):284-96.

[62] Mapstone M, Cheema AK, Fiandaca MS, Zhong X, Mhyre TR, MacArthur LH, et al. Plasma phospholipids identify antecedent memory impairment in older adults. Nat Med. 2014 Apr;20(4):415-8.

[63] Han X, Rozen S, Boyle SH, Hellegers C, Cheng H, Burke JR, et al. Metabolomics in early Alzheimer's disease: identification of altered plasma sphingolipidome using shotgun lipidomics. PLoS One. 2011;6(7):e21643.

[64] Mielke MM, Haughey NJ, Bandaru VV, Weinberg DD, Darby E, Zaidi N, et al. Plasma sphingomyelins are associated with cognitive progression in Alzheimer's disease. J Alzheimers Dis. 2011;27(2):259-69.

[65] Oresic M, Hyotylainen T, Herukka SK, Sysi-Aho M, Mattila I, Seppanan-Laakso T, et al. Metabolome in progression to Alzheimer's disease. Transl Psychiatry. 2011;1:e57.

[66] Spann NJ, Garmire LX, McDonald JG, Myers DS, Milne SB, Shibata N, et al. Regulated accumulation of desmosterol integrates macrophage lipid metabolism and inflammatory responses. Cell. 2012 Sep 28;151(1):138-52.

[67] Hu X, Wang Y, Hao LY, Liu X, Lesch CA, Sanchez BM, et al. Sterol metabolism controls T(H)17 differentiation by generating endogenous RORgamma agonists. Nat Chem Biol. 2015 Feb;11(2):141-7.

[68] Sato Y, Suzuki I, Nakamura T, Bernier F, Aoshima K, Oda Y. Identification of a new plasma biomarker of Alzheimer's disease using metabolomics technology. J Lipid Res. 2012 Mar;53(3):567-76.

[69] Jansen LA. Ethical concerns relating to the detection and treatment of ovarian cancer. Gynecol Oncol. 2002 Jan;84(1):1-3.

[70] Jansen M, Wang W, Greco D, Bellenchi GC, di Porzio U, Brown AJ, et al. What dictates the accumulation of desmosterol in the developing brain? FASEB J. 2013 Mar; 27(3):865-70.

[71] Vance JE. Dysregulation of cholesterol balance in the brain: contribution to neurodegenerative diseases. Dis Model Mech. 2012 Nov;5(6):746-55.

[72] Karasinska JM, Hayden MR. Cholesterol metabolism in Huntington disease. Nat Rev Neurol. 2011 Oct;7(10):561-72.

[73] Popp J, Meichsner S, Kolsch H, Lewczuk P, Maier W, Kornhuber J, et al. Cerebral and extracerebral cholesterol metabolism and CSF markers of Alzheimer's disease. Biochem Pharmacol. 2013 Jul 1;86(1):37-42.

[74] Sato Y, Bernier F, Yamanaka Y, Aoshima K, Oda Y, Ingelsson M, et al. Reduced plasma desmosterol/cholesterol and longitudinal cognitive decline in Alzheimer's dis-

ease. Alzheimer's & Dementia: Diagnosis, Assessment & Disease Monitoring. 2014; (in press).

[75] Swaminathan S, Shen L, Risacher SL, Yoder KK, West JD, Kim S, et al. Amyloid pathway-based candidate gene analysis of [(11)C]PiB-PET in the Alzheimer's Disease Neuroimaging Initiative (ADNI) cohort. Brain Imaging Behav. 2012 Mar;6(1):1-15.

[76] Booij BB, Lindahl T, Wetterberg P, Skaane NV, Saebo S, Feten G, et al. A gene expression pattern in blood for the early detection of Alzheimer's disease. J Alzheimers Dis. 2011;23(1):109-19.

[77] Fehlbaum-Beurdeley P, Sol O, Desire L, Touchon J, Dantoine T, Vercelletto M, et al. Validation of AclarusDx, a blood-based transcriptomic signature for the diagnosis of Alzheimer's disease. J Alzheimers Dis. 2012;32(1):169-81.

[78] Lunnon K, Sattlecker M, Furney SJ, Coppola G, Simmons A, Proitsi P, et al. A blood gene expression marker of early Alzheimer's disease. J Alzheimers Dis. 2013;33(3): 737-53.

[79] Lunnon K, Ibrahim Z, Proitsi P, Lourdusamy A, Newhouse S, Sattlecker M, et al. Mitochondrial dysfunction and immune activation are detectable in early Alzheimer's disease blood. J Alzheimers Dis. 2012;30(3):685-710.

[80] Chong MS, Goh LK, Lim WS, Chan M, Tay L, Chen G, et al. Gene expression profiling of peripheral blood leukocytes shows consistent longitudinal downregulation of TOMM40 and upregulation of KIR2DL5A, PLOD1, and SLC2A8 among fast progressors in early Alzheimer's disease. J Alzheimers Dis. 2013;34(2):399-405.

[81] Zampetaki A, Willeit P, Drozdov I, Kiechl S, Mayr M. Profiling of circulating microRNAs: from single biomarkers to re-wired networks. Cardiovasc Res. 2012 Mar 15;93(4):555-62.

[82] Guo H, Ingolia NT, Weissman JS, Bartel DP. Mammalian microRNAs predominantly act to decrease target mRNA levels. Nature. 2010 Aug 12;466(7308):835-40.

[83] Filipowicz W, Bhattacharyya SN, Sonenberg N. Mechanisms of post-transcriptional regulation by microRNAs: are the answers in sight? Nat Rev Genet. 2008 Feb;9(2): 102-14.

[84] Lu M, Zhang Q, Deng M, Miao J, Guo Y, Gao W, et al. An analysis of human microRNA and disease associations. PLoS One. 2008;3(10):e3420.

[85] Esquela-Kerscher A, Slack FJ. Oncomirs - microRNAs with a role in cancer. Nat Rev Cancer. 2006 Apr;6(4):259-69.

[86] Vickers KC, Palmisano BT, Shoucri BM, Shamburek RD, Remaley AT. MicroRNAs are transported in plasma and delivered to recipient cells by high-density lipoproteins. Nat Cell Biol. 2011 Apr;13(4):423-33.

[87] Gallo A, Tandon M, Alevizos I, Illei GG. The majority of microRNAs detectable in serum and saliva is concentrated in exosomes. PLoS One. 2012;7(3):e30679.

[88] Michael A, Bajracharya SD, Yuen PS, Zhou H, Star RA, Illei GG, et al. Exosomes from human saliva as a source of microRNA biomarkers. Oral Dis. 2010 Jan;16(1):34-8.

[89] Wang D, Qiu C, Zhang H, Wang J, Cui Q, Yin Y. Human microRNA oncogenes and tumor suppressors show significantly different biological patterns: from functions to targets. PLoS One. 2010;5(9).

[90] Arroyo JD, Chevillet JR, Kroh EM, Ruf IK, Pritchard CC, Gibson DF, et al. Argonaute2 complexes carry a population of circulating microRNAs independent of vesicles in human plasma. Proc Natl Acad Sci U S A. 2011 Mar 22;108(12):5003-8.

[91] Turchinovich A, Weiz L, Langheinz A, Burwinkel B. Characterization of extracellular circulating microRNA. Nucleic Acids Res. 2011 Sep 1;39(16):7223-33.

[92] Xu J, Wu C, Che X, Wang L, Yu D, Zhang T, et al. Circulating microRNAs, miR-21, miR-122, and miR-223, in patients with hepatocellular carcinoma or chronic hepatitis. Mol Carcinog. 2011 Feb;50(2):136-42.

[93] Roth P, Wischhusen J, Happold C, Chandran PA, Hofer S, Eisele G, et al. A specific miRNA signature in the peripheral blood of glioblastoma patients. J Neurochem. 2011 Aug;118(3):449-57.

[94] Malumbres R, Sarosiek KA, Cubedo E, Ruiz JW, Jiang X, Gascoyne RD, et al. Differentiation stage-specific expression of microRNAs in B lymphocytes and diffuse large B-cell lymphomas. Blood. 2009 Apr 16;113(16):3754-64.

[95] Dong Y, Wu WK, Wu CW, Sung JJ, Yu J, Ng SS. MicroRNA dysregulation in colorectal cancer: a clinical perspective. Br J Cancer. 2011 Mar 15;104(6):893-8.

[96] Li J, Wang Y, Yu W, Chen J, Luo J. Expression of serum miR-221 in human hepatocellular carcinoma and its prognostic significance. Biochem Biophys Res Commun. 2011 Mar 4;406(1):70-3.

[97] Delay C, Hebert SS. MicroRNAs and Alzheimer's Disease Mouse Models: Current Insights and Future Research Avenues. Int J Alzheimers Dis. 2011;2011:894938.

[98] Long JM, Ray B, Lahiri DK. MicroRNA-153 physiologically inhibits expression of amyloid-beta precursor protein in cultured human fetal brain cells and is dysregulated in a subset of Alzheimer disease patients. J Biol Chem. 2012 Sep 7;287(37): 31298-310.

[99] Long JM, Lahiri DK. MicroRNA-101 downregulates Alzheimer's amyloid-beta precursor protein levels in human cell cultures and is differentially expressed. Biochem Biophys Res Commun. 2011 Jan 28;404(4):889-95.

[100] John B, Enright AJ, Aravin A, Tuschl T, Sander C, Marks DS. Human MicroRNA targets. PLoS Biol. 2004 Nov;2(11):e363.

[101] Patel N, Hoang D, Miller N, Ansaloni S, Huang Q, Rogers JT, et al. MicroRNAs can regulate human APP levels. Mol Neurodegener. 2008;3:10.

[102] Hebert SS, Horre K, Nicolai L, Papadopoulou AS, Mandemakers W, Silahtaroglu AN, et al. Loss of microRNA cluster miR-29a/b-1 in sporadic Alzheimer's disease correlates with increased BACE1/beta-secretase expression. Proc Natl Acad Sci U S A. 2008 Apr 29;105(17):6415-20.

[103] Geekiyanage H, Jicha GA, Nelson PT, Chan C. Blood serum miRNA: non-invasive biomarkers for Alzheimer's disease. Exp Neurol. 2012 Jun;235(2):491-6.

[104] Mizuno H, Nakamura A, Aoki Y, Ito N, Kishi S, Yamamoto K, et al. Identification of muscle-specific microRNAs in serum of muscular dystrophy animal models: promising novel blood-based markers for muscular dystrophy. PLoS One. 2011;6(3):e18388.

[105] Cuk K, Zucknick M, Heil J, Madhavan D, Schott S, Turchinovich A, et al. Circulating microRNAs in plasma as early detection markers for breast cancer. Int J Cancer. 2013 Apr 1;132(7):1602-12.

[106] Schipper HM, Maes OC, Chertkow HM, Wang E. MicroRNA expression in Alzheimer blood mononuclear cells. Gene Regul Syst Bio. 2007;1:263-74.

[107] Cogswell JP, Ward J, Taylor IA, Waters M, Shi Y, Cannon B, et al. Identification of miRNA changes in Alzheimer's disease brain and CSF yields putative biomarkers and insights into disease pathways. J Alzheimers Dis. 2008 May;14(1):27-41.

[108] Kumar P, Dezso Z, MacKenzie C, Oestreicher J, Agoulnik S, Byrne M, et al. Circulating miRNA biomarkers for Alzheimer's disease. PLoS One. 2013;8(7):e69807.

[109] Lin L, Lesnick TG, Maraganore DM, Isacson O. Axon guidance and synaptic maintenance: preclinical markers for neurodegenerative disease and therapeutics. Trends Neurosci. 2009 Mar;32(3):142-9.

[110] Gallo G. Tau is actin up in Alzheimer's disease. Nat Cell Biol. 2007 Feb;9(2):133-4.

[111] Wu F, Yao PJ. Clathrin-mediated endocytosis and Alzheimer's disease: an update. Ageing Res Rev. 2009 Jul;8(3):147-9.

[112] Chacon PJ, Garcia-Mejias R, Rodriguez-Tebar A. Inhibition of RhoA GTPase and the subsequent activation of PTP1B protects cultured hippocampal neurons against amyloid beta toxicity. Mol Neurodegener. 2011;6(1):14.

[113] Saunders AM, Strittmatter WJ, Schmechel D, George-Hyslop PH, Pericak-Vance MA, Joo SH, et al. Association of apolipoprotein E allele epsilon 4 with late-onset familial and sporadic Alzheimer's disease. Neurology. 1993 Aug;43(8):1467-72.

[114] Harold D, Abraham R, Hollingworth P, Sims R, Gerrish A, Hamshere ML, et al. Genome-wide association study identifies variants at CLU and PICALM associated with Alzheimer's disease. Nat Genet. 2009 Oct;41(10):1088-93.

[115] Hollingworth P, Harold D, Sims R, Gerrish A, Lambert JC, Carrasquillo MM, et al. Common variants at ABCA7, MS4A6A/MS4A4E, EPHA1, CD33 and CD2AP are associated with Alzheimer's disease. Nat Genet. 2011 May;43(5):429-35.

[116] McGuinness B, Passmore P. Can statins prevent or help treat Alzheimer's disease? J Alzheimers Dis. 2010;20(3):925-33.

[117] Tan L, Yu JT, Tan MS, Liu QY, Wang HF, Zhang W, et al. Genome-wide serum microRNA expression profiling identifies serum biomarkers for Alzheimer's disease. J Alzheimers Dis. 2014;40(4):1017-27.

[118] McDermott AM, Kerin MJ, Miller N. Identification and validation of miRNAs as endogenous controls for RQ-PCR in blood specimens for breast cancer studies. PLoS One. 2013;8(12):e83718.

[119] Chen ZH, Zhang GL, Li HR, Luo JD, Li ZX, Chen GM, et al. A panel of five circulating microRNAs as potential biomarkers for prostate cancer. Prostate. 2012 Sep 15;72(13):1443-52.

[120] Dickerson BC, Wolk DA. Biomarker-based prediction of progression in MCI: Comparison of AD signature and hippocampal volume with spinal fluid amyloid-beta and tau. Front Aging Neurosci. 2013;5:55.

[121] Leidinger P, Backes C, Deutscher S, Schmitt K, Mueller SC, Frese K, et al. A blood based 12-miRNA signature of Alzheimer disease patients. Genome Biol. 2013;14(7):R78.

[122] Galimberti D, Villa C, Fenoglio C, Serpente M, Ghezzi L, Cioffi SM, et al. Circulating miRNAs as Potential Biomarkers in Alzheimer's Disease. J Alzheimers Dis. 2014 Jul 7.

[123] Jarry J, Schadendorf D, Greenwood C, Spatz A, van Kempen LC. The validity of circulating microRNAs in oncology: five years of challenges and contradictions. Mol Oncol. 2014 Jun;8(4):819-29.

[124] Kim YK, Yeo J, Kim B, Ha M, Kim VN. Short structured RNAs with low GC content are selectively lost during extraction from a small number of cells. Mol Cell. 2012 Jun 29;46(6):893-5.

[125] Zhang X, Azhar G, Wei JY. The expression of microRNA and microRNA clusters in the aging heart. PLoS One. 2012;7(4):e34688.

[126] Kirschner MB, Edelman JJ, Kao SC, Vallely MP, van Zandwijk N, Reid G. The Impact of Hemolysis on Cell-Free microRNA Biomarkers. Front Genet. 2013;4:94.

[127] Blondal T, Jensby Nielsen S, Baker A, Andreasen D, Mouritzen P, Wrang Teilum M, et al. Assessing sample and miRNA profile quality in serum and plasma or other biofluids. Methods. 2013 Jan;59(1):S1-6.

[128] Cheng HH, Yi HS, Kim Y, Kroh EM, Chien JW, Eaton KD, et al. Plasma processing conditions substantially influence circulating microRNA biomarker levels. PLoS One. 2013;8(6):e64795.

[129] Leshkowitz D, Horn-Saban S, Parmet Y, Feldmesser E. Differences in microRNA detection levels are technology and sequence dependent. RNA. 2013 Apr;19(4):527-38.

[130] Yin S, Ho CK, Shuman S. Structure-function analysis of T4 RNA ligase 2. J Biol Chem. 2003 May 16;278(20):17601-8.

[131] Mestdagh P, Hartmann N, Baeriswyl L, Andreasen D, Bernard N, Chen C, et al. Evaluation of quantitative miRNA expression platforms in the microRNA quality control (miRQC) study. Nat Methods. 2014 Aug;11(8):809-15.

[132] Meyer SU, Pfaffl MW, Ulbrich SE. Normalization strategies for microRNA profiling experiments: a 'normal' way to a hidden layer of complexity? Biotechnol Lett. 2010 Dec;32(12):1777-88.

[133] Pradervand S, Weber J, Thomas J, Bueno M, Wirapati P, Lefort K, et al. Impact of normalization on miRNA microarray expression profiling. RNA. 2009 Mar;15(3):493-501.

[134] Ikram MK, Cheung CY, Wong TY, Chen CP. Retinal pathology as biomarker for cognitive impairment and Alzheimer's disease. J Neurol Neurosurg Psychiatry. 2012 Sep;83(9):917-22.

[135] Chen Y, Shi S, Zhang J, Gao H, Liu H, Wang J, et al. [Diagnostic value of AD7C-NTP for patients with mild cognitive impairment due to Alzheimer's disease]. Zhonghua Yi Xue Za Zhi. 2014 Jun 3;94(21):1613-7.

[136] Youn YC, Park KW, Han SH, Kim S. Urine neural thread protein measurements in Alzheimer disease. J Am Med Dir Assoc. 2011 Jun;12(5):372-6.

[137] Ma L, Chen J, Wang R, Han Y, Zhang J, Dong W, et al. Alzheimer-associated urine neuronal thread protein level increases with age in a healthy Chinese population. J Clin Neurosci. 2014 Aug 21.

[138] Watt AD, Perez KA, Rembach AR, Masters CL, Villemagne VL, Barnham KJ. Variability in blood-based amyloid-beta assays: the need for consensus on pre-analytical processing. J Alzheimers Dis. 2012;30(2):323-36.

[139] Thambisetty M, Lovestone S. Blood-based biomarkers of Alzheimer's disease: challenging but feasible. Biomark Med. 2010 Feb;4(1):65-79.

[140] Josephs KA, Petersen RC, Knopman DS, Boeve BF, Whitwell JL, Duffy JR, et al. Clinicopathologic analysis of frontotemporal and corticobasal degenerations and PSP. Neurology. 2006 Jan 10;66(1):41-8.

[141] Norton MC, Smith KR, Ostbye T, Tschanz JT, Corcoran C, Schwartz S, et al. Greater risk of dementia when spouse has dementia? The Cache County study. J Am Geriatr Soc. 2010 May;58(5):895-900.

[142] Honjo K, van Reekum R, Verhoeff NP. Alzheimer's disease and infection: do infectious agents contribute to progression of Alzheimer's disease? Alzheimers Dement. 2009 Jul;5(4):348-60.

[143] Itzhaki RF, Wozniak MA, Appelt DM, Balin BJ. Infiltration of the brain by pathogens causes Alzheimer's disease. Neurobiol Aging. 2004 May-Jun;25(5):619-27.

Chapter 9

# New Frontiers in Alzheimer's Disease Diagnosis

Franc Llorens, Sabine Nuhn, Christoph Peter,
Inga Zerr and Katharina Stoeck

Additional information is available at the end of the chapter

http://dx.doi.org/10.5772/59652

## 1. Introduction

Alzheimer´s disease (AD) is the most prevalent form of dementia accounting for 60-70% of all cases worldwide. As the world's population ages the incidence of AD is expected to increase rapidly turning into a global epidemic disease with incalculable sociological and economic consequences. In 2006, the prevalence of AD worldwide was calculated in 26.6 million and it is estimated that by 2050 current prevalence will be triplicated or quadruplicated, affecting 1 out of 85 persons worldwide [1, 2]. An accurate diagnosis and a timely detection are critical for improving the physical, clinical, emotional and financial impacts of the disease. However, this aim is far to be achieved and several studies indicate that less than 35 percentage of people living with AD or related dementias are correctly diagnosed [3, 4]. As a consequence, between 18% and 67% of the dementia patients are treated with a potentially inappropriate medication [5].

In this dramatic scenario, new technical, methodological and notional approaches are explored in order to overcome the inherent limitations in AD clinical diagnosis. Indeed, the identification of reliable diagnostic tools in AD remains impeded by the clinical, neuropathological and molecular overlap existing between AD and other types of dementia such as Mild Cognitive Impairment (MCI), or mixed forms of dementia, such as Vascular Dementia (VaD), Frontotemporal Lobar Degeneration (FTLD) or Lewy Body Dementia (LBD), and by the high AD heterogeneity according to disease onset, progression and duration [6-8].

Since the complexity of this scenario impairs the use of current diagnostic tools for a correct data interpretation, in the recent years, new strategies such as the integrated and combined use of neuropsychological profiles, imaging and biological fluids biomarkers have been developed, improving current diagnosis classification [9-11] and predicting the conversion from MCI to AD [12, 13].

Despite recent solid advances in the topic, up to date, no single diagnostic tool or combination of diagnostic tools can unequivocally confirm AD diagnosis. Indeed absolute confirmation and definite AD diagnostic still requires histopathologic analysis on the post-mortem brain certifying the presence of the pathologic disease hallmarks such as β-amyloid plaques and neurofibrillary tangles.

Since AD is a progressive disease and no treatment is available to recover neuronal integrity, the inaccuracy of AD early diagnosis and prognosis makes early therapeutic intervention difficult and impedes the prevention of neurodegeneration and cognitive dysfunction.

Identification of disease specific clinical, imaging and biochemical-based tools at early stages will help to greater extent to an early treatment which may restrain the disease progression. Additionally, a thorough understanding of the role of biomarkers in AD disease and their modulated levels in AD patients will facilitate the comprehension of their role in AD etiopathology and would help to establish a link between diagnostic and therapeutic fields. Therefore, the ultimate goal is to develop early and reliable diagnosis methods to establish an appropriate and prompt treatment. Indeed this aspect is imperative to maximize the efficiency of potential therapies and decrease symptomatology before pathological changes spread throughout the brain and massive death of neurons has already occurred. Finally, it should also be taken into consideration that the development of successful epidemiological risk assessment and diagnosis programs, including a routinely monitoring of disease progression, will need to be established through the development of new methodologies and protocols at low cost and with non-invasive approaches.

The present chapter summarizes the most recent findings in the field of AD, including neuropsychological profiles and brain and biological fluids biomarkers, which are currently paving the way for new focused approaches in AD diagnosis and prognosis.

## 2. Diagnostic criteria/Clinical and research criteria

According to the International Classification of Diseases (ICD-10) and the Diagnostic and Statistical Manual of Mental Disorders of the American Psychiatric Association (DSM IV) dementia is defined as a a worsening of cognitive function from a preexisting individual level. The major symptom is decline in memory and should be followed by at least one dysfunction in another major cognitive core skill, severe enough to impair a person's ability to perform everyday activities. The cognitive impairments should be irreversible and not be attributable to e.g. a delirium or another psychiatric disorder and must be present for at least 6 month.

Moreover, the German Society of Psychiatry, Psychotherapy and Neurology (DGPPN) as well as the German Neurological Society (DGN) refer to a subtle change in personality and behavior in the process of dementia [14]. The criteria of the American National Institute of Neurological and Communicative Disorders and Stroke/Alzheimer's disease and Related Disorders Association (NINCDS/ADRDA) are more often referred to in the literature, which differentiate the degree of diagnostic accuracy in "possible" or "probable dementia" [15, 16].

Based on the latter, commonly accepted dementia criteria, a "probable Alzheimer's dementia" (AD dementia) is diagnosed by signs of dementia on clinical examination and neuropsychological tests whereby the memory impairment should be followed by another deficit in an additional cognitive skill. In alternative there is impairment in two cognitive skills with a recognized progression and without evidence of a reduced consciousness.

The age at onset should range between 40 and 90 years and other reasons for the cognitive decline, e.g. treatable causes, should have been carefully ruled out in the diagnostic work up.

The clinical criteria of a "possible Alzheimer's dementia" comprise a dementia syndrome of untypical clinical presentation or duration in absence of other recognizable factors causative of dementia, or if there is a progressive cognitive deficit without a recognized underlying cause.

Exclusion criteria are referred to as sudden onset, focal neurological signs (hemiparesis, hemianopsia) at onset as well as early appearance of gait disorders or epileptic fits.

This categorization is kept according to different revisions of the NINCDS/ADRDA-criteria [16, 17]. Additionally, next to deficits in episodic memory, detection of specific biomarkers in the cerebrospinal fluid (CSF) and imaging (Magnetic Resonance Imaging (MRI) and/or Emission Computed Tomography (PET) is suggested which can increase sensitivity of AD diagnosis.

Further supporting results are, e.g., a progressive worsening of specific cognitive function, disabling in all-day activities, and occurrence of behavioral changes, a positive family history of AD (especially if neuropathologically confirmed), a normal CSF result (basic analysis) and unspecific electroencephalogram (EEG) changes.

A diagnosis of AD is compatible with plateaus during disease course, side symptoms as depression, aggressive behavior, paranoia etc., neurological symptoms in progressed disease state (myoclonus, gait problems, epileptic fits) and a normal Computerized Tomography (CT)-scan [14].

While both terminologies: "probable AD", "possible AD" are proposed for the clinical setting, a third category of "probable and possible AD" was suggested for research purposes. Recent research criteria for clinical AD diagnosis include next to mnestic deficits an occurrence of deficits in non-mnestic function, e.g., language, visual-spatial orientation, executive function. Furthermore, an early diagnosis of AD is proposed already during prodromal stages of dementia, which refer to the clinical picture of a mild cognitive impairment (MCI) [18].

A MCI is a recognized risk factor for AD. Yet, there are presently no commonly agreed criteria [14]. According to international consensus criteria, MCI is considered a condition between normal and demented, a worsening of cognitive function (on self-observation or observation by others) that can be demonstrated on neuropsychological tests, a worsening of cognitive function during an observational time period during disease as well as conserved or only minimally impaired dysfunction in complex all-day activities [19]. The difference between MCI and dementia is based mostly on well-functioning in all-day activities. Standard measurements for cognitive function comprise 1-1.5 standard deviation below the age- and education-matched age group and a mini-mental status test of 24 or above points [18, 20].

The prevalence and conversion rates are variable according to the distinct examination setting. In the clinical setting the annual conversion rate from MCI to AD has been calculated at around 10 percent [14, 21].

At present 4 different MCI subtypes are characterized: amnestic single domain, amnestic multiple domains, non-amnestic single domain and non-amnestic multiple domains [20], whereas the probability to develop AD is highest in MCI with memory deficits [14, 21].

## 3. Neuropsychological profiles

### 3.1. The neuropsychological profile of AD

AD is generally characterized by a slowly progressive preclinical (pre-symptomatical) state over several years, an approximately 1-2 years lasting pre-dementia phase until development of dementia, which can be categorized into 3 states (mild, medium, severe) [22, 23].

The progressive cognitive deficits hereby parallel neuropathological changes in the brain, whereby cognitive deficits vary individually. The degree of disease severeness refers to cognition and life skills, whereby transition of states can merge. A mild dementia is considered when complex tasks cannot be performed anymore, but an independent life organisation is still possible. A medium-state dementia is referred to if an independent life organisation is impaired but possible with help and observation of family and care-givers. In severe dementia constant guidance and help is required, an independent life organisation is not possible anymore.

At early stages of AD deficits are predominantly characterized by impairment of declarative memory, visual-spatial orientation and lexical-semantic language. Emotionally, in social contacts as well as in personality, patients with AD appear normal for a long period of time ("facade"). They tend to trivialize their deficits. When they recognize cognitive dysfunction, AD patients often describe themselves to be more forgetful without further specification.

*Memory impairment* (representative brain areas: hippocampus, gyrus parahippocampalis and adjusted temporomedial areas) affects the ability to encode and recapitulate novel memory contents for a longer period of time, whereas the short time memory and the working memory are mostly unaffected in early stages. The procedural memory often keeps unaffected. In the clinical setting progressive memory deficits often appear in forgetfulness of novel information, in repetitive phrases, difficulties in maintaining complex tasks (strands), e.g. forgetting where the keys/money have been stored, which can lead to paranoid reactions. Neuropsychological characterisations are a slow learning curve, rapid forgetfulness, recency-effects due to deficits in encoding, impaired and prolonged memorising, intrusions and a reduced discrimination-ability, non-profit of context cues as well as deficits in orientation in time [22].

http://dx.doi.org/10.5772/59652

In further disease progression according to a time-associated gradient (first in- last out) also long term memories (semantic and biographical memory) are impaired, with affection of identity and personality in medium and severe AD stages [23].

Deficits of the *visual-spatial orientation* (representative brain areas: parietal lobes) are often associates with important all-day activities: writing, calculating, reading the clock, getting dressed or basic orientation in space. This can overlap with memory deficits and deficits in planning skills. Firstly affected are untrained complex skills, e.g., drawing, clock drawing (mispositioning of the minute hand, confusion of hour/minute hand), reading street maps, orientation in unknown buildings, filling in documents. Drawings can show simplifications, repetitions, altered angles, "closing-in" and loss of perspective. Well established and trained skills, e.g., reading, signing a paper, getting dressed, are mainly affected in medium disease stage. A sensitive parameter that can be valuable in early AD diagnosis but also as a parameter of disease progression is clock reading as a trained skill [24, 25].

Deficits in visual-spatial orientation with massive impairment in complex visual awareness are the main characteristic and leading symptom of the *posterior cortical atrophy* (affected brain region: atrophy of the parietal and occipital lobe). The posterior cortical atrophy is a recognised variant of AD with early onset, early visual agnosia and prosopagnosia, whereas memory is less impaired in the beginning [23]. Depending on the affected projection system (occipital-parietal or occipital-temporal) problems of analysing visual-spatial information: e.g., space, depth, movement, position and orientation (dorsal visual route/"where-system") or problems in analysing of shapes/structures, colours, objects, faces and complex space-topographical scenes (ventral visual route/"what system") can occur. Both systems are tightly connected [26, 27].

Affection of *language* (affected brain region: Wernicke area) is characterized by initial difficulties in finding the right words, which is compensated by strategies of avoidance and paraphrases as well as by difficulties in naming of less frequently used objects. The patients tend to make semantic-superior and semantic-associative mistakes (dog=animal, pyramid=Egypt or also volcano=vesuvius). Syntax, articulation and prosody are unaffected.

Material that they read is less often understood, the understanding of complex facts or contents in the figurative sense (collocations) is declining. Verbal fluency is reduced, whereas the semantic is more affected than the phonematic [28]. During disease, language becomes progressively poor of content, stays however relatively fluent with difficulties in word finding as well as with imprecise, diffuse and less informative comments, drifting from topic, talking cross purposes and setting phrases. This results in abrupt sentences, mistakes of syntax, phonematic paraphrases and in problems of speech comprehension for simple comments. In the final stages a total loss of speech occurs [23].

Next to the 3 main symptoms, disturbances in *executive function* (affected brain region: prefrontal cortex) appear. Executive functions comprise: problem solving thinking, monitoring, planning and conducting of complex tasks, working memory, cognitive fluidity and flexibility. Besides a reduced word fluidity and flexibility also abilities in planning can be impaired early. Especially the so-called set-shifting abilities, that require a permanent shift in alertness, are affected at early stages [29].

*Attention* is tightly associated with executive function. This is especially required in complex tasks. Deficits in attention initially present very discretely, e.g. in dual task-questions (pre-frontal cortex, anterior cingulum).

During disease progression, also alertness is impaired which presence of a more rapid exhaustion.

During medium stages all components of attention are majorly affected [22]. Last but not least, apraxia (affected brain region: parietal lobe) and agnosia (affected brain region: occipital lobe and both basal temporal neocortex) can occur already during early and middle stages of dementia. Simple movements are not possible any longer, inaccurate moves cannot be corrected, this can present as, e.g., body-part-as object-mistakes (ideomotoric apraxia), impairment of planning and conducting of sequential tasks (ideatoric apraxia), recognition of line drawing is inhibited.

Cognitive-related *impairment of all-day activities* affects complex instrumental skills in early stages of dementia, e.g. using new instruments, filling in written documents, later on using familiar devices and basal all-day abilities deteriorate progressively.

*Psychiatric side symptoms* such as anxiety, agitation, excitability, aggressive behaviour or paranoia are not frequently present in early stages, but appear more often in middle and late stages of disease. There is a higher vulnerability for states of disorientation already in the preclinical stage, e.g. after hospital admissions, drug intolerance, malnutrition. Also depressive mood changes as well as reduction of daily activities are considered early signs [23].

*Depression* is the most frequent psychiatric side symptom and accounts for about 30% of the patients, especially during early disease stage and here from the degree of presentation rather mild. However, depression is considered a main psychiatric disease in the elderly. In general, depressed patients can articulate their symptoms more precisely; they can manage their all-day activities in a better way and demonstrate during neuropsychological testing self-doubts and complain about deficits in concentration. The mood is continuously suppressed and a lack of motivation is more exhibited.

The onset of cognitive deterioration is more distinct in patients with depression, whereas in patients with AD this occurs more gradually. The deficits can affect the whole spectrum of cognition, whereby executive dysfunction (predominantly flexibility) and problems with attention dominate. However, also memory deficits are described [30]. In detailed observation of single tasks aspects, e.g. in recalls of wordlists, primacy more than recency effects are shown, and recall is generally better.

While demented patients guess more often and describe things, depressed patients react with omissions and hesitant answers. Orientation is widely intact and confabulation, aphasic and apractic elements don't occur [22, 31].

http://dx.doi.org/10.5772/59652

### 3.2. The neuropsychological examination

Major tasks and aims of a neuropsychological examination comprise 1) determination and quantification of impaired cognitive function and resources as well as their consequences for maintaining all-day life, 2) assessment on changes of cognitive dysfunctions in progressive or reversible disease conditions, 3) differential diagnosis and securing of diagnosis as well as 4) evaluation of therapeutic benefits.

An important detail of the examination is a thorough interview with exploration of the clinical history, self-observation and observation of others, orientation, current mood situation (psychiatric side symptoms), as well as observation of behaviour during both interview and test situation. A final judgement is built from the test results with reference to emotional and motivational processes, a qualitative mistake analysis, and observation of behaviour during tests and interview, the resulting information derived from the interview and an evaluation of all-day competences during course of disease.

Neuropsychological testing represents an essential diagnostic tool in dementia diagnosis. It should be thoroughly performed and comprise the essential key competences. An "overtesting" should be avoided. In general, the choice of tests should orientate according to the individual differential diagnosis that is being questioned, the capacity of the individual patient and the time that is available.

Consecutively, a choice of test procedures is presented, that have been established in dementia diagnosis. As some of them cannot be administered solely for securing the diagnosis, a combination of several test procedures should be used.

For assessment of cognitive deficits in AD both screening methods as well as standardized psychometric tests are applied. Presumably, the most practical screening test in the clinical setting is the MMSE (Mini-Mental-State-Examination) according to Folstein et al. [32]. It comprises the examination of orientation in time and space, retentiveness and memory, attention and working memory, language (reading, writing, naming, speech comprehension, reading and meaning comprehension) as well as visual-spatial competences. The test takes usually approximately 10-12 minutes, the analysis results from a simple summation of points. At maximum 30 points can be achieved. The specificity ranges at 87 percent and the sensitivity at 82 percent [33]. However screening tests- as the mentioned MMSE- are only suitable, using cut off levels, for overviewing and determining severity of the dementia and for follow-up during disease course.

The MMSE is not acceptably sensitive in early onset dementia and does not allow, amongst other due to missing age and education correction, a satisfactory differentiation between "healthy" and "ill". For quantification of disease severity standard values of interpretation are provided, that can vary easily. Alternatively also CDR (Clinical Dementia Rating) or GDS (Global Deterioration Scale) can be applied. A general drop in points of around 3 MMSE points per year substantiates the suspected diagnosis of AD [34].

The *DemTect (Dementia Detection Test)*, likewise a screening test, focuses more precisely on Alzheimer-specific impairments with its task of word-list learning and delayed recall.

Furthermore it comprises more tasks on executive functions (working memory, word fluidity and cognitive flexibility). At maximum 18 points can be obtained. The DemTect is economic in time (8-12 minutes), it encloses a rough age correction (< 60 / ≥ 60 years) and presents with a high sensitivity for early stage AD and MCI [35].

After introduction in 1986 in the USA from the *Consortium to Establish a Registry for AD*, the newly established *CERAD test battery* has received great acceptance also in German-speaking countries. This novel neuropsychiatric testing tool has developed into a standardized dementia test procedure which aims to decipher cognitive dysfunction typical of AD [34, 36]. Analysed skills are: semantic fluidity (naming animals), naming of black and white drawings, verbal compliance and retentiveness (word list), delayed recall and recognition as well as constructive praxis (to copy something) and figural memory. The test battery also includes the MMSE. The results of a huge multicentre-validation study performed in German-speaking countries (n=1100), show that the variables: verbal fluidity, word list, memory, recall of wordlist, discrimination ability and recall of constructive praxis majorly contributed to the discriminability from healthy elderly persons to AD patients with a sensitivity of 87 percent and a specificity of 98 percent. Severe differences in profiles of AD patients, patients with vascular dementia and mixed dementia could not be obtained. A better discrimination was attained between AD patients, patients with depression and mild impairments. Both patients with depression and MCI ranged between Healthy and AD [36, 37].

To trace better on subcortical dysfunction, since 2005 additional tasks were included that aim to quantify on cognitive processing speed and flexibility (Trail making test A and B) as well as phonematic word fluidity tasks (words with initial letter "s") (CERAD-Plus). The whole test duration ranges between 30-45 minutes. The raw score are age- and education-matched (school and professional education) and also gender-matched. They are designated as z-levels as a measure of deviation to normal. The CERAD-Plus test battery allows a qualitative assessment on cognitive ability, on evaluation of disease severity and a follow up on repeated testing.

However, at present a parallel test version is not available, thus it is recommended to use an alternative test for memorising word lists when test intervals are on short-term. In suspicion of other underlying dementia causes further psychometric tests can be applied.

As an additional screening instrument for calculation of disease severity and for follow-up, the *clock-drawing test* is often recommended [38]. Next to visual-spatial abilities the test requires abilities in planning and semantic memory. The assessment includes, e.g. the integrity of the clock face, the presence of the clock hands, problems of drawing and conceptual difficulties. The sensitivity accounts for 90 percent, the specificity ranges at 56 percent. A qualitative evaluation is reasonable as well as the observation while drawing the clock face. In a qualitative feature analysis for securing the AD diagnosis in differentiation to patients with depression and healthy subjects (n=205, patients of a memory clinic) only errors occurred solely in patients with AD (with exception of one): in disorganised stereograms, only one clock-hand, mixing of numbers (1-12 with 12-24), mixing of minutes- and clock-hands, false or altered order of numbers and inability to write numbers [39].

In mind of the low specificity of the clock drawing test, Schmidtke et al. suggest an additional *clock reading test* with respect that it doesn't require higher executive function. The clock reading test is culture-, language-, education- and gender-independent, however shows a slight age-effect. It is easy to use and quickly analysable by a simple point system. Both in AD and LBD abnormalities are detected early and in comparison to healthy persons the sensitivity ranges at 82 percent, the specificity at 70 percent [24, 25].

In suspicion of an *apractic dysfunction*, a corresponding examination is informally possible, while allowing the patient to mimic easy gestures or mimic using distinct utensils (e.g. hammer, saw and scissors). As long as the patient is unable to perform the movements according to verbal request, one should allow him (to exclude problems with language comprehension) to imitate the demanded movements. For assessment of an ideatoric apraxia the patient is asked, e.g. to prepare a letter for shipment.

In order to examine *all-day competences* there are different tests available, e.g. the ADL-/ IADL-scale (Activities of Daily Living /Instrumental Activities of Daily Living), the Bayer-ADL-scale (Bayer Activities of Daily Living) or the FAQ (Functional Activities Questionnaire) which evaluate distinct functions partially very detailed. These tests are completed in general by relatives or by the interviewer [40-42]. Hereby, the FAQ has proven more sensitive compared to the IADL (85% to 57%) in the differentiation of "demented" and "normal". The specificity ranged at 81 percent [42].

Psychiatric side symptoms, e.g. *depression*, are assessed early during the neuropsychiatric interview. As needed additional depression scales can be used, e.g. the Geriatric Depression scale (GDS) or the Beck Depression Inventar (BDI), that are available also in short profile [43]. The input of depression scales depends on each situation and on the cognitive capacity of the patient. It should not lead to extend the usual time of the whole neuropsychiatric test situation.

## 4. Diagnostic imaging methods in AD

### 4.1. Computerized Tomography (CT)

Computerized Tomography (CT) is helpful in the detection of atrophy as well as other focal processes in brain and spinal cord, however it is not sufficient to substantiate AD diagnosis. Based on the low tissue contrast in comparison to magnetic resonance imgaging (MRI), CT serves well in the diagnostic classification of dementia syndromes. Advantages compared to MRI include a shorter time of investigation, low costs and a broad distribution [44]. In addition, CT allows an uncomplicated monitoring of critically ill patients.

With progressing age, brain volume decreases due to dying neurons and decline in water content. The annual atrophy rate ranges at around 0.24 % of total brain volume and is visible by the expansion of the ventricular system [45].

In AD, patients show a progressive brain atrophy in advancing disease which lies above the age matched population. This is demonstrated by enlargement of sulci and a dilatation of the ventricular system. Hereby, the dilatation of the ventricular system points to a subcortical tissue loss whereas the enlargement of the outer CSF interspaces points to cortical tissue loss [46]. The senso-motoric and the primary-visual cortex stay unaffected.

### 4.2. Magnetic Resonance Imaging (MRI)

MRI allows a high-contrast presentation of neuro-anatomical structures, pathological processes as well as of functional changes in brain activity. With progressive age a higher exchange rate of fluids exists between the ventricular system and the brain parenchyma. This is visible in T2- and Fluid-attenuated inversion recovery (FLAIR)-sequences by signal alterations in the ependyma of the anterior horns [47]. Intermittent, subcortical and central signal increases in the white matter (white-matter-lesions) increase with progressive age. Additionally brain iron accumulation can be detected in basal ganglia by increasing signal changes in T2-sequences.

Already in early AD stages MRI can display brain atrophy patterns. These can predominamtly be located in the medial temporal lobe, in the hippocampus and the gyrus parahippocampalis. Also, the entorhinal cortex, the amygdala, basal ganglia as well as thalamus and the parietal cortex can be involved [44]. An important role in the early detection of AD plays the Nucleus basalis Meynert. The voxel-based morphometry (VBM) reduces the weaknesses of predominantly investigator-dependent manual volumetry [48]. Modern computer techniques allow the spatial recognition of specific brain regions or the whole brain [49]. Hereby the volume of the typically affected brain region is exactly displayed and is comparable to that of other control groups. The majority of published studies show that patients with a MCI present with a smaller hippocampal volume than healthy controls and patients with AD have a smaller hippocampal volume in comparison to patients with MCI [50]. Patients with MCI hold an elevated risk for the development of AD [51]. Typical AD changes can also occur after brain trauma and long-lasting epilepsy.

Functional MRI (fMRI) has the potential to demonstrate cerebral blood flow as well as oxygen use of certain brain areas in response to specific stimuli or while processing certain cognitive tasks.

Due to the inherent magnetic properties of blood, represented by hemoglobin and deoxyhemoglobin, different patterns of activiation are visible [44].

Despite of the high spatial resolution, this method presents with a high sensitivity for minor head movements. Studies of AD patients show a decrease of activitiy in the hippocampus, the parahippocampal areas as well as in the parietal and pre-frontal cortex in comparison to healthy control groups. Furthermore, fMRI is useful in monitoring of medical treatment in AD patients.

### 4.3. Emission computed tomography (SPECT and PET)

Imaging via single photon emission computed tomography (SPECT) and positron emission computed tomography (PET) allows the detection of local hemodynamic and metabolic dysfunction. After intravenous injection of a radioactive tracer and uptake in brain, the tracer localizes at the region of regional acitivity and images are taken. As the tracers often have short radioactive half life, the radioactive decay (emission of positrons) can be measured.

SPECT imaging shows the regional cerebral blood flow (rCBF) at rest by the regional uptake of glucose as an expression of neuronal activity. Hereby functional abnormalities can already be detected before symptom onset. The tracers $^{99m}$Tc-HMPAO and $^{99m}$Tc-ECD are mostly used in clinical practise. Due to their lipophilic character the tracers reach the cells in the first minutes after injection proportionately to rCBF [52]. The typical SPECT image in AD is characterized by a reduced rCBF in the medial and superior temporal lobes as well as in the posterior cingulum and precuneus without a reduced striatal DAT-binding [53]. Due to a very low spatial resolution of SPECT the diagnostic accuracy is lower than PET [54]. However application can be meaningful in clinical practise in order to differentiate other dementia causes.

PET imaging illustatrates a regional dysfunction of glucose metabolism via application of $^{18}$F-FDG. Patients with AD demonstrate here, according to SPECT, a typical nuclide-distribution pattern of neuronal loss. Over 85 % of PET diagnosed AD patients could be neuropathologically verified [53]. At early AD disease stage and before symptom onset, a temporoparietal metabolic dysfunction is visible by voxel-based (volumetric pixel) analysis. Also patients with a genetic risk for development of AD show early decreases in signal activity [55]. As PET is the most efficient method for diagnostic verification of an AD, it has meanwhile established to a standard tool in dementia research [56].

For further diagnostic approaches the tracer $^{11}$C-PIB was developed, which allows detection and distribution of Aß-plaques *in vivo* [57]. Next to an efficient diagnostic procedure and early disease recognition the dimension of AD dementia can be illustrated.

## 5. Biomarkers in peripheral tissues

Biomarkers are used as indicators of normal and pathogenic processes in a broad range of tissues, especially in peripheral tissues, which facilitates the accessibility of testing samples with minimal invasive methods. Despite substantial progress has been made in the area of biomarker development to confirm the diagnosis at early-clinical AD stages, less is known about the potential role of biomarkers in peripheral tissues in the prediction of AD [58]. Since it has been demonstrated for decades the existence of biochemical changes in the brain preceding the clinical AD onset (up to 20 years in advance) [59, 60] it is suggested that these changes may be also indirectly reflected in biological fluids. However, no tests are currently available to confirm an early AD diagnosis prior to clinical or symptomatic manifestations. The ongoing standardization efforts and quality control programs in biomarkers analysis, the development of tests in fully automated instruments, the combined detection of the well-established core biomarkers, the discovery of new regulated molecules improving current sensibility and sensitivity and the analysis of novel promising biomarkers in large independent cohorts will boost biomarker´s performance and facilitate the introduction of new AD diagnosis and prognosis tests in biological fluids in clinical routine.

### 5.1. CSF

CSF is the prime target among biological fluids in the search of specific biomarkers related to neurological disorders. The easy accessibility to this biofluid and its singular biophysic-chemical characteristics make CSF ideal for biomarkers investigation. On one hand, CSF is not a very complex fluid, being composed of a restricted amount of metabolites [61], which facilitates technical screening for regulated molecules. On the other hand, the direct contact between CSF and the extracellular space of the brain puts CSF in a valuable position to be considered as a potential indicator of the pathological processes occurring in the brain during different disease stages. This last aspect has not been analysed in depth since real comparisons and correlations are cumbersome and can only be formally made when using CSF and brain tissues from the same patients and the same disease stages.

The performance of CSF biomarkers as a diagnostic tool has greatly improved in parallel with the improvement of detection methodologies such as new generation proteomic technologies and high-throughput transcriptomic methodologies (deep-sequencing, microarrays and quantitative PCR panels), which eased and expanded the possibilities to measure full expression signature in a single assay enabling the inference of networks and biological functions associated to deregulated datasets. Indeed, current data indicate the existence of deregulated levels of proteins, peptides, small RNAs, mitochondrial DNA and a broad range of metabolites in the CSF of AD samples. In addition new outcomes are expected from worldwide undergoing large longitudinal studies in very-well defined cohorts [62].

#### *5.1.1. Protein biomarkers*

In recent years, a number of reports have exploited proteomic techniques to study the levels of selected proteins and peptides in the CSF of healthy and diseased individuals. Current data indicate that proteins and peptides such as β-amyloid (Aβ1-42/Aβ42 and Aβ1-40/Aβ40), total tau and phosphorylated tau (p-tau) meet the criteria to discriminate AD from individuals suffering from other types of dementias, as well as from healthy individuals and are considered as the core AD biomarkers [63]. According to different studies these biomarkers meet the consensus recommendations on AD biomarkers that should have >80% sensitivity and >80% specificity [64]. Importantly, core AD biomarkers molecules correlate with neuropathological hallmarks of AD, such as the presence of extracellular amyloid plaques (Aβ peptides), axonal degeneration (tau protein) and neuronal tangles (p-tau).

Three main observations unveil the clinical relevance of these molecules. Firstly, their appropriate sensibility and sensitivity have been successfully validated by independent large-scale multicentre studies [65-69], although these studies also point out that biomarkers measurements present significant inter-laboratory variations [70]. Secondly, Aβ42, tau and p-tau have been validated as predictors of AD in patients with MCI [71-74]. Lastly, longitudinal studies indicate that, at least, Tau and Aβ42 in CSF reflect the underlying disease state in early clinical and late stages of AD.

#### 5.1.1.1. *Aβ peptides*

Aβ42 along with Aβ40 is secreted into the extracellular space and biological fluids, including CSF, as consequence of the proteolytic activity of proteinases on the Amyloid precursor protein (APP). Both peptides are found in senile plaques but their intracellular production, aggregation rates and proposed pathogenic functions are significantly distinct [75-77].

A consistent decrease in Aβ42 levels has been observed in the CSF of patients suffering from AD in several studies [78-80] but also in Subcortical White-matter Dementia (SWD) [81] and in Down Syndrome (DS) [82]. Reduced Aβ42 levels in AD are suggested to reflect either sequestration of Aβ42 in senile plaques, since Aβ42 CSF levels inversely correlate with the presence of senile plaques [83], or due to non-detectable Aβ42 oligomers in the assay, although alternative explanations may be plausible. In FTD, Aβ42 levels are significantly lower than in control samples, but higher than in AD cases [81, 84]. Aβ42 sensitivity and specificity in AD samples ranges from 78 to 100% (mean 85,6%) and from 67 to 100% (mean 88,5%), respectively [78]. A recent meta-analysis of 50 analytical studies indicates that CSF Aβ42 concentrations are significantly lower in AD when compared to MCI, FTD, PD and VaD but only moderately lower when compared to LBD [85].

Contrary to what is observed with Aβ42, Aβ40 and Aβ38 levels are not altered in the CSF of AD patients [79, 86, 87], but a significant decrease in Aβ40 levels is observed in FTLD when compared to AD and control cases [88]. In addition, Aβ40 levels, and more markedly Aβ38 levels, are decreased in FTD when compared to control samples [89].

A growing body of evidence suggests the superior performance of Aβ42/Aβ40 ratio when compared to Aβ42 alone using different analytic assays [79, 90, 91]. Importantly Aβ42/Aβ40 ratio is able to predict the conversion from MCI patients to AD when compared to cognitively stable MCI patients and MCI patients who developed other forms of dementia [79]. Aβ42/Aβ40 ratio is also able to discriminate better AD from VaD, LBD and non-AD dementia than Aβ42 alone and equally AD from FTD and non-AD dementia than the combination of Aβ42, p-tau and total tau [92]. Multiple studies also show an increased sensitivity and specificity in the use of Aβ ratio when compared to Aβ42/tau ratio, although the performance of combined biomarker analysis in AD diagnosis and prognosis is still a matter under discussion [93-96].

In addition to the regulated levels of monomeric Aβ species in the CSF of AD patients, encouraging observations have been reported in the potential diagnostic and prognostic role of BACE1, one of the main enzymes involved in the pathological cleave of the APP. Several independent observations indicate the presence of higher BACE1 levels and activity in the CSF of MCI and AD samples when compared to controls [97-100]. BACE1 activity is also increased in CJD samples [101] suggesting common pathological mechanisms among both diseases. Importantly, BACE1 correlate with classical AD biomarker's profile, brain atrophy in AD cases [102] and ApoE4 genotype [99], the latter being associated with an increased Aβ peptide *ex vivo* production [103]. In addition, specific BACE1 inhibitors dramatically reduce the presence of Aβ peptides in the CSF of AD patients [104] pointing out for a direct correlation between brain Aβ peptide processing and Aβ CSF levels.

#### *5.1.1.2. Aβ oligomers*

Recent studies demonstrated the presence of increased levels of Aβ oligomeric species in the CSF of AD patients when compared to controls using a broad range of methodological approaches [105-110]. Indeed, the analysis of individual Aβ oligomeric species is gaining experimental momentum due to their potential specific role in AD pathogenesis. Aβ40 oligomers levels are found to be increased in the CSF of AD patients at different disease severity stages, and a combined analysis of Aβ40 oligomers and monomeric Aβ42 greatly improved sensitivity and specificity to 95% and 90%, respectively [108]. Although the pathogenic role of Aβ40 in AD is still under discussion Aβ40 deposits have been reported both in control and AD brains [111, 112]. Aβ40-positive senile plaques with amyloid core are frequently associated with microglia in contrast to Aβ42-positive plaques [111], suggesting a role of microglia in the generation and aggregation of Aβ40 species in diseased brain. However, the different ability of Aβ fibrils and oligomers to react with microglia suggests a more complex scenario [113].

Aβ42 oligomers are increased in the CSF of AD patients [114] and the ratio of Aβ oligomers to Aβ42 is significantly elevated in AD patients [115]. Interestingly, the increased levels of Aβ42 oligomers in the CSF of MCI and AD samples may explain decreased levels of monomeric Aβ42. The recent development of the protein misfolding cyclic amplification assay (PMCA), based on the seeding activity of Aβ oligomers catalysing the polymerization of the monomeric Aβ, permits the discrimination of AD samples from other neurodegenerative non-degenerative neurological diseases with a sensitivity of 90% and specificity of 92% [109]. The use of Aβ-PMCA as a prognostic tool for detection of MCI still needs to be established. Importantly, detection of Aβ oligomers in the CSF is highly dependent on the native or disaggregated state of these oligomers [114, 116].

The finding that regulated levels of Aβ oligomer species are present in the CSF of AD patients' biofluids has a tremendous translational interest, since growing evidences indicate that soluble Aβ oligomers rather than aggregated Aβ plaques are more likely to be the main pathogenic agents of disease [117-119]. Consequently, preliminary data indicate that the analysis of Aβ oligomers, combined with levels of soluble Aβ peptides, may be relevant disease predictors and valuable tools for the analysis of AD progression.

#### *5.1.1.3. Tau*

The levels of total tau in the CSF, contrary to Aβ42 levels, increase with age [120]. Increments in tau levels have also been described in the CSF of AD and MCI patients in a broad range of several studies [121, 122] ranging from moderate to severe depending on the methodology and cohort used [78]. It is believed that deregulated tau may be reflecting the neuronal and axonal damage present in brain tissue and, as a consequence, the presence of increased tau levels is not a specific event for AD. Accordingly, transient tau increments have been also reported in acute stroke [123], and the most increased tau levels are observed in prion diseases such as in CJD, where massive neuronal cell death is present [124, 125]. Higher CSF tau is also associated with smaller brain volume in individuals with AD [126]. On the other hand, neurological diseases with minor neuronal loss and other dementias such as VaD, LBD and alcoholic dementia reflect minor or no significant changes in the levels of tau protein in the CSF, and tauopathies such as FTD also present inconsistent data [121, 127, 128].

A meta-analysis from different studies comparing tau levels in different dementia samples found that, although tau levels in AD are significantly increased when compared to controls, tau concentrations are moderately elevated in LBD, FTLD and VaD impeding a clear stratification between disease groups. Nevertheless, tau levels are useful to differentiate VaD from stroke [129] and, as expected, only CJD is characterized by extremely increased tau values, resulting in a sensitivity and specificity over 90% [130].

The improved performance of tau when analysed together with other AD biomarkers has been widely demonstrated [131, 132]. The combined use of Aβ42 and tau discriminates better between controls and AD and is very useful to predict MCI progression [69, 133]. A recent study also showed that decreased Aβ42 and increased tau levels are able to discriminate LBD from PD patients in spite of both being synucleopathies [134]. In the same line of evidences, combination of α-synuclein levels and Aβ42/tau ratios improves the diagnostic accuracy of PD [135].

A broad range of studies also demonstrated the helpfulness of the combined analysis of tau with non-AD core biomarkers. Assessment of tau and neuronal thread protein raises specificity and sensitivity for AD when compared to the individual analysis of both proteins [136]. Similarly, integrated analysis of tau and the regional cerebral blood flow in the posterior cingulate cortex discriminates MCI progressing to AD from non-progressive MCI [137]. The combined analysis of tau is also valuable for discriminating other diseases besides AD. As an example, the merged analysis of tau and midbrain-to-pons atrophy is reported to be useful for early identification of progressive supranuclear palsy (PSP), discriminating PSP cases from controls and patients suffering from corticobasal syndrome (CBS) and FTD [138].

*5.1.1.4. Phospho-tau*

Similarly to total tau, p-tau levels are increased in AD samples, although higher variability on its specificity and sensibility is reported when compared to the non-phosphorylated tau form [78, 127]. Several considerations should be done in this regard.

On one hand, the number of studies analysing p-tau levels is not as large as those performed for its non-phosphorylated form. In addition, sensitivity and sensibility may depend on the analysed phosphorylation site, although sensitivity for AD seems equal for at least the three main epitopes used in clinical diagnosis [139]. Importantly, results from a meta-analysis study indicate that tau phosphorylated at the Threonine 181 levels are able to discriminate AD from other dementias and MCI [140].

On the other hand, the utility of p-tau in the differential AD diagnosis against other neurodegenerative diseases is advantageous over total tau since p-tau levels reflect AD pathogenesis [141]. Indeed, p-tau levels in the CSF may reflect the levels of tau phosphorylation in AD brains. Tau is more increased in the CSF of sCJD patients than in AD, while p-tau is only modestly increased in sCJD [142]. In addition, tau levels are increased in neurological diseases such as in acute ischemic stroke, while p-tau levels remains unaltered [123]. Indeed, tau phosphorylation is physiologically regulated during several biological processes such as neuronal development, while tau levels usually remain more stable. Therefore, a direct correlation between total tau and p-tau levels cannot be established, and several lines of evidence indicate that p-tau levels are differently regulated, not only in AD, but also in other neurodegenerative diseases. In this regard, the main tau kinase, Glycogen synthase kinase 3 (GSK3) is assumed to be hyperactivated in AD brain, inducing pathogenic tau hyperphosphorylation, aggregation and formation of the intracellular NFTs. Although a direct correlation between GSK3 activity and tangle formation in AD is still under discussion [143], GSK3 levels and activity are markedly reduced in sCJD brain [144]. Thus, the distinct regulation of tau phosphorylation in the brain of AD and CJD, may explain the different p-tau/tau ratios observed in both diseases, which permits a differential diagnosis [145].

Recently it has been observed that patients suffering from rpAD present highly increased p-tau levels in the CSF [146] when compared to controls and classical AD patients. Since it is estimated that rpAD may be accounting for 10-30% of all AD cases, it is urgently needed to establish if lack of disease stratification may lead to misinterpretation of p-tau analysis between rapidly progressive and classical AD forms. In this regard, a combination of high CSF tau without proportionally elevated p-tau-181 is associated with a faster rate of cognitive decline [147]. In this regard, longitudinal studies indicates that a combination of low Aβ42 and high tau and p-tau levels is highly predictive of MCI progression and cognitive decline rate [74, 148].

*5.1.1.5. Inflammatory cytokines*

A common feature in the Central Nervous System of neurodegenerative diseases is the presence of chronic neuroinflammation associated with an exacerbated gliosis [149]. The role of a chronic and sustained inflammation in neurodegeneration is still a matter of debate as neuroinflammation has been suggested to play both detrimental and protective functions depending on disease stage, brain region, activation of anti-inflammatory mechanisms and cellular milieu among others [150]. Besides these considerations point out a critical role of neuroinflammation in the molecular mechanisms linked to AD pathology [151] and a broad range of inflammatory cytokines and immune response mediators are increased in the CSF of AD patients. A correlation between inflammatory markers and biomarkers of neurodegeneration has been described [152], and consequently, neurodegenerative disorders with high inflammatory chronic profiles such as prion diseases [153] present higher inflammatory-related deregulations in the CSF [154, 155]. However, the specific inflammatory profile observed in different types of dementia and at different disease stages indicates that inflammatory biomarkers could be used as surrogate markers for AD diagnosis and prognosis.

The anti-inflammatory cytokine TGFβ–1 is consistently upregulated in AD cases [156, 157]. Interestingly, during the progression from MCI to AD, a pro-inflammatory state is proposed since MCI patients who progressed to AD showed higher TNFα and lower TGFβ–1 and Aβ42 levels than control individuals or those non progressing to AD [158]. These data are in agreement with increased levels of the acute-phase C-reactive protein (CRP) and IL-6 in the CSF of MCI patients when compared to AD patients, indicating that inflammatory mechanisms are already progressing even before changes in core AD biomarkers such as Aβ42 and tau can be detected in the CSF [159].

In relation to this, a comparative analysis between Amnestic Mild Cognitive Impairment (aMCI) and MS patients indicated that pro-inflammatory cytokines and CD45+ lymphocytes are present in the same levels in both diseases. Taking into account that MS can be considered the most representative neuroinflammatory disease, these observations indicate that inflammatory mechanisms may be crucial for AD etiopathology.

In this regard, the pro-inflammatory cytokine osteopontin (OPN), also known as the secreted phosphoprotein 1 (SPP1) and involved in macrophage recruitment to inflammatory sites and cytokine production [160], is also elevated in the CSF of AD patients and in MCI patients developing AD. OPN levels correlate with cognitive decline and with increased levels in early disease phases [161, 162]. OPN has also been found elevated in the CSF during attacks of MS [163].

In addition, the major acute-phase protein SAP (Serum amyloid P component) has lower levels in MCI patients who progressed to AD than in those who did not progress to AD [164], suggesting that low SAP levels are linked to an increased risk of progression to AD.

Alternative promising inflammatory-biomarkers have been proposed. On one hand, lipocalin 2, whose levels are decreased in the CSF of MCI and AD patients and increased in brain regions with associated AD pathology [165]. On the other hand, the astrocytic marker YKL-40, has been reported to be increased in AD at early stages of the disease [166-169] and in FTD and aMCI patients [166]. In addition YKL-40 levels correlate positively with the classical core biomarkers tau and p-tau [166].

#### *5.1.1.6. MicroRNAs*

microRNAs (miRNA) are endogenous small non-coding RNAs (20-22 nucleotides) that are involved in post-transcriptional gene regulation by targeting mRNAs for cleavage or translational repression [170]. miRNAs have emerged as key regulators of various aspects of neuronal development and dysfunction. Deregulated small RNA signatures, especially miRNAs, have been observed in the brain of a broad range of neurodegenerative diseases such as AD, PD, HD or ALS [171, 172] and experimental evidences ascribe a functional role to miRNAs in the pathogenic molecular mechanisms leading to neurodegeneration [173-175]. With the advent of high-throughput technologies, full transcriptomic signatures can be provided not only from tissues, but also from samples with small amounts of starting material such as biological fluids and associated exosomes [176-178]. In this regard, more than 100 circulating miRNAs are deregulated in pathological conditions [179] and some of them have been proposed as potential biomarkers for disease diagnosis and prognosis, mainly in cancer and neurodegenerative diseases. Regarding the levels of circulating miRNAs in AD, several studies already reported changes when compared to control samples. A recent pilot study in two different cohorts showed that hsa-miR-27a-3p expression is reduced in the CSF of AD patients [180]. Decreased levels of this miRNA correlate with high tau and low Aβ amyloid levels. A second study analysed a selected group of miRNA candidates and observed that miRNAs 34a, 125b and

146a levels were significantly lower in the CSF of AD patients when compared to control cases, while the levels of the miRNAs 29a and 29b were significantly higher [181]. In an independent study low levels of miRNA-146a were also detected in the CSF of AD patients [182]. In this regard the expression of miRNA-146a is increased in AD [183] and CJD brains [184], in AD mice models [185] and in scrapie mice [184]. miRNA-146a expression in AD mice models also correlates with senile plaque density and synaptic pathology [185]. This miRNA is induced by the interleukin IL-1β, modulating the expression of IL-6 and the cyclooxygenase COX-2 and acting as a negative regulator of the astrocyte-mediated inflammatory response [186, 187]. In addition miRNA-146a negatively regulates TLR signalling to prevent exacerbated inflammation, thus, it seems to play a key role in the modulation of the neuropathology associated to chronic inflammation in neurodegenerative diseases. Whether the regulation of miRNAs in CSF is a consequence of neuronal cell damage or a modulated pathogenic response is still a matter of discussion.

In summary, all preliminary studies argue for the presence of deregulated levels of miRNAs in the CSF of AD patients with potential translational value. Exclusion of blood contamination effects, standardization of the assays, together with cross-disease and technical validation in larger cohorts need to be carried out to assess the potential role of miRNAs signatures as specific diagnostic and prognosis biomarker tool in AD and to define new diagnostic therapeutic opportunities related to the miRNA field.

#### *5.1.1.7. Mitochondrial DNA*

A pioneering study demonstrated that asymptomatic patients at risk of AD and symptomatic AD patients exhibit a significant decrease in the levels of circulating cell-free mtDNA in the CSF [188]. Data were generated by qPCR and digital droplet PCR and validated in an independent cohort of patients. Interestingly, this decrease is disease-specific, as mtDNA levels in the CSF of FTLD patients remain unchanged. Since decreased levels of mtDNA precede the appearance of the classical AD biomarkers such as Aβ42, mtDNA is an excellent potential preclinical AD biomarker. Further studies in larger cohorts including rpAD and CJD samples will determinate the clinical use of mtDNA analysis as a prognosis AD biomarker.

#### *5.1.1.8. Metabolic profile*

The use of analytic technologies such as Nuclear magnetic resonance and Liquid chromatography–mass spectrometry to analyse the metabolic signatures of biological fluids deserves special attention [189]. The metabolic profile in human CSF samples of AD patients and age-matched healthy controls unveils the presence of a significant presence of deregulated metabolites in AD cases [190]. Among them, higher corticols levels are found in AD cases, which correlate with AD progression and severity. In addition, the same study proved that combined analysis of different metabolites may increase sensitivity and specificity above 80%.

A second metabolic profile study identified the deregulated metabolic pathways in the CSF of MCI and AD patients [191]. The number of altered pathways increased with disease severity. Among them, Krebs cycle was significantly affected in MCI and cholesterol and sphingolipids transport was altered in AD. A high percentage of altered pathways in the CSF were also deregulated in plasma from the same individuals (30% in MCI and 60% in AD, respectively). Deregulated pathways performing the best disease discrimination were biosynthesis and metabolism of cortisone and prostaglandin 2.

Finally, a third study using metabolomics in the CSF of MCI and AD patients demonstrated the presence of elevated methionine (MET), 5-hydroxyindoleacetic acid (5-HIAA), vanillyl-mandelic acid, xanthosine and glutathione levels in AD patients and elevated 5-HIAA, MET, hypoxanthine and other metabolites in MCI patients when compared to healthy controls. Metabolite ratios revealed changes within tryptophan, MET and purine pathways [192], showing a partial overlap between MCI and AD.

Metabolomics is a promising tool for AD diagnosis indicating a slightly lower or similar performance when compared to classical AD biomarkers such as tau and Aβ42 depending on the study. Further analysis in large independent cohorts, technical updates as well as a combination of metabolic profiling with classical or alternative biomarkers will define the potential use of high throughput metabolic analysis in the AD diagnostic field. Besides, metabolite signatures may help to unveil the progression mechanisms and pathways leading to different dementia stages.

### 5.2. Blood

Despite the description of altered levels of several molecules in the blood levels of several molecules in the blood of AD patients as AD clinical biomarkers. Direct analysis in blood or blood-derived serum or plasma samples presents a broad range of advantages over CSF analysis. Blood extraction is minimally invasive and sample is easily collected, processed and stored over time. However, variations in the levels of blood metabolites may be reflecting a broad spectrum of changes not directly related to the neurodegenerative process. In addition, the dynamic range of the changes are lower than in CSF obtaining, most of the times, inconsistent data. Additionally, contrary to CSF, blood is a very complex fluid composed of different types of metabolites and cell types that present significant oscillations in response to external factors not related to pathogenic events. The analysis of specific blood cells could be an alternative approach to link potential biomarkers levels with AD pathology, being a field under intense study.

#### *5.2.1. Protein biomarkers*

The core CSF AD biomarkers present minimal alterations in plasma. Aβ40 levels are higher in AD than in controls, although a high overlap is observed between groups. No changes have been observed for Aβ42, and Aβ40 and both Aβ40 and Aβ42 levels showed no association with cognitive decline [86]. Albeit some partial overlap between groups, tau levels in plasma are increased in AD when compared to control and MCI patients. Interestingly, tau levels cannot differentiate non-progressive from AD progressive MCI patients and there is a lack of correlation between CSF and plasma tau levels [193].

High-throughputs proteomic studies have tried to report the complex deregulated signatures between control and AD samples. A 2D-Mass spectrometry-based study detected a deregulated set of proteins in AD plasma complement factor H precursor and $\alpha$-2-macroglobulin, which were validated and correlated with disease severity [194]. Independent multi-analyte profiling studies also demonstrated the presence of deregulated levels of proteins in MCI and AD samples when compared to controls both in serum and plasma. Among them some hits are related to AD pathogenesis such as the apoE [195, 196] as well as a broad range of inflammatory mediators [196, 197]. In an array-based ELISA study, 18 signalling proteins were able to distinguish AD from control samples with high accuracy (90%) and to predict MCI to AD progression [198], although the validation of this dataset has been ambiguous [199, 200]. The observation of a high variability between independent analyses indicates that further validations by independent methodologies in different cohorts need to be performed before resolving the clinical relevance of high-throughput blood-based analysis.

Alternative plasma biomarkers include the brain-reactive autoantibodies, present in sera irrespective of the presence of any pathology. This finding led to the analysis of the potential AD-specific autoantibody signature, which has been suggested to possess diagnostic value due to its ability to distinguish AD cases from controls, PD and breast cancer samples [201].

### *5.2.2. microRNAs*

miRNA signature from CSF is only slightly more stable when compared to serum, suggesting that both biofluids are appropriate for the screening analysis of small RNAs [202]. Therefore, several studies addressed the potential deregulated miRNA signature in blood-derived AD samples. Using a microarray and qPCR validation approach the miR-125b, miR-23a and miR-26b were downregulated in the serum of AD cases when compared to non-inflammatory and inflammatory neurological controls and to FTD cases [203]. miR-125b presented the best accuracy discriminating AD from other groups. The same study observed that miR-125b and miR-26b levels were also diminished in the CSF of AD patients. An independent validation study was able to replicate downregulation of miR-125b in AD serum [204].

In a different approach, using RNA-sequencing and qPCR validation, downregulated levels of the miR-98-5p, miR-885-5p, miR-483-3p, miR-342-3p, miR-191-5p and let-7d-5p in the serum of AD cases were reported. The miR-342-3p showed the best sensitivity and specificity and correlated with cognitive decline [205]. However, downregulated levels of miR-342-3p in biological fluids are also a common hallmark in cancer [206]. Using a similar approach a 12 blood-based miRNA signatures was suggested to discriminate AD patients from controls and samples from patients suffering from different neurodegenerative diseases with high diagnostic accuracies [207]. Nonetheless, the different sample origin impedes a formal comparison between disease group's studies. The analysis of peripheral blood mononuclear cells identified upregulated levels of miR-34a, miR-181b in AD cells [208].

Despite the promising future of miRNA as biomarkers tools of clinical relevance, several considerations needs to be done. Lack of validation among current available studies, even when using similar platform, indicates that sample collection and methodology needs further standardization. In addition, high-throughput data need to be cross-validated in longitudinal studies using different cohorts and selected miRNAs validated in multicentre studies. Under these conditions miRNA in blood-related samples may serve as prognostic and diagnostic through the analysis of miRNA signatures alone or combined with the analysis of classical AD biomarkers.

# 6. Conclusion

The use of combined analysis of current AD diagnostic tools is gaining experimental momentum due to its demonstrated value as a better prognostic and diagnostic tool when compared to individual assessments. As most promising candidates, CSF markers as well as methods of in vivo neuroimaging have been identified. Among them, we can find structural MRI, $^{18}$F-FDG-PET and novel in vivo amyloid-PET imaging [209, 210]. In longitudinal studies it was shown that with the help of these biomarkers AD could be diagnosed already in mild symptomatic states with high accuray allowing a predictability of its development [210]. Investigations of patients with genetic AD have demonstrated already 15 years prior to the onset of dementia significant pathological alterations in distinct biomarkers [211, 212].

Although these results are only assignable in a limited way to sporadic AD, the latter study provides impressive evidence on the long preclinical course of AD.

Current diagnostic concepts should therefore apply not at first when AD dementia has developed, but support explicitly the application of biomarkers at distinct stages of AD as it was shown that biomarkers become positive already at early and presymptomatic stages [213, 214].

In conclusion, differential diagnosis of a dementia syndrom requires esides clinical history and neuropsychological testing, analysis of metabolites in biological fluids as well as imaging methods. All these diagnostic approaches will not only allow an explanation towards the underlying cause of dementia but will also be useful in monitoring disease treatment and progression. The detection of AD at an early stage is hereby essential, as a further disease progression can be influenced positively by early initiation of treatment.

Integration of data generated during the last decades should be used to build up a worldwide rational algorithm based in the use of standardized, economically affordable methodologies and easily accessible samples.

### Nomenclature

AD: Alzheimer's disease, rpAD: rapidly progressive Alzheimer's disease, CJD: Creutzfeldt-Jakob disease, aMCI: Amnestic Mild Cognitive Impairment, MCI: Mild cognitive impairment, FTLD: Frontotemporal Lobe Degeneration, FTD: Frontotemporal Dementia, CSF: Cerebrospinal Fluid, PD: Parkinson Disease, HD: Huntington Disease, ELISA: Enzyme-Linked Immuno-Sorbent Assay, MS: Multiple Sclerosis, SWD: Subcortical White-matter Dementia, MMSE: Mini–mental state examination, APP: Amyloid precursor protein, DS: Down Syndrome, CRP:

C-reactive protein, PSP: progressive supranuclear palsy, CBS: corticobasal syndrome; NINCDS/ADRDA: American National Institute of Neurological and Communicative Disorders and Stroke /Alzheimer's disease and Related Disorders Association; DGPPN: German Society of Psychiatry, Psychotherapy and Neurology; DGN: German Neurological Society; MRI: Magnetic Resonance Imaging, PET: Emission Computed Tomography; SPECT: single photon emission computed tomography; EEG: Electroencephalogram; CT; Computerized Tomography; CDR: Clinical Dementia Rating; GDS: Global Deterioration Scale; ADL-/IADL: Activities of Daily Living /Instrumental Activities of Daily Living; VBM: voxel-based morphometry; FLAIR; Fluid-attenuated inversion recovery; rCBF: regional cerebral blood flow.

## Acknowledgements

The study was supported by the EU grants JPND-DEMTEST (Biomarker based diagnosis of rapid progressive dementias-optimization of diagnostic protocols, 01ED1201A) and PRIORITY (Protecting the food chain from prions, FP7-KBBE-2007-2A) and by funds from the Federal Ministry of Health (grant no. 1369-341] and from the German Center for Neurodegenerative Diseases (DZNE).

## Author details

Franc Llorens[1,2], Sabine Nuhn[1], Christoph Peter[1], Inga Zerr[1,2] and Katharina Stoeck[1]

1 Department of Neurology, Clinical Dementia Center, University Medical School, Georg-August University, Göttingen, Germany

2 German Center for Neurodegenerative Diseases (DZNE) – Göttingen, Germany

## References

[1] Hebert LE, Scherr PA, Bienias JL, Bennett DA, Evans DA. Alzheimer disease in the US population: prevalence estimates using the 2000 census. *Arch Neurol* 2003 Aug; 60:1119-1122.

[2] Brookmeyer R, Johnson E, Ziegler-Graham K, Arrighi HM. Forecasting the global burden of Alzheimer's disease. *Alzheimers Dement* 2007 Jul;3:186-191.

[3] Boise L, Neal MB, Kaye J. Dementia assessment in primary care: results from a study in three managed care systems. *J Gerontol A Biol Sci Med Sci* 2004 Jun;59:M621-M626.

[4] Boustani M, Peterson B, Hanson L, Harris R, Lohr KN. Screening for dementia in primary care: a summary of the evidence for the U.S. Preventive Services Task Force. *Ann Intern Med* 2003 Jun 3;138:927-937.

[5] Gaugler JE, Ascher-Svanum H, Roth DL, Fafowora T, Siderowf A, Beach TG. Characteristics of patients misdiagnosed with Alzheimer's disease and their medication use: an analysis of the NACC-UDS database. *BMC Geriatr* 2013;13:137.

[6] Komarova NL, Thalhauser CJ. High degree of heterogeneity in Alzheimer's disease progression patterns. *PLoS Comput Biol* 2011 Nov;7:e1002251.

[7] Koedam EL, Lauffer V, van der Vlies AE, van der Flier WM, Scheltens P, Pijnenburg YA. Early-versus late-onset Alzheimer's disease: more than age alone. *J Alzheimers Dis* 2010;19:1401-1408.

[8] Schmidt C, Redyk K, Meissner B, et al. Clinical features of rapidly progressive Alzheimer's disease. *Dement Geriatr Cogn Disord* 2010;29:371-378.

[9] de Leon MJ, Mosconi L, Blennow K, et al. Imaging and CSF studies in the preclinical diagnosis of Alzheimer's disease. *Ann N Y Acad Sci* 2007 Feb;1097:114-145.

[10] Walhovd KB, Fjell AM, Brewer J, et al. Combining MR imaging, positron-emission tomography, and CSF biomarkers in the diagnosis and prognosis of Alzheimer disease. *AJNR Am J Neuroradiol* 2010 Feb;31:347-354.

[11] Boutoleau-Bretonniere C, Lebouvier T, Delaroche O, et al. Value of neuropsychological testing, imaging, and CSF biomarkers for the differential diagnosis and prognosis of clinically ambiguous dementia. *J Alzheimers Dis* 2012;28:323-336.

[12] Shaffer JL, Petrella JR, Sheldon FC, et al. Predicting cognitive decline in subjects at risk for Alzheimer disease by using combined cerebrospinal fluid, MR imaging, and PET biomarkers. *Radiology* 2013 Feb;266:583-591.

[13] Edwards M, Balldin VH, Hall J, O'Bryant S. Combining Select Neuropsychological Assessment with Blood-Based Biomarkers to Detect Mild Alzheimer's Disease: A Molecular Neuropsychology Approach. *J Alzheimers Dis* 2014 Jun 10.

[14] Deutsche Gesellschaft für Psychiatrie PuNDDGfND. Demenzen. S3-Leitlinie, 2009.

[15] McKhann G, Drachman D, Folstein M, Katzman R, Price D, Stadlan EM. Clinical diagnosis of Alzheimer's disease: report of the NINCDS-ADRDA Work Group under the auspices of Department of Health and Human Services Task Force on Alzheimer's Disease. *Neurology* 1984 Jul;34:939-944.

[16] McKhann GM, Knopman DS, Chertkow H, et al. The diagnosis of dementia due to Alzheimer's disease: recommendations from the National Institute on Aging-Alzheimer's Association workgroups on diagnostic guidelines for Alzheimer's disease. *Alzheimers Dement* 2011 May;7:263-269.

[17] Dubois B, Feldman HH, Jacova C, et al. Research criteria for the diagnosis of Alzheimer's disease: revising the NINCDS-ADRDA criteria. *Lancet Neurol* 2007 Aug; 6:734-746.

[18] Albert MS, Dekosky ST, Dickson D, et al. The diagnosis of mild cognitive impairment due to Alzheimer's disease: recommendations from the National Institute on Aging-Alzheimer's Association workgroups on diagnostic guidelines for Alzheimer's disease. *Alzheimers Dement* 2011 May;7:270-279.

[19] Winblad B, Palmer K, Kivipelto M, et al. Mild cognitive impairment--beyond controversies, towards a consensus: report of the International Working Group on Mild Cognitive Impairment. *J Intern Med* 2004 Sep;256:240-246.

[20] Petersen RC. Clinical practice. Mild cognitive impairment. *N Engl J Med* 2011 Jun 9;364:2227-2234.

[21] Loewenstein D. Assessment of Alzheimer´s Disease. Handbook on the Neuropsychology of Aging and Dementia. Springer, 2013:271-280.

[22] Jahn T. Neuropsychologie der Demenz. Lautenbacher S, Gauggel (Hrsg.): Neuropsychologie psychischer Störungen. Springer, 2010:360-381.

[23] Schmidtke K. Otto, M. Demenzen. Wallesch, CW, Förstl, H (Hrsg.) Thieme, 2012:203-227.

[24] Schmidtke K, Olbrich S. The Clock Reading Test: validation of an instrument for the diagnosis of dementia and disorders of visuo-spatial cognition. *Int Psychogeriatr* 2007 Apr;19:307-321.

[25] Schmidtke K. Neuropsychologische Untersuchung bei Patienten mit Demenzverdacht. In: Hüll M, ed., 26 ed Nervenheilkunde, 2007:651-658.

[26] Tsai PH, Teng E, Liu C, Mendez MF. Posterior cortical atrophy: evidence for discrete syndromes of early-onset Alzheimer's disease. *Am J Alzheimers Dis Other Demen* 2011 Aug;26:413-418.

[27] Groh-Bordin C. Störungen der Visuellen Raumwahrnehmung und Raumkognition. In: Kerkhoff G, ed. Sturm, W. et al. (Hrsg.): Lehrbuch der Klinischen Neuropsychologie, Springer, 2009:500-512.

[28] Monsch AU, Bondi MW, Butters N, Salmon DP, Katzman R, Thal LJ. Comparisons of verbal fluency tasks in the detection of dementia of the Alzheimer type. *Arch Neurol* 1992 Dec;49:1253-1258.

[29] Engel S. Kognitives Screening. In: Mück A LFR, ed. Demenzerkrankungen. Deutscher Ärzte-Verlag Mahlberg R, Gutzmann (Hrsg.). 2009.

[30] Beblo T. Neuropsychologie affektiver Störungen. Neuropsychologie psychischer Störungen. 2. Auflage Lautenbacher, S, Gauggel, S (Hrsg.). 2010:211-218.

[31] Beblo T. Neuropsychologie der Depression. In: Lautenbacher S, ed. Göttingen: Hogrefe, 2006.

[32] Folstein MF, Folstein SE, McHugh PR. "Mini-mental state". A practical method for grading the cognitive state of patients for the clinician. *J Psychiatr Res* 1975 Nov; 12:189-198.

[33] Anthony JC, LeResche L, Niaz U, Von Korff MR, Folstein MF. Limits of the 'Mini-Mental State' as a screening test for dementia and delirium among hospital patients. *Psychol Med* 1982 May;12:397-408.

[34] Ivemeyer D. Demenztests in der Praxis. In: Zerfaß R, ed. München: Urban & Fischer, 2006.

[35] Kalbe E, Kessler J, Calabrese P, et al. DemTect: a new, sensitive cognitive screening test to support the diagnosis of mild cognitive impairment and early dementia. *Int J Geriatr Psychiatry* 2004 Feb;19:136-143.

[36] Aebi C. Validierung der neuropsychologischen Testbatterie CERAD-NP. Eine Multi-Center Studie. Dissertation, Bassel 2002.: 2002.

[37] Barth S. Neuropsychologische Profile in der Demenzdiagnostik: Eine Untersuchung mit der CERAD-NP-Testbatterie. In: Schönknecht PPJSJ, ed. Fortschritte Neurologie Psychiatrie : 2005:1-9.

[38] Shulman KI. Clock-drawing: is it the ideal cognitive screening test? *Int J Geriatr Psychiatry* 2000 Jun;15:548-561.

[39] Schröder MR et al. Merkmalsanalyse von Uhrzeichnungen als Beitrag zur Diagnostik der Demenz vom Alzheimer Typ. In: Hasse-Sander IMHHRMHJ, ed., 12 ed Zeitschrift für Gerontopsychologie & -psychiatrie, 1999:55-66.

[40] Lawton MP, Brody EM. Assessment of older people: self-maintaining and instrumental activities of daily living. *Gerontologist* 1969;9:179-186.

[41] Erzigkeit H, Lehfeld H, Pena-Casanova J, et al. The Bayer-Activities of Daily Living Scale (B-ADL): results from a validation study in three European countries. *Dement Geriatr Cogn Disord* 2001 Sep;12:348-358.

[42] Pfeffer RI, Kurosaki TT, Harrah CH, Jr., Chance JM, Filos S. Measurement of functional activities in older adults in the community. *J Gerontol* 1982 May;37:323-329.

[43] Yesavage JA, Brink TL, Rose TL, et al. Development and validation of a geriatric depression screening scale: a preliminary report. *J Psychiatr Res* 1982;17:37-49.

[44] Ortiz-Teran L. Currently Available Neuroimaging Approaches in Alzheimer Disease (AD) Early Diagnosis. In: et al, ed. Suzanne de La Monte (Hg.): The Clinical Spectrum of Alzheimer's Disease -The Charge Toward Comprehensive Diagnostic and Therapeutic Strategies: InTech., 2011.

[45] de Leon MJ, George AE, Golomb J, et al. Frequency of hippocampal formation atrophy in normal aging and Alzheimer's disease. *Neurobiol Aging* 1997 Jan;18:1-11.

[46] Wallesch C. Demenzen. 2., überarbeitete und erweiterte Auflage. Stuttgart: Thieme (Referenzreihe Neurologie Herausgegeben von G. Deuschl, H.C. Diener, H.C. Hopf)., 2012.

[47] Reiser M. Radiologie. 3., vollst. überarb. u. erw. Aufl. In: et al, ed. Stuttgart: Thieme (Duale Reihe)., 2011.

[48] Kinkingnehun S, Sarazin M, Lehericy S, Guichart-Gomez E, Hergueta T, Dubois B. VBM anticipates the rate of progression of Alzheimer disease: a 3-year longitudinal study. *Neurology* 2008 Jun 3;70:2201-2211.

[49] Thompson PM, Hayashi KM, de Zubicaray GI, et al. Mapping hippocampal and ventricular change in Alzheimer disease. *Neuroimage* 2004 Aug;22:1754-1766.

[50] Becker JT, Davis SW, Hayashi KM, et al. Three-dimensional patterns of hippocampal atrophy in mild cognitive impairment. *Arch Neurol* 2006 Jan;63:97-101.

[51] Apostolova LG, Steiner CA, Akopyan GG, et al. Three-dimensional gray matter atrophy mapping in mild cognitive impairment and mild Alzheimer disease. *Arch Neurol* 2007 Oct;64:1489-1495.

[52] Farid K, Caillat-Vigneron N, Sibon I. Is brain SPECT useful in degenerative dementia diagnosis? *J Comput Assist Tomogr* 2011 Jan;35:1-3.

[53] Mosconi L, Berti V, Glodzik L, Pupi A, De SS, de Leon MJ. Pre-clinical detection of Alzheimer's disease using FDG-PET, with or without amyloid imaging. *J Alzheimers Dis* 2010;20:843-854.

[54] Matsuda H. Cerebral blood flow and metabolic abnormalities in Alzheimer's disease. *Ann Nucl Med* 2001 Apr;15:85-92.

[55] Duran FL, Zampieri FG, Bottino CC, Buchpiguel CA, Busatto GF. Voxel-based investigations of regional cerebral blood flow abnormalities in Alzheimer's disease using a single-detector SPECT system. *Clinics (Sao Paulo)* 2007 Aug;62:377-384.

[56] Herholz K, Carter SF, Jones M. Positron emission tomography imaging in dementia. *Br J Radiol* 2007 Dec;80 Spec No 2:S160-S167.

[57] Morris JC, Roe CM, Grant EA, et al. Pittsburgh compound B imaging and prediction of progression from cognitive normality to symptomatic Alzheimer disease. *Arch Neurol* 2009 Dec;66:1469-1475.

[58] Blennow K, Zetterberg H, Fagan AM. Fluid biomarkers in Alzheimer disease. *Cold Spring Harb Perspect Med* 2012 Sep;2:a006221.

[59] Price JL, Morris JC. Tangles and plaques in nondemented aging and "preclinical" Alzheimer's disease. *Ann Neurol* 1999 Mar;45:358-368.

[60] Davies L, Wolska B, Hilbich C, et al. A4 amyloid protein deposition and the diagnosis of Alzheimer's disease: prevalence in aged brains determined by immunocytochemistry compared with conventional neuropathologic techniques. *Neurology* 1988 Nov;38:1688-1693.

[61] Cutler RW, Spertell RB. Cerebrospinal fluid: a selective review. *Ann Neurol* 1982 Jan; 11:1-10.

[62] Fagan AM. CSF Biomarkers of Alzheimer's Disease: Impact on Disease Concept, Diagnosis, and Clinical Trial Design. Advances in Geriatry 2014.

[63] Blennow K, Hampel H, Weiner M, Zetterberg H. Cerebrospinal fluid and plasma biomarkers in Alzheimer disease. *Nat Rev Neurol* 2010 Mar;6:131-144.

[64] Consensus report of the Working Group on: "Molecular and Biochemical Markers of Alzheimer's Disease". The Ronald and Nancy Reagan Research Institute of the Alzheimer's Association and the National Institute on Aging Working Group. *Neurobiol Aging* 1998 Mar;19:109-116.

[65] Mattsson N, Zetterberg H, Hansson O, et al. CSF biomarkers and incipient Alzheimer disease in patients with mild cognitive impairment. *JAMA* 2009 Jul 22;302:385-393.

[66] Kanai M, Matsubara E, Isoe K, et al. Longitudinal study of cerebrospinal fluid levels of tau, A beta1-40, and A beta1-42(43) in Alzheimer's disease: a study in Japan. *Ann Neurol* 1998 Jul;44:17-26.

[67] Shoji M, Matsubara E, Murakami T, et al. Cerebrospinal fluid tau in dementia disorders: a large scale multicenter study by a Japanese study group. *Neurobiol Aging* 2002 May;23:363-370.

[68] Visser PJ, Verhey F, Knol DL, et al. Prevalence and prognostic value of CSF markers of Alzheimer's disease pathology in patients with subjective cognitive impairment or mild cognitive impairment in the DESCRIPA study: a prospective cohort study. *Lancet Neurol* 2009 Jul;8:619-627.

[69] Shaw LM, Vanderstichele H, Knapik-Czajka M, et al. Cerebrospinal fluid biomarker signature in Alzheimer's disease neuroimaging initiative subjects. *Ann Neurol* 2009 Apr;65:403-413.

[70] Mattsson N, Zetterberg H, Blennow K. Lessons from Multicenter Studies on CSF Biomarkers for Alzheimer's Disease. *Int J Alzheimers Dis* 2010;2010.

[71] Hampel H, Teipel SJ, Fuchsberger T, et al. Value of CSF beta-amyloid1-42 and tau as predictors of Alzheimer's disease in patients with mild cognitive impairment. *Mol Psychiatry* 2004 Jul;9:705-710.

[72] Herukka SK, Hallikainen M, Soininen H, Pirttila T. CSF Abeta42 and tau or phosphorylated tau and prediction of progressive mild cognitive impairment. *Neurology* 2005 Apr 12;64:1294-1297.

[73] Hansson O, Zetterberg H, Buchhave P, Londos E, Blennow K, Minthon L. Association between CSF biomarkers and incipient Alzheimer's disease in patients with mild cognitive impairment: a follow-up study. *Lancet Neurol* 2006 Mar;5:228-234.

[74] Snider BJ, Fagan AM, Roe C, et al. Cerebrospinal fluid biomarkers and rate of cognitive decline in very mild dementia of the Alzheimer type. *Arch Neurol* 2009 May; 66:638-645.

[75] Hartmann T, Bieger SC, Bruhl B, et al. Distinct sites of intracellular production for Alzheimer's disease A beta40/42 amyloid peptides. *Nat Med* 1997 Sep;3:1016-1020.

[76] Hampel H, Shen Y, Walsh DM, et al. Biological markers of amyloid beta-related mechanisms in Alzheimer's disease. *Exp Neurol* 2010 Jun;223:334-346.

[77] Hoshi M, Sato M, Matsumoto S, et al. Spherical aggregates of beta-amyloid (amylospheroid) show high neurotoxicity and activate tau protein kinase I/glycogen synthase kinase-3beta. *Proc Natl Acad Sci U S A* 2003 May 27;100:6370-6375.

[78] Blennow K. Cerebrospinal fluid protein biomarkers for Alzheimer's disease. *NeuroRx* 2004 Apr;1:213-225.

[79] Hansson O, Zetterberg H, Buchhave P, et al. Prediction of Alzheimer's disease using the CSF Abeta42/Abeta40 ratio in patients with mild cognitive impairment. *Dement Geriatr Cogn Disord* 2007;23:316-320.

[80] Vanmechelen E, Vanderstichele H, Hulstaert F, et al. Cerebrospinal fluid tau and beta-amyloid(1-42) in dementia disorders. *Mech Ageing Dev* 2001 Nov;122:2005-2011.

[81] Sjogren M, Minthon L, Davidsson P, et al. CSF levels of tau, beta-amyloid(1-42) and GAP-43 in frontotemporal dementia, other types of dementia and normal aging. *J Neural Transm* 2000;107:563-579.

[82] Tamaoka A, Sekijima Y, Matsuno S, Tokuda T, Shoji S, Ikeda SI. Amyloid beta protein species in cerebrospinal fluid and in brain from patients with Down's syndrome. *Ann Neurol* 1999 Dec;46:933.

[83] Strozyk D, Blennow K, White LR, Launer LJ. CSF Abeta 42 levels correlate with amyloid-neuropathology in a population-based autopsy study. *Neurology* 2003 Feb 25;60:652-656.

[84] Riemenschneider M, Wagenpfeil S, Diehl J, et al. Tau and Abeta42 protein in CSF of patients with frontotemporal degeneration. *Neurology* 2002 Jun 11;58:1622-1628.

[85] Tang W, Huang Q, Wang Y, Wang ZY, Yao YY. Assessment of CSF Abeta as an aid to discriminating Alzheimer's disease from other dementias and mild cognitive impairment: A meta-analysis of 50 studies. *J Neurol Sci* 2014 Jul 15.

[86] Mehta PD, Pirttila T, Mehta SP, Sersen EA, Aisen PS, Wisniewski HM. Plasma and cerebrospinal fluid levels of amyloid beta proteins 1-40 and 1-42 in Alzheimer disease. *Arch Neurol* 2000 Jan;57:100-105.

[87] Schoonenboom NS, Mulder C, Van Kamp GJ, et al. Amyloid beta 38, 40, and 42 species in cerebrospinal fluid: more of the same? *Ann Neurol* 2005 Jul;58:139-142.

[88] Pijnenburg YA, Schoonenboom SN, Mehta PD, et al. Decreased cerebrospinal fluid amyloid beta (1-40) levels in frontotemporal lobar degeneration. *J Neurol Neurosurg Psychiatry* 2007 Jul;78:735-737.

[89] Gabelle A, Roche S, Geny C, et al. Decreased sAbetaPPbeta, Abeta38, and Abeta40 cerebrospinal fluid levels in frontotemporal dementia. *J Alzheimers Dis* 2011;26:553-563.

[90] Lewczuk P, Lelental N, Spitzer P, Maler JM, Kornhuber J. Amyloid-beta 42/40 Cerebrospinal Fluid Concentration Ratio in the Diagnostics of Alzheimer's Disease: Validation of Two Novel Assays. *J Alzheimers Dis* 2014 Jul 30.

[91] Shoji M, Matsubara E, Kanai M, et al. Combination assay of CSF tau, A beta 1-40 and A beta 1-42(43) as a biochemical marker of Alzheimer's disease. *J Neurol Sci* 1998 Jun 30;158:134-140.

[92] Spies PE, Slats D, Sjogren JM, et al. The cerebrospinal fluid amyloid beta42/40 ratio in the differentiation of Alzheimer's disease from non-Alzheimer's dementia. *Curr Alzheimer Res* 2010 Aug;7:470-476.

[93] Wiltfang J, Esselmann H, Bibl M, et al. Amyloid beta peptide ratio 42/40 but not A beta 42 correlates with phospho-Tau in patients with low- and high-CSF A beta 40 load. *J Neurochem* 2007 May;101:1053-1059.

[94] Lewczuk P, Esselmann H, Otto M, et al. Neurochemical diagnosis of Alzheimer's dementia by CSF Abeta42, Abeta42/Abeta40 ratio and total tau. *Neurobiol Aging* 2004 Mar;25:273-281.

[95] Bombois S, Duhamel A, Salleron J, et al. A new decision tree combining Abeta 1-42 and p-Tau levels in Alzheimer's diagnosis. *Curr Alzheimer Res* 2013 May 1;10:357-364.

[96] Parnetti L, Chiasserini D, Eusebi P, et al. Performance of abeta1-40, abeta1-42, total tau, and phosphorylated tau as predictors of dementia in a cohort of patients with mild cognitive impairment. *J Alzheimers Dis* 2012;29:229-238.

[97] Holsinger RM, McLean CA, Collins SJ, Masters CL, Evin G. Increased beta-Secretase activity in cerebrospinal fluid of Alzheimer's disease subjects. *Ann Neurol* 2004 Jun; 55:898-899.

[98] Zhong Z, Ewers M, Teipel S, et al. Levels of beta-secretase (BACE1) in cerebrospinal fluid as a predictor of risk in mild cognitive impairment. *Arch Gen Psychiatry* 2007 Jun;64:718-726.

[99] Ewers M, Zhong Z, Burger K, et al. Increased CSF-BACE 1 activity is associated with ApoE-epsilon 4 genotype in subjects with mild cognitive impairment and Alzheimer's disease. *Brain* 2008 May;131:1252-1258.

[100] Zetterberg H, Andreasson U, Hansson O, et al. Elevated cerebrospinal fluid BACE1 activity in incipient Alzheimer disease. *Arch Neurol* 2008 Aug;65:1102-1107.

[101] Holsinger RM, Lee JS, Boyd A, Masters CL, Collins SJ. CSF BACE1 activity is increased in CJD and Alzheimer disease versus (corrected) other dementias. *Neurology* 2006 Aug 22;67:710-712.

[102] Ewers M, Cheng X, Zhong Z, et al. Increased CSF-BACE1 activity associated with decreased hippocampus volume in Alzheimer's disease. *J Alzheimers Dis* 2011;25:373-381.

[103] Ye S, Huang Y, Mullendorff K, et al. Apolipoprotein (apo) E4 enhances amyloid beta peptide production in cultured neuronal cells: apoE structure as a potential therapeutic target. *Proc Natl Acad Sci U S A* 2005 Dec 20;102:18700-18705.

[104] Menting KW, Claassen JA. beta-secretase inhibitor; a promising novel therapeutic drug in Alzheimer's disease. *Front Aging Neurosci* 2014;6:165.

[105] Fukumoto H, Tokuda T, Kasai T, et al. High-molecular-weight beta-amyloid oligomers are elevated in cerebrospinal fluid of Alzheimer patients. *FASEB J* 2010 Aug; 24:2716-2726.

[106] Santos AN, Ewers M, Minthon L, et al. Amyloid-beta oligomers in cerebrospinal fluid are associated with cognitive decline in patients with Alzheimer's disease. *J Alzheimers Dis* 2012;29:171-176.

[107] Holtta M, Hansson O, Andreasson U, et al. Evaluating amyloid-beta oligomers in cerebrospinal fluid as a biomarker for Alzheimer's disease. *PLoS One* 2013;8:e66381.

[108] Gao CM, Yam AY, Wang X, et al. Abeta40 oligomers identified as a potential biomarker for the diagnosis of Alzheimer's disease. *PLoS One* 2010;5:e15725.

[109] Salvadores N, Shahnawaz M, Scarpini E, Tagliavini F, Soto C. Detection of misfolded Abeta oligomers for sensitive biochemical diagnosis of Alzheimer's disease. *Cell Rep* 2014 Apr 10;7:261-268.

[110] Pitschke M, Prior R, Haupt M, Riesner D. Detection of single amyloid beta-protein aggregates in the cerebrospinal fluid of Alzheimer's patients by fluorescence correlation spectroscopy. *Nat Med* 1998 Jul;4:832-834.

[111] Fukumoto H, Asami-Odaka A, Suzuki N, Iwatsubo T. Association of A beta 40-positive senile plaques with microglial cells in the brains of patients with Alzheimer's disease and in non-demented aged individuals. *Neurodegeneration* 1996 Mar;5:13-17.

[112] Gravina SA, Ho L, Eckman CB, et al. Amyloid beta protein (A beta) in Alzheimer's disease brain. Biochemical and immunocytochemical analysis with antibodies specific for forms ending at A beta 40 or A beta 42(43). *J Biol Chem* 1995 Mar 31;270:7013-7016.

[113] Ferrera D, Mazzaro N, Canale C, Gasparini L. Resting microglia react to Abeta42 fibrils but do not detect oligomers or oligomer-induced neuronal damage. *Neurobiol Aging* 2014 May 29.

[114] Englund H, Degerman GM, Brundin RM, et al. Oligomerization partially explains the lowering of Abeta42 in Alzheimer's disease cerebrospinal fluid. *Neurodegener Dis* 2009;6:139-147.

[115] Herskovits AZ, Locascio JJ, Peskind ER, Li G, Hyman BT. A Luminex assay detects amyloid beta oligomers in Alzheimer's disease cerebrospinal fluid. *PLoS One* 2013;8:e67898.

[116] Sancesario GM, Cencioni MT, Esposito Z, et al. The load of amyloid-beta oligomers is decreased in the cerebrospinal fluid of Alzheimer's disease patients. *J Alzheimers Dis* 2012;31:865-878.

[117] Haass C, Selkoe DJ. Soluble protein oligomers in neurodegeneration: lessons from the Alzheimer's amyloid beta-peptide. *Nat Rev Mol Cell Biol* 2007 Feb;8:101-112.

[118] Shankar GM, Li S, Mehta TH, et al. Amyloid-beta protein dimers isolated directly from Alzheimer's brains impair synaptic plasticity and memory. *Nat Med* 2008 Aug; 14:837-842.

[119] Lesne S, Koh MT, Kotilinek L, et al. A specific amyloid-beta protein assembly in the brain impairs memory. *Nature* 2006 Mar 16;440:352-357.

[120] Sjogren M, Vanderstichele H, Agren H, et al. Tau and Abeta42 in cerebrospinal fluid from healthy adults 21-93 years of age: establishment of reference values. *Clin Chem* 2001 Oct;47:1776-1781.

[121] Humpel C. Identifying and validating biomarkers for Alzheimer's disease. *Trends Biotechnol* 2011 Jan;29:26-32.

[122] Andreasen N, Minthon L, Davidsson P, et al. Evaluation of CSF-tau and CSF-Abeta42 as diagnostic markers for Alzheimer disease in clinical practice. *Arch Neurol* 2001 Mar;58:373-379.

[123] Hesse C, Rosengren L, Andreasen N, et al. Transient increase in total tau but not phospho-tau in human cerebrospinal fluid after acute stroke. *Neurosci Lett* 2001 Jan 19;297:187-190.

[124] Stoeck K, Sanchez-Juan P, Gawinecka J, et al. Cerebrospinal fluid biomarker supported diagnosis of Creutzfeldt-Jakob disease and rapid dementias: a longitudinal multicentre study over 10 years. *Brain* 2012 Oct;135:3051-3061.

[125] Buerger K, Otto M, Teipel SJ, et al. Dissociation between CSF total tau and tau protein phosphorylated at threonine 231 in Creutzfeldt-Jakob disease. *Neurobiol Aging* 2006 Jan;27:10-15.

[126] Fagan AM, Head D, Shah AR, et al. Decreased cerebrospinal fluid Abeta(42) correlates with brain atrophy in cognitively normal elderly. *Ann Neurol* 2009 Feb; 65:176-183.

[127] Zetterberg H, Blennow K, Hanse E. Amyloid beta and APP as biomarkers for Alzheimer's disease. *Exp Gerontol* 2010 Jan;45:23-29.

[128] Andreasen N, Vanmechelen E, Van d, V, et al. Cerebrospinal fluid tau protein as a biochemical marker for Alzheimer's disease: a community based follow up study. *J Neurol Neurosurg Psychiatry* 1998 Mar;64:298-305.

[129] Kaerst L, Kuhlmann A, Wedekind D, Stoeck K, Lange P, Zerr I. Cerebrospinal fluid biomarkers in Alzheimer's disease, vascular dementia and ischemic stroke patients: a critical analysis. *J Neurol* 2013 Nov;260:2722-2727.

[130] van Harten AC, Kester MI, Visser PJ, et al. Tau and p-tau as CSF biomarkers in dementia: a meta-analysis. *Clin Chem Lab Med* 2011 Mar;49:353-366.

[131] De R, V, Galloni E, Marcon M, et al. Analysis of combined CSF biomarkers in AD diagnosis. *Clin Lab* 2014;60:629-634.

[132] Holtzman DM. CSF biomarkers for Alzheimer's disease: current utility and potential future use. *Neurobiol Aging* 2011 Dec;32 Suppl 1:S4-S9.

[133] Sunderland T, Linker G, Mirza N, et al. Decreased beta-amyloid1-42 and increased tau levels in cerebrospinal fluid of patients with Alzheimer disease. *JAMA* 2003 Apr 23;289:2094-2103.

[134] Kaerst L, Kuhlmann A, Wedekind D, Stoeck K, Lange P, Zerr I. Using cerebrospinal fluid marker profiles in clinical diagnosis of dementia with Lewy bodies, Parkinson's disease, and Alzheimer's disease. *J Alzheimers Dis* 2014;38:63-73.

[135] Parnetti L, Farotti L, Eusebi P, et al. Differential role of CSF alpha-synuclein species, tau, and Abeta42 in Parkinson's Disease. *Front Aging Neurosci* 2014;6:53.

[136] Kahle PJ, Jakowec M, Teipel SJ, et al. Combined assessment of tau and neuronal thread protein in Alzheimer's disease CSF. *Neurology* 2000 Apr 11;54:1498-1504.

[137] Okamura N, Arai H, Maruyama M, et al. Combined Analysis of CSF Tau Levels and ((123)I)Iodoamphetamine SPECT in Mild Cognitive Impairment: Implications for a Novel Predictor of Alzheimer's Disease. *Am J Psychiatry* 2002 Mar;159:474-476.

[138] Borroni B, Malinverno M, Gardoni F, et al. A combination of CSF tau ratio and midsaggital midbrain-to-pons atrophy for the early diagnosis of progressive supranuclear palsy. *J Alzheimers Dis* 2010;22:195-203.

[139] Hampel H, Buerger K, Zinkowski R, et al. Measurement of phosphorylated tau epitopes in the differential diagnosis of Alzheimer disease: a comparative cerebrospinal fluid study. *Arch Gen Psychiatry* 2004 Jan;61:95-102.

[140] Tang W, Huang Q, Yao YY, Wang Y, Wu YL, Wang ZY. Does CSF p-tau help to discriminate Alzheimer's disease from other dementias and mild cognitive impairment? A meta-analysis of the literature. *J Neural Transm* 2014 May 10.

[141] Hampel H, Blennow K, Shaw LM, Hoessler YC, Zetterberg H, Trojanowski JQ. Total and phosphorylated tau protein as biological markers of Alzheimer's disease. *Exp Gerontol* 2010 Jan;45:30-40.

[142] Sanchez-Juan P, Green A, Ladogana A, et al. CSF tests in the differential diagnosis of Creutzfeldt-Jakob disease. *Neurology* 2006 Aug 22;67:637-643.

[143] Kremer A, Louis JV, Jaworski T, Van LF. GSK3 and Alzheimer's Disease: Facts and Fiction... *Front Mol Neurosci* 2011;4:17.

[144] Llorens F, Zafar S, Ansoleaga B, et al. Subtype and regional regulation of prion biomarkers in sporadic Creutzfeldt-Jakob disease. *Neuropathol Appl Neurobiol* 2014 Aug 18.

[145] Riemenschneider M, Wagenpfeil S, Vanderstichele H, et al. Phospho-tau/total tau ratio in cerebrospinal fluid discriminates Creutzfeldt-Jakob disease from other dementias. *Mol Psychiatry* 2003 Mar;8:343-347.

[146] Schmidt C, Haik S, Satoh K, et al. Rapidly progressive Alzheimer's disease: a multicenter update. *J Alzheimers Dis* 2012;30:751-756.

[147] Kester MI, van der Vlies AE, Blankenstein MA, et al. CSF biomarkers predict rate of cognitive decline in Alzheimer disease. *Neurology* 2009 Oct 27;73:1353-1358.

[148] Visser PJ, Verhey F, Knol DL, et al. Prevalence and prognostic value of CSF markers of Alzheimer's disease pathology in patients with subjective cognitive impairment or mild cognitive impairment in the DESCRIPA study: a prospective cohort study. *Lancet Neurol* 2009 Jul;8:619-627.

[149] Amor S, Peferoen LA, Vogel DY, et al. Inflammation in neurodegenerative diseases--an update. *Immunology* 2014 Jun;142:151-166.

[150] Aguzzi A, Barres BA, Bennett ML. Microglia: scapegoat, saboteur, or something else? *Science* 2013 Jan 11;339:156-161.

[151] Akiyama H, Barger S, Barnum S, et al. Inflammation and Alzheimer's disease. *Neurobiol Aging* 2000 May;21:383-421.

[152] Alcolea D, Carmona-Iragui M, Suarez-Calvet M, et al. Relationship Between beta-Secretase, Inflammation and Core Cerebrospinal Fluid Biomarkers for Alzheimer's Disease. *J Alzheimers Dis* 2014 May 12.

[153] Llorens F, Lopez-Gonzalez I, Thune K, et al. Subtype and regional-specific neuroinflammation in sporadic creutzfeldt-jakob disease. *Front Aging Neurosci* 2014;6:198.

[154] Stoeck K, Bodemer M, Zerr I. Pro- and anti-inflammatory cytokines in the CSF of patients with Creutzfeldt-Jakob disease. *J Neuroimmunol* 2006 Mar;172:175-181.

[155] Stoeck K, Bodemer M, Ciesielczyk B, et al. Interleukin 4 and interleukin 10 levels are elevated in the cerebrospinal fluid of patients with Creutzfeldt-Jakob disease. *Arch Neurol* 2005 Oct;62:1591-1594.

[156] Swardfager W, Lanctot K, Rothenburg L, Wong A, Cappell J, Herrmann N. A meta-analysis of cytokines in Alzheimer's disease. *Biol Psychiatry* 2010 Nov 15;68:930-941.

[157] Rota E, Bellone G, Rocca P, Bergamasco B, Emanuelli G, Ferrero P. Increased intrathecal TGF-beta1, but not IL-12, IFN-gamma and IL-10 levels in Alzheimer's disease patients. *Neurol Sci* 2006 Apr;27:33-39.

[158] Tarkowski E, Andreasen N, Tarkowski A, Blennow K. Intrathecal inflammation precedes development of Alzheimer's disease. *J Neurol Neurosurg Psychiatry* 2003 Sep; 74:1200-1205.

[159] Schuitemaker A, Dik MG, Veerhuis R, et al. Inflammatory markers in AD and MCI patients with different biomarker profiles. *Neurobiol Aging* 2009 Nov;30:1885-1889.

[160] Wang KX, Denhardt DT. Osteopontin: role in immune regulation and stress responses. *Cytokine Growth Factor Rev* 2008 Oct;19:333-345.

[161] Comi C, Carecchio M, Chiocchetti A, et al. Osteopontin is increased in the cerebrospinal fluid of patients with Alzheimer's disease and its levels correlate with cognitive decline. *J Alzheimers Dis* 2010;19:1143-1148.

[162] Sun Y, Yin XS, Guo H, Han RK, He RD, Chi LJ. Elevated osteopontin levels in mild cognitive impairment and Alzheimer's disease. *Mediators Inflamm* 2013;2013:615745.

[163] Bornsen L, Khademi M, Olsson T, Sorensen PS, Sellebjerg F. Osteopontin concentrations are increased in cerebrospinal fluid during attacks of multiple sclerosis. *Mult Scler* 2011 Jan;17:32-42.

[164] Verwey NA, Schuitemaker A, van der Flier WM, et al. Serum amyloid p component as a biomarker in mild cognitive impairment and Alzheimer's disease. *Dement Geriatr Cogn Disord* 2008;26:522-527.

[165] Naude PJ, Nyakas C, Eiden LE, et al. Lipocalin 2: novel component of proinflammatory signaling in Alzheimer's disease. *FASEB J* 2012 Jul;26:2811-2823.

[166] Alcolea D, Carmona-Iragui M, Suarez-Calvet M, et al. Relationship Between beta-Secretase, Inflammation and Core Cerebrospinal Fluid Biomarkers for Alzheimer's Disease. *J Alzheimers Dis* 2014 Jan 1;42:157-167.

[167] Perrin RJ, Craig-Schapiro R, Malone JP, et al. Identification and validation of novel cerebrospinal fluid biomarkers for staging early Alzheimer's disease. *PLoS One* 2011;6:e16032.

[168] Craig-Schapiro R, Perrin RJ, Roe CM, et al. YKL-40: a novel prognostic fluid biomarker for preclinical Alzheimer's disease. *Biol Psychiatry* 2010 Nov 15;68:903-912.

[169] Antonell A, Mansilla A, Rami L, et al. Cerebrospinal Fluid Level of YKL-40 Protein in Preclinical and Prodromal Alzheimer's Disease. *J Alzheimers Dis* 2014 Jul 2.

[170] Krol J, Loedige I, Filipowicz W. The widespread regulation of microRNA biogenesis, function and decay. *Nat Rev Genet* 2010 Sep;11:597-610.

[171] Gascon E, Gao FB. Cause or Effect: Misregulation of microRNA Pathways in Neurodegeneration. *Front Neurosci* 2012;6:48.

[172] Maciotta S, Meregalli M, Torrente Y. The involvement of microRNAs in neurodegenerative diseases. *Front Cell Neurosci* 2013;7:265.

[173] Lehmann SM, Kruger C, Park B, et al. An unconventional role for miRNA: let-7 activates Toll-like receptor 7 and causes neurodegeneration. *Nat Neurosci* 2012 Jun; 15:827-835.

[174] Salta E, De SB. Non-coding RNAs with essential roles in neurodegenerative disorders. *Lancet Neurol* 2012 Feb;11:189-200.

[175] Eacker SM, Dawson TM, Dawson VL. Understanding microRNAs in neurodegeneration. *Nat Rev Neurosci* 2009 Dec;10:837-841.

[176] Cheng L, Quek CY, Sun X, Bellingham SA, Hill AF. The detection of microRNA associated with Alzheimer's disease in biological fluids using next-generation sequencing technologies. *Front Genet* 2013;4:150.

[177] McAlexander MA, Phillips MJ, Witwer KW. Comparison of Methods for miRNA Extraction from Plasma and Quantitative Recovery of RNA from Cerebrospinal Fluid. *Front Genet* 2013;4:83.

[178] Pritchard CC, Cheng HH, Tewari M. MicroRNA profiling: approaches and considerations. *Nat Rev Genet* 2012 May;13:358-369.

[179] Weiland M, Gao XH, Zhou L, Mi QS. Small RNAs have a large impact: circulating microRNAs as biomarkers for human diseases. *RNA Biol* 2012 Jun;9:850-859.

[180] Sala FC, Lau P, Salta E, et al. Reduced expression of hsa-miR-27a-3p in CSF of patients with Alzheimer disease. *Neurology* 2013 Dec 10;81:2103-2106.

[181] Kiko T, Nakagawa K, Tsuduki T, Furukawa K, Arai H, Miyazawa T. MicroRNAs in plasma and cerebrospinal fluid as potential markers for Alzheimer's disease. *J Alzheimers Dis* 2014;39:253-259.

[182] Muller M, Kuiperij HB, Claassen JA, Kusters B, Verbeek MM. MicroRNAs in Alzheimer's disease: differential expression in hippocampus and cell-free cerebrospinal fluid. *Neurobiol Aging* 2014 Jan;35:152-158.

[183] Lukiw WJ, Zhao Y, Cui JG. An NF-kappaB-sensitive micro RNA-146a-mediated inflammatory circuit in Alzheimer disease and in stressed human brain cells. *J Biol Chem* 2008 Nov 14;283:31315-31322.

[184] Lukiw WJ, Dua P, Pogue AI, Eicken C, Hill JM. Upregulation of micro RNA-146a (miRNA-146a), a marker for inflammatory neurodegeneration, in sporadic Creutzfeldt-Jakob disease (sCJD) and Gerstmann-Straussler-Scheinker (GSS) syndrome. *J Toxicol Environ Health A* 2011;74:1460-1468.

[185] Li YY, Cui JG, Hill JM, Bhattacharjee S, Zhao Y, Lukiw WJ. Increased expression of miRNA-146a in Alzheimer's disease transgenic mouse models. *Neurosci Lett* 2011 Jan 3;487:94-98.

[186] Iyer A, Zurolo E, Prabowo A, et al. MicroRNA-146a: a key regulator of astrocyte-mediated inflammatory response. *PLoS One* 2012;7:e44789.

[187] Boldin MP, Taganov KD, Rao DS, et al. miR-146a is a significant brake on autoimmunity, myeloproliferation, and cancer in mice. *J Exp Med* 2011 Jun 6;208:1189-1201.

[188] Podlesniy P, Figueiro-Silva J, Llado A, et al. Low cerebrospinal fluid concentration of mitochondrial DNA in preclinical Alzheimer disease. *Ann Neurol* 2013 Nov; 74:655-668.

[189] Schlotterbeck G, Ross A, Dieterle F, Senn H. Metabolic profiling technologies for biomarker discovery in biomedicine and drug development. *Pharmacogenomics* 2006 Oct; 7:1055-1075.

[190] Czech C, Berndt P, Busch K, et al. Metabolite profiling of Alzheimer's disease cerebrospinal fluid. *PLoS One* 2012;7:e31501.

[191] Trushina E, Dutta T, Persson XM, Mielke MM, Petersen RC. Identification of altered metabolic pathways in plasma and CSF in mild cognitive impairment and Alzheimer's disease using metabolomics. *PLoS One* 2013;8:e63644.

[192] Kaddurah-Daouk R, Zhu H, Sharma S, et al. Alterations in metabolic pathways and networks in Alzheimer's disease. *Transl Psychiatry* 2013;3:e244.

[193] Zetterberg H, Wilson D, Andreasson U, et al. Plasma tau levels in Alzheimer's disease. *Alzheimers Res Ther* 2013;5:9.

[194] Hye A, Lynham S, Thambisetty M, et al. Proteome-based plasma biomarkers for Alzheimer's disease. *Brain* 2006 Nov;129:3042-3050.

[195] Hu WT, Holtzman DM, Fagan AM, et al. Plasma multianalyte profiling in mild cognitive impairment and Alzheimer disease. *Neurology* 2012 Aug 28;79:897-905.

[196] Doecke JD, Laws SM, Faux NG, et al. Blood-based protein biomarkers for diagnosis of Alzheimer disease. *Arch Neurol* 2012 Oct;69:1318-1325.

[197] O'Bryant SE, Xiao G, Barber R, et al. A serum protein-based algorithm for the detection of Alzheimer disease. *Arch Neurol* 2010 Sep;67:1077-1081.

[198] Ray S, Britschgi M, Herbert C, et al. Classification and prediction of clinical Alzheimer's diagnosis based on plasma signaling proteins. *Nat Med* 2007 Nov;13:1359-1362.

[199] Bjorkqvist M, Ohlsson M, Minthon L, Hansson O. Evaluation of a previously suggested plasma biomarker panel to identify Alzheimer's disease. *PLoS One* 2012;7:e29868.

[200] Soares HD, Chen Y, Sabbagh M, Roher A, Schrijvers E, Breteler M. Identifying early markers of Alzheimer's disease using quantitative multiplex proteomic immunoassay panels. *Ann N Y Acad Sci* 2009 Oct;1180:56-67.

[201] Nagele E, Han M, Demarshall C, Belinka B, Nagele R. Diagnosis of Alzheimer's disease based on disease-specific autoantibody profiles in human sera. *PLoS One* 2011;6:e23112.

[202] Burgos K, Malenica I, Metpally R, et al. Profiles of extracellular miRNA in cerebrospinal fluid and serum from patients with Alzheimer's and Parkinson's diseases correlate with disease status and features of pathology. *PLoS One* 2014;9:e94839.

[203] Galimberti D, Villa C, Fenoglio C, et al. Circulating miRNAs as Potential Biomarkers in Alzheimer's Disease. *J Alzheimers Dis* 2014 Jul 7.

[204] Tan L, Yu JT, Liu QY, et al. Circulating miR-125b as a biomarker of Alzheimer's disease. *J Neurol Sci* 2014 Jan 15;336:52-56.

[205] Tan L, Yu JT, Tan MS, et al. Genome-wide serum microRNA expression profiling identifies serum biomarkers for Alzheimer's disease. *J Alzheimers Dis* 2014;40:1017-1027.

[206] Wang Q, Li P, Li A, et al. Plasma specific miRNAs as predictive biomarkers for diagnosis and prognosis of glioma. *J Exp Clin Cancer Res* 2012;31:97.

[207] Leidinger P, Backes C, Deutscher S, et al. A blood based 12-miRNA signature of Alzheimer disease patients. *Genome Biol* 2013;14:R78.

[208] Schipper HM, Maes OC, Chertkow HM, Wang E. MicroRNA expression in Alzheimer blood mononuclear cells. *Gene Regul Syst Bio* 2007;1:263-274.

[209] Hampel H, Lista S, Teipel SJ, et al. Perspective on future role of biological markers in clinical therapy trials of Alzheimer's disease: a long-range point of view beyond 2020. *Biochem Pharmacol* 2014 Apr 15;88:426-449.

[210] Hampel H, Frank R, Broich K, et al. Biomarkers for Alzheimer's disease: academic, industry and regulatory perspectives. *Nat Rev Drug Discov* 2010 Jul;9:560-574.

[211] Vos SJ, Xiong C, Visser PJ, et al. Preclinical Alzheimer's disease and its outcome: a longitudinal cohort study. *Lancet Neurol* 2013 Oct;12:957-965.

[212] Bateman RJ, Xiong C, Benzinger TL, et al. Clinical and biomarker changes in dominantly inherited Alzheimer's disease. *N Engl J Med* 2012 Aug 30;367:795-804.

[213] Jack CR, Jr., Knopman DS, Jagust WJ, et al. Hypothetical model of dynamic biomarkers of the Alzheimer's pathological cascade. Lancet Neurol 2010 Jan;9:119-128.

[214] Jack CR, Jr., Knopman DS, Jagust WJ, et al. Tracking pathophysiological processes in Alzheimer's disease: an updated hypothetical model of dynamic biomarkers. Lancet Neurol 2013 Feb;12:207-216.

Section 4

# Clinical Aspects

Chapter 10

# Genetic, Biochemical and Histopathological Aspects of Familiar Alzheimer's Disease

Genaro Gabriel Ortiz, Fermín P. Pacheco-Moisés,
Erika D. González-Renovato, Luis Figuera,
Miguel A. Macías-Islas, Mario Mireles-Ramírez,
L. Javier Flores-Alvarado, Angélica Sánchez-López,
Dhea G. Nuño-Penilla, Irma E. Velázquez- Brizuela,
Juan P. Sánchez-Luna and Alfredo Célis de la Rosa

Additional information is available at the end of the chapter

## 1. Introduction

Alzheimer's disease (AD) is the most common cause of dementia among people over 65 years. In industrialized countries it is the fourth leading cause of death; in our country and although there are no figures on the epidemiological dimension of this disease, statistical projections of Latin American countries with similar socio-economic conditions, estimated to affect approximately 350,000 Mexicans. This disease is slowly progressive and is characterized by progressive dementia with profound memory loss, decreased ability to perform routine tasks, difficulties in judgment, disorientation, personality changes, difficulty in learning, and loss of language skills. On average, its duration is 8-12 years in which there is a period of 2-3 years when the symptoms are very subtle and often goes unnoticed. Although protocols have carefully designed clinical diagnosis, diagnostic certainty of Alzheimer's disease is about 85% and it was confirmed by post-mortem brain examination.

The EA is inseparably between clinical symptoms of dementia and the presence of specific lesions in selected areas of the cerebral cortex and hippocampus. The neuropathological findings in the disease exhibited protein deposits manifest as neuritic plaques; consisting of extracellular deposits composed of amyloid β (β-amyloid plaques). Also showed neurofibrillary interneuronal tangles consisting of cytoskeletal protein tau, and granulo-vaculoar degeneration (figures 6-9), reduction and dysfunction of synapses, neuronal death and reduction in overall brain volume. AD typically affects the hippocampus and adjacent structures, memory deficits are typically among the earliest and most pronounced signs of AD. When pathological changes spread beyond the hippocampus, other cognitive areas also become affected [1-5]

It is possible to distinguish two different types of AD based upon age onset and familial aggregation: familiar AD (FAD) and late-onset AD (LOAD). FAD is characterized by Mendelian inheritance (autosomal dominant) and early onset (<60 years). FAD represents about 5–10% of all AD cases [5], LOAD is characterized by later onset >60 years) and complex patterns of inheritance. Although they differ in age onset, both forms of the disease are defined by the same pathological features; neuronal loss and the presence of beta-amyloid plaques and neurofibrillary tangles (figure 6, 7). Plaques are extracellular deposits of insoluble amyloid proteins while tangles are intracellular aggregations of hyperphosphorilated tau protein. AD has a characteristic onset, is very gradual and insidious, this is a particularity that distinguishes the pathology from other forms of dementia [9].

Genetic factors, including risk factors are related to AD. In a minority of hereditary disease appears so in a pattern of autosomal dominant inheritance. Chromosomes 21, 14 and 1 are associated with some familial forms of early onset; Moreover, the late-onset familial forms appear linked to chromosomes 12 and 19. Sporadic cases, most cannot be explained from a genetic point of view, although they have stated hypotheses that the action of toxic agents or unidentified infectious affecting genetic aspects (figure 1) [9-11].

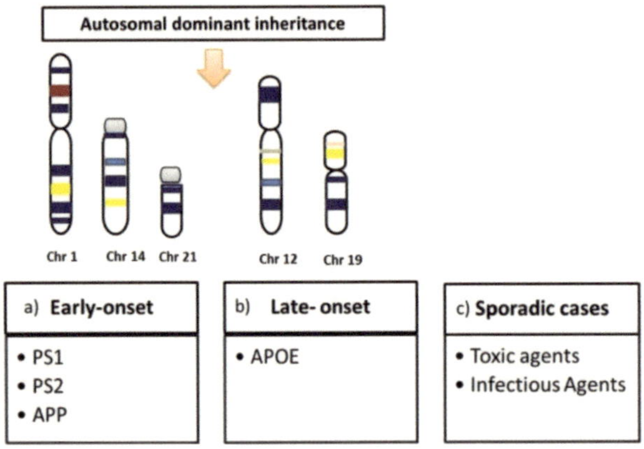


**Figure 1.** Genetic Factors Related to Alzheimer's Dementia

Genetic factors related to Alzheimer's dementia.

**a.** Chromosomes 1, 14 and 21 are associated with Early-onset forms. These genes are linked to mutations on Presenilin-1 (PS1), Presenilin-2 (PS2) and Amiloid precursor protein (APP), numerous studies has demonstrated that changes in these proteins predisposes individuals to familial Alzheimer disease.

**b.** Chromosomes 14 and 19 are associated with late-onset forms. Chromosome 19 are linked to mutations on Apolipoprotein E, specially isoform 4 (APOE4)

c. Others form Of Alzheimer's dementia cannot be explained from a genetic point of view, including sporadic cases [11-13].

Mutations in different genes located on chromosomes 14 and 1, responsible for the disease of early onset familial Alzheimer (EOAD), in a portion of patients show penetrance (proportion of individuals that show the phenotype) about 100 % with autosomal dominant inheritance. In the EOAD, autosomal dominant mutations in three genes; APP encoding amyloid precursor protein, PSEN1 and PSEN2 encoding presenilin 1 and 2, lead to increased production of beta amyloid [8]. The presenilin mutations, especially PS1 (~85%), are much more common in early onset familial AD than APP mutation [14]. It has demonstrated the existence of a locus on chromosome 14 (14q 24.3) in a group of families with EOAD. Using positional cloning the gene designated S 182, which contains 14 exons and encodes the synthesis of a protein of 467 amino acids (aa) called presenilin 1 (PS-1) (figure 1) containing from 6 to 9 transmembrane domains, and two hydrophilic regions was isolated that are oriented towards the cytosol; at least over 90 different mutations found in the gene of the PS-1 to chromosome 14 mutations (include: His163Arg, Ala246Glu, Leu286Val and Cys410Tyr) most display complete penetrance, but a common mutation is Glu318Gly and this predisposes individuals to familial Alzheimer disease. All except one are missense and represent about 30-50% of cases of EAFP. PSEN-1 mutations are usually associated with very aggressive EOAD, with duration of dementia of about 5 years [6]. PSEN-2 gene mutations are very rare. The ages at onset of EOAD are thought to vary (PSEN-1 25–60, APP 40–65 and PSEN-2 45–84. It is quite possible that other genes with mutations leading to EOAD will be found [14-18].

The first gene associated with late forms family was identified in a family sample by applying a new method of genetic analysis. The identified Apo E locus is located on the long arm of chromosome 19 (figure 2).

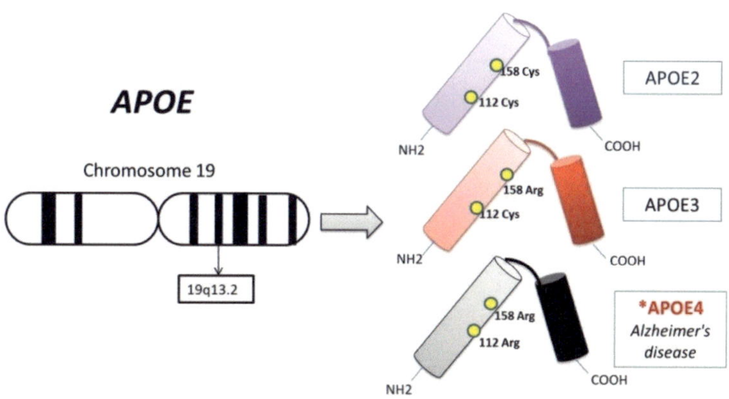


**Figure 2.** Association Between Apo E Isoforms and Alzheimer's Disease

The *APOE* gene is located on the long arm of **chromosome 19** at position 13.2. There are 3 different alleles of the *APOE* gene, producing 3 major isoforms, Known as *ApoE2* (cys112, cys158), *ApoE3* (cys112, arg158), and *ApoE4* (arg112, arg158). The APOE4 isoform of increases an individual's risk for developing late-onset Alzheimer disease [19,20].

Numerous studies have reported association between Apo E (locus) and EOAD, and sporadic cases. The relationship between Apo E and AD is set by the overrepresentation of one of the common protein isoforms in the group of patients. Of the 3 major isoforms, known as E2, E3 and E4, E4 are frequently associated with the onset of the disease [19]. The hypothesis of the existence of a locus that could explain some of the cases EOAD was confirmed in 1992, in which several groups pre-sented evidence of a locus on chromosome 14; this was named, along with S 182, PS-1 or AD3. The role of the PS-1 gene in the body is unknown. Homology with family proteins Notch/lin-12 indicates that it may play an important role in signal transduction, and it is stated that the process involved in apoptosis. The gene of the PS-1 is expressed in different regions of the brain, skeletal muscle, kidney, pancreas, placenta and heart. Processing produces two fragments, this process occurs naturally and is under control. An increase of the amount of PS-1 produced by the cells, *in vitro*, is not accompanied by increase in the concentration of the fragments. Of the 10 exons which holds the PS-1 gene, most of the mutations are linked to exon 5 (comprising the transmembrane domain 1 and 2) and exon 8 (comprising the trans-membrane domain 6 and 7). The effects on the PS-1 gene, in the 2 sites mentioned above, show a significant difference with respect to age at onset of the disease when compared to each other. Patients with mutations in the transmembrane domain (TD) 6 and 7, having an average age of onset higher than those with mutations in the DT 1 and 2.14 [12,13]

All mutations, except one, are missense, resulting in a change of one aa by another. The mutation known as D9 is one of the exceptions, and described in many families of diverse origin (English, Japanese, Australian, Latin's). Involvement cause removal of exon 9, the reading frame is not altered processing and disposal site and the corresponding fragments. The mutation has the remarkable feature that is expressed in almost all families, spastic paraparesia; a phenotype that does not seem to occur with any other mutation. In an English family mutation was detected in codon 141 of the PS-1 gene with incomplete penetrance. The involvement was manifested in a change of Iso by Val, the disease started with an average age of onset of 55 years. The mutations cause about 2% of all EOEA, and occur less frequently than those found in the PS-1 gene. Only found two missense mutations with incomplete penetrance [12].

Another gene, called STM-2, was isolated families descendants of German settlers installed in the Volga region in Russia. The STM-2 gene encodes a 448 aa protein called presenilin 2 (PS-2), PS-2 contained 12 exons, 10 of which were coding exons, and that the primary transcript encodes a 448 amino acid polypeptide with 67 (80%) of homology to PS1 gene in some regions. This protein has been identified as part of the enzymatic complex that cleaves amyloid beta peptide from APP. The affected families had a missense mutation at codon 141, resulting in a change of aspartic (Asp) by Iso. In these families had been excluded linkage to chromosomes 14 and 21. The PS-2 gene also contains 12 exons, and the protein for which it encodes contains from 6 to 9 DT [12,13].

The PS-2 transmembrane protein has 67% homology to the sequence of aa from the PS-1, and therefore depending homology. The PS-2 is localized in the endoplasmic reticulum with the hydrophilic domains oriented towards the cytoplasm (figure 3).

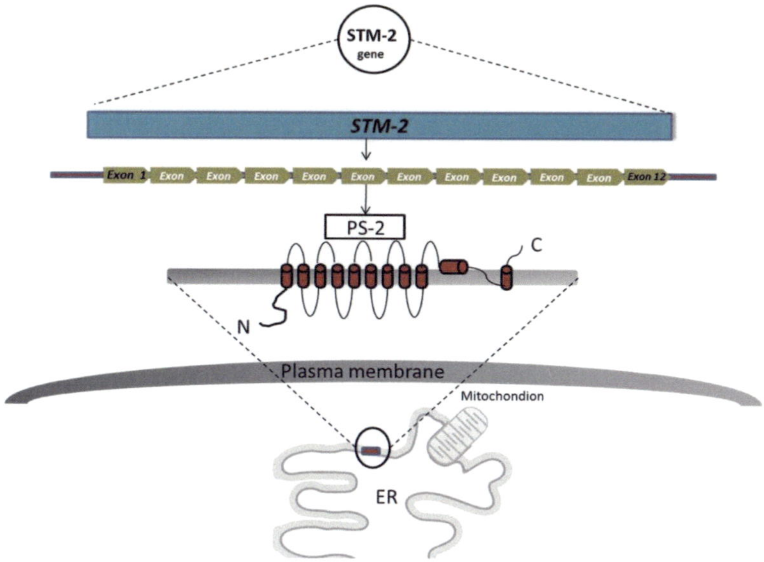


**Figure 3.** The Membrane Topology of PS2

The PS-2 protein is derived from the STM-2 gene from 12 exons. The ten-transmembrane-domain model of PS2 with one hydrophobic region and 10 associated to the membrane of the endoplasmic reticulum.

The homology between PS-1 and PS-2 is particularly focused on the DT. The amino-terminal domain and the domain located between exons 8 and 10, have the lowest degree of homology and are supposed to be where the functional specificity of each of the proteins resides. Another mutation that is associated with EOEA is located at codon 239 and is manifested in a change of methionine (Met) by Val. As can be seen, the mutation sites are different from those presented in the PS-1, characterized by incomplete penetrance. It is thought that mutations in the gene of the PS-2 may cause an increase in apoptotic activity and consequently accelerating the process of neurodegeneration. In EOEA families with mutations in the PS-1 gene the average age of onset is much younger (45 years, range 29 to 62 years) that family with mutations in the PS-2 gene (52 years, range between 40 and 88 years).

Neuritic plaques, extracellular structures observable in AD are composed of amyloid beta peptide (ßA) and other elements such as glia and astrocytes (figures 6-9). The main constituent is ßA peptide natural product of the metabolism of amyloid precursor protein (APP). The study of families in the Volga allowed to demonstrate that the total amount of long ßA peptide (aa 42-43) and short (39-40 aa) were significantly lower in the case of mutations in the PS-2 gene mutations compared the PS-1 gene. Experiments *in vivo* have suggested that the PS-1 mutant altered proteolytic processing of APP at the C-terminal peptide SSA to favor deposition ßA long peptide (more insoluble and form faster kinetic characteristics). The relationship between PS-1 and EA does not seem clear; however, studies from fibroblasts and plasma from patients who have inherited mutations in this gene, demonstrating that the effect of these changes is to increase the ßA 42 peptide in the plasma. The mechanism by which PS-1 exerts its effect in AD is unknown. Mutations in the protein produce the same effect as the effects on the PPA. Presenilins are involved indirectly with a gamma-secretase, an enzymatic complex that processes of the PPA, and may be triggering or mediating its activity (figure 4) [12,13].

The presence of extracellular amyloid-peptide-containing neuritic plaques and intracellular neurofibrillary tangles and the loss of synapses in defined regions of the brain are the hallmarks associated with both familial and sporadic AD postmortem pathology.

In this chapter we reviewed the genetic, molecular, biochemical, and histopathological aspects of familiar AD (EOAD) linked to chromosomes 1, 14 and 19 and especially those found in a region of the state of Jalisco, Mexico.

## 2. Detection of EOAD

Detect EOAD is more complicated than LOAD [9], as their main symptom not always starts with memory loss, but with other symptoms such as vision problems, motor or speech, mood swings, irritability, disorientation even in familiar places, difficulty in learning and reasoning, lack of initiative and isolation. People who have it take longer and be diagnosed, as some of these symptoms are related to stress or depression. Early of AD detection is very important for the patient. Family environment can accelerate disease because the stress, is misunderstanding, lack of patience, affected by worsening symptoms, while good weather and a quiet home life makes slow the progression of symptoms (figure 5). Family members who have been able to detect early Alzheimer's must be psychologically and emotionally prepared to live with the disease [21-23].

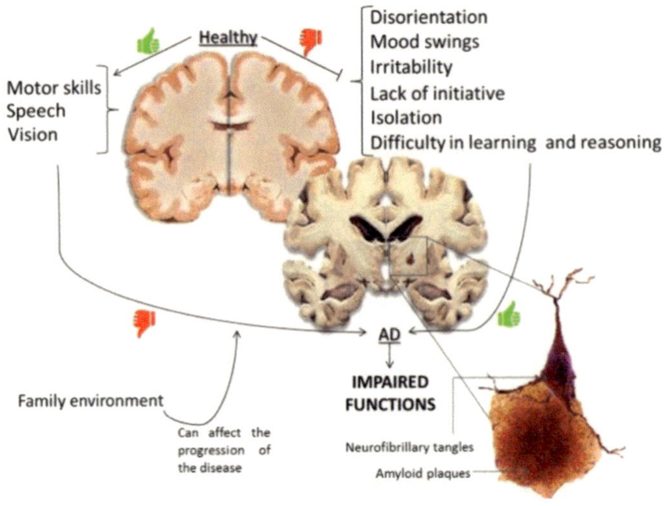


**Figure 4.** Symptomatology in Alzheimer´s Disease *versus* Helathy Control

During the initial stage, clinical data are diverse, but can be mentioned as the most significant: progressive memory loss, and changes in personality and behavior. Another common finding in EOAD is language difficulty (aphasia) such as naming which is commonly detected my persons close to the patients. Common findings that develop by the progression of AD are depression, headaches, seizures, myoclunus, Babinsky reflex, grasp reflex, extra-pyramidal signs and Parkinsonism. Being a progressive disease, the disease is progressive, and clinical signs and symptoms may vary from patient to patient; also the evolution of a patient with EOAD has been studied, it is believed that there are differences according between FAD and non NFAD; that patients with FAD compared to NFAD presented more frequent non-memory symptoms like visuospatial deficit. FAD present more memory deficit tan NFAD at the moment of the initial clinic visit. FAD has more tendencies to develop more headaches, myoclonus, gait abnormalities and pseudobulbar affect. Healthy control presents unaltered motor skills, speech and vision functions. However, in Alzheimer´s Disease patient's motor skills, speech and vision functions are impaired, while disorientation, mood swings, irritability, lack of initiative, isolation and difficulty in learning and reasoning is also present. On the other hand family environment can affect the progression of the symptomatology of the disease.

The age of onset difference between FAD and NFAD is that FAD develops 14 years earlier and the MMSE score is lower than NFAD. Initial clinic visits from patients with cognitive deterioration are to be focused on the disease onset, course and symptoms. A powerful tool for the clinical insight is the Mini- Mental State Examination (MMSE) which will help to know the cognitive status of the individual (Screening). There modifying factors that have been related to the progression of AD like is the level of school attendance, history of headaches and seizures. Now a day it is important to follow the guidelines to pursue a genetic testing of the most common mutations in AD allowing clinicians evaluate and manage patients with early onset dementias.

## 3. Risk factors in early life

The risk of dementia and Alzheimer's disease starts from the maternal womb. Fetal malnutrition, low birth weight and not breastfeeding may have long-term negative consequences. It has been shown that these and other conditions related to the early age of life, increased susceptibility to several chronic diseases, particularly cardiovascular disease and its risk factors (e.g. hyperinsulinemia, diabetes, atherosclerosis, hypertension, lipid disorders). The socioeconomic conditions are associated with other handicaps: nutrition, environmental stimulation, access to education, neuron-developmental, body growth, and subsequent cognitive performance. Several studies have used anthropometric as height indices, the length of the leg and arm, head circumference as markers of neurodevelopment in the first years of life and have found an inverse association with dementia and AD in later life.

The educational attainment has been the most studied factor. In most studies, low educational attainment is associated consistently with increased risk of cognitive impairment and dementia. There are multiple explanations for the association between low IQ and dementia:

1. Education produces a selection bias, since people with more education may show better performance on cognitive tests

2. Education is associated with other factors such as socioeconomic status early age, nutrition, IQ and adult life as an occupation, health and better lifestyles

3. Education increases cognitive reserve offering a potentiating neuroprotection and inducing long term [11-13].

## 4. Genetics and Alzheimer

Some genes were associated with AD: on chromosome 21 gene encoding the β-amyloid precursor protein, on chromosome 14 gene presenilin 1 (PS1), on the chromosome 1 gene for presenilin 2 (PS2), on chromosome 17 gene coding for protein, and chromosome 19 in the apolipoprotein E (ApoE). Four alleles of ApoE, which is believed to play an important role in AD is the ApoE type 4 are known ApoE4 allele has been seen as a risk factor for AD, with an attributable risk estimated 45 to 60%. Thus the approach to the diagnosis of probable AD also includes the study of ApoE.

Mutations in different genes located on chromosomes 14 and 1, responsible for EOAD of, in a portion of patients show a penetration (proportion of individuals that show the phenotype) about 100% with autosomal dominant. It has demonstrated the existence of a locus on chromosome 14 (14q 24.3) in a group of families with EOAD. Using the positional cloning the gene designated S 182, which contains 14 exons and encodes the synthesis of a protein of 467 amino acids (aa) called presenilin 1 (PS-1) containing from 6 to 9 transmembrane domains and two hydrophilic regions was isolated that are oriented towards cytosol [5,6] [table 1].

### 4.1. The Amyloid Precursor Protein (APP)

The amyloid precursor protein is a member of a family to understand her two similar proteins, APLP1 and APLP2. The APP is present in dendrites, cell bodies and axons of neurons and neuronal function is unknown. APP is synthesized in the rough endoplasmic reticulum, Golgi glycosylated and released into the membrane as a transmembrane protein, leaving the portion containing 613-671 β amyloid partially included in the membrane. The APP gene is located on chromosome 21; several investigators have identified many families of patients in whom the disease is declared prematurely, mutations in the APP gene located in different parts of the same: thus, a Swedish family found a double mutation at codons 670 and 671, and in other families, a mutation at codon 717 is detected. In these families, only those who show these mutations suffer from Alzheimer's disease, which proves without any doubt that there is a relationship between APP metabolism and Alzheimer's disease. The APP can experience a different metabolism to generate as a final product or other fragments. In the non-amyloidogenic pathway, APP secretase short region within the amyloid form a COOH-terminal 83 amino acid residues or appas called fragment CT83. In the amyloidogenic pathway, two enzymes called β-secretase or BACE and γ-secretase cleaved APP at the N terminal of the peptide sequence in endosomal compartments Aß, while the $\gamma$ -secretase cleaves the C-terminal sequence ab on cell surface or near it. Two types of $\gamma$ -secretase that are called presenilin-1 and presenilin-2: PS1 and PS1. These enzymes are currently the subject of extensive studies, because its blockade by drugs theoretically decrease the formation of β-amyloid [14, 15].

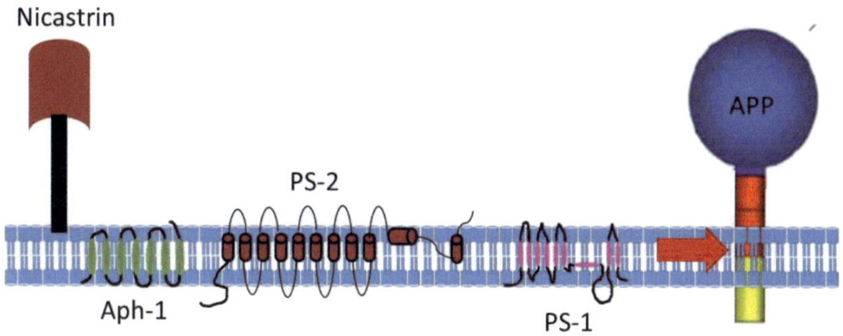


**Figure 5.** $\gamma$ – Secretase Complex

The $\gamma$-secretase complex is composed of four membrane proteins: nicastrin, aph-1, PS-2, and presenilin (1 or 2). The actual catalytic site is in presenilin. Cleavage of APP and other substrates occurs in the membrane. Presenilins are involved indirectly with the complex.

More than 90 different mutations have been found in the gene for the PS-1 on chromosome 14. All mutations but one are missense and represent about 30-50% of cases of another gene, in this case located on chromosome 1 was found was using the same strategy that isolated the PS-1. Gene, called STM-2, was isolated families descended from German settlers installed in the Volga region in Russia (ref). STM-2 gene encodes a 448 aa protein called presenilin 2 (PS-2), named after the latter has homology (over 80%) compared to the PS-1 gene in some regions (ref.). The mutations cause about 2% of total EOAD and occur less frequently than those found in the PS-1 gene. Only found two missense mutations penetrance incomplete [16].

The first gene associated with late forms family was identified in a family sample by applying a new method of genetic analysis. The identified Apo E locus is located on the long arm of chromosome 19. Numerous studies have reported association between Apo E (locus) and EOAD, and sporadic cases. The relationship between Apo E and EA iș set by the over-representation of one common protein isoforms in the group of patients. Of the 3 major isoforms, known as E2, E3 and E4, E4 is often found associated with the appearance of the disease [13].

This table exhibited examples of some important mutations per gene; number of gene mutations identified are also shown in table.

| Mutations in PSEN1 gene | | | | |
|---|---|---|---|---|
| **Number of Mutations in gene** | **Mutations** | **Exon/Domain** | **Onset** | **General description of Clinical data** |
| 185 mutations described in 405 families | Thr116Asn | 5/ HL-I | Early Autosomal dominant heritance | • Progressive memory loss<br>• Changes in personality and behavior.<br>• Language difficulty<br>• Depression<br>• Headaches<br>• Seizures<br>• Myoclunus<br>• Babinsk reflex<br>• Grasp reflex<br>• Cerebellar signs |
| | Met139Val | 5/ TM-II | | |
| | Met146Leu | 5/ TM-II | | |
| | Thr291Pro | 9/ HL-VI (MA) | | |
| | Leu171Pro | 6/ TM-III | | |
| | Ala431Glu | 12/ HL-VIII | | |
| **Mutations in PSEN2 gene** | | | | |
| **Number of Mutations in gene** | **Mutations** | **Exon/Domain** | **Onset** | |
| 13 mutationes describen in 22 families | Ala85Val | 4/ N-term | Early Autosomal dominant heritance | |
| | Thr122Pro | 5/ HL-1 | | |
| | Thr122Arg | 5/ HL-1 | | |
| | Ser130Leu | 5/ HL-1 | | |
| | Asn141Ile | 5/ TM-II | | |
| | Val148Ile | 5/ TM-II | | |
| **Mutations in APP gene** | | | | |
| **Number of Mutations in gene** | **Mutations** | **Exon/Domain** | **Onset** | |
| 33 mutations described in 90 families | Ala692Gly | 17/ N-term | Late | |
| | Glu693Gln | 17/ N-term | | |
| | Ile716Phe | 17/ TM-I | | |
| | Val717Leu | 17/ TM-I | | |
| | Leu723Pro | 17/ TM-I | | |
| | Ile716Val | 17/ TM-I | | |
| **Mutations in APOe gene** | | | | |
| **Number of Mutations in gene** | **Mutations** | **Exon/Domain** | **Onset** | |
| 88 mutations described | -293 (G/T) | Promoter region | Late | |
| | -427 (T/C) | Promoter region | | |
| | -491 (A/T) | Promoter region | | |

**Table 1.** Mutations

### 4.2. Presenilin (PS-1 and PS-2)

The hypothesis of the existence of a locus that could explain some of the cases EAFP was confirmed in 1992, in which several groups pre-sat evidence of a locus on chromosome 14; this was named, along with S 182, PS-1 or AD3. The role of the PS-1 gene in the organism is unknown. Its homology to proteins of the Notch / lin-12 family suggests that it may play a role in signal transduction, and it is stated that the process involved in gene apoptosis. The PS-1 is expressed in different regions of brain, skeletal muscle, kidney, pancreas, placenta and the heart. Its processing produces 2 fragments, this process occurs naturally and is under control. An increase of the amount of PS-1 produced by the cells, *in vitro*, is not accompanied by increase in the concentration of the fragments. Of the 14 exons which holds the PS-1 gene, most of the mutations are linked to exon 5 (comprising the transmembrane domain 1 and 2) and exon 8 (comprising the transmembrane domain 6 and 7); the effects on the PS-1 gene, in the 2 sites mentioned above show a significant difference with respect to age at onset of the disease when compared to each other, patients with mutations in the transmembrane domain (DT) 6 and 7, with a mean age of onset higher than those with mutations in the DT 1 and 2 [16-17].

All mutations, except one, are missense, resulting in a change of a from one another. The mutation known as D9 is one of the exceptions, and described in many families of diverse origin (English, Japanese, Australian and Latin´s). Involvement causes the elimination of exon 9 (the deletion occurs); do not changes the reading frame processing and disposal site and the corresponding fragments. The mutation has the remarkable feature that is expressed in almost all families, spastic paraparesy, and a phenotype that is not apparent with any other mutation. In an England family a mutation was detected in codon 141 of PS-1 gene with incomplete penetrance. The involvement is manifested in a change of Iso by Val, the disease began with an average age of onset of 55 years [16-17].

The STM 2 gene (located on chromosome 1), also known as AD 4, PS-2, the affected families had a missense mutation at codon 141, resulting in a change of aspartic acid (Asp) by Iso. In these families ligations were excluded chromosomes 14 and 21. The PS-2 gene also contains 10 exons, and the protein for which it encodes contains 6 to 9 DT. The PS-2 transmembrane protein has 67% homology to the sequence of aa from the PS-1, and therefore, the homology in función. PS-2 is localized in the endoplasmic reticulum with the hydrophilic domains oriented cytoplasm. The homology between PS-1 and PS-2 is particularly focused on the DT. The amino-terminal domain and the domain located between exons 8 and 10, has the lowest degree of homology and which is supposed to be the functional specificity of each of the living proteins (ref.). Another mutation that is associated with the EOAD is located at codon 239 and is manifested in a change of methionine (Met) to Valina (Val) (ref.). As can be seen, the mutation sites are different from those presented in the PS-1, characterized by a penetration incomplete. This data support that mutations in the gene of the PS-2 cause an increase in apoptotic activity, and therefore accelerate neurodegeneration.

In EOAD families with mutations in the PS-1 gene the average age of onset is much younger (45 years, range 29 to 62 years) that families with mutations in the PS-2 gene (52 years, range between 40 and 88 years) (ref.).

Senile plaques, extracellular structures observable in AD, are formed by the amyloid beta peptide (ßA) and other elements such as glia and astrocytes. The main constituent is ßA peptide natural product of the metabolism of amyloid precursor protein (APP) (Figure 7). The study of families in the Volga possible to show that the total amount of long ßA peptide (aa 42-43) and short (39-40 aa) were significantly lower in the case of mutations in the PS-2 gene mutations compared in PS-1 (figure2) Gene *in vivo* experiments have suggested that the mutated PS-1 alters the proteolytic processing of APP at the C-terminal peptide ßA to favor the deposition of peptide ßA long (more insoluble form and kinetic properties more fast), the relationship between PS-1 and EA does not seem clear; however, studies from fibroblasts and plasma from patients with inherited mutations in this gene, show that the effect of these changes is to increase the peptide ßA 42 in plasma. The mechanism by the that PS-1 exerts its effect in AD; mutations in the protein produce the same effect that the damages in the PPA. Presenilins are involved in an indirect way with gama-secretase, an enzyme that processes of the PPA. The PS-2 mutated gene causes the disease, and also makes it through the common mechanism to which reference was made earlier, that is, increasing the concentration of peptide ßA 42. Transgenic animals carrying the PS-1 mutation, have 2 times ßA peptide 42 in the brain tissue compared to normal mice. Although mutations in the APP gene and the PS-1 and PS-2 genes have a dramatic effect, they are only responsible for 50% of cases of EOAD. They represent 5% of all cases in the general population. Men and women who inherit two copies (one from each parent) of the gene, called ApoE4, are at very high risk of developing Alzheimer. However, the two copies of ApoE4 is rare, affecting only 2 percent of the population, while about 15 percent of people carry a single copy of this version of the gene. This gene affects a protein involved in the transport of cholesterol in cholesterol-the cells is a crucial component of all cell membranes, including nerve cells. Nerve cells are constantly responding to experience, through the development, improvement, reduction or elimination of their electrochemical contact with other nerve cells. For all these processes, efficient transport of cholesterol is critical. Only about 10-15 percent of the population carries one copy of E4, over 50 percent of people who develop Alzheimer's disease are carriers E4. However, the increased risk of E4 seems confined largely to women.

Functional magnetic resonance imaging was used to examine the connections in the network of the brain's memory and has been shown that in older women with the E4 variant, this network of interconnected brain regions which usually share a synchronized pattern activity-shows a loss of sync, a pattern typically seen in Alzheimer's patients. In healthy elderly women (but not men) with at least one E4 allele, activity in a brain area called precuneus seems out of sync with other regions whose activation patterns in general are closely coordinated

We performed genetic and Spanish-language neuropsychological control; Mexican persons without dementia known to be at 50% risk of inheriting one of two *PSEN1* mutations. Early declines in performance on the Trail Making Test, delayed recall of a 10-word list, the Wechsler Adult Intelligence Scale Block Design Test, and total MMSE score in these subjects. In a previous work (ref) we explore the sub-items on the MMSE that best differentiate *PSEN1* mutation carriers (MCs) and non-carriers (NCs) and explore the relationship of age and education to these scores. Neuropsicological data exhibited MCs performed worse than NCs on the Mini-Mental State Examination. In multiple linear regression analyses a question frequently asked is: if APOE4 carriers had different results in function evaluations affected by

Alzheimer's disease, including episodic memory, working memory, mental speed, reaction time and vocabulary reading. As expected, performance in all tests (except for reading vocabulary, which tends to stay with age) declined by age groups, a sign of normal cognitive aging. But the APOE4 did not affect performance, indicating that people with APOE4 age normally in those cognitive functions, at least between 20 and 64 years old. According to the researchers, this finding suggests that APOE4 increases the risk of Alzheimer's later in life by an unknown process that accelerates or intensifies normal cognitive changes [24-27].

### 4.3. Beta-Amyloid (Aß)

Discovered in 1984 by Glenner et al., Is a peptide of 39-42 amino acids originating from the called amyloid precursor protein (APP) by the action of peptidadas called secretases. There are two major types of b-amyloid called amyloid-b and b-amyloid 1-40 1-42 according to the number of amino acids present. APP is a transmembrane protein having 770 aminácidos and located on different cell types. On its extracellular portion, the APP has several regions with neurotrophic activity.

Senile plaques in the brain parenchyma and vessel amyloid deposits are composed primarily amyloid beta peptide (Aß). Although the accumulation of Aß is common in non-demented elderly individuals in EA this accumulation is usually higher and / or faster. Currently, genetic evidence, in vitro experiments and in animal models suggest that the accumulation of brain Aß oligomers as might be an important development factor cognitivo deterioration; hence the removal of Aß in the brain is one of the therapeutic strategies for AD currently undergoing clinical trial. Aß is one of the normal internal proteolysis products transmembrane protein called APP (amyloid precursor protein). Excessive accumulation of Aß in AD could be explained by several mechanisms, some of them converging. Include increased production of Aß, kinetics of aggregation or self-assembly and quick removal of faulty brain as a result of: 1 an abnormally slow transport from the interstitial fluid into the cerebral spinal fluid (perivascular drainage) or plasma (transport through capillaries) and 2 deficiente proteolytic degradation. Excess production or the greater tendency of Aß oligomerization may explain the rapid deposition of Aß in some rare hereditary forms of AD, caused by mutations in APP or presenilin genes called 1 and 2, components of the secretase complex responsible for the generation of Aß. Instead, poor elimination could be relevant in the normal brain aging and may be magnified in the most common forms of AD called sporadic. Beyond a well-defined, as the inheritance of one or two e4 alleles of apolipoprotein E, a risk factor for sporadic AD probably has multiple risk factors include head trauma, ischemic events, hypertension, insulin resistance, among others, and a complex pathogenesis that is still far from being understood [14-15].

### 4.4. Tau protein

Tau belongs to the family of microtubule-associated proteins (MAPs) and normally binds to and stabilizes microtubules (MTs) in neurons. Tau protein has four different domains: the N-terminal, the proline rich, the microtubule-binding and the C-terminal domain. In the adult human brain six tau isoforms are expressed by different splicing of the same tau mRNA; they vary in the number of microtubule-binding domains (having either three or four) and in the number and size of N-terminal inserts [2]. Tau can be post-translationally modified in several ways (e.g. glycosylation, ubiquitination and oxidation), but phosphorylation is by far the most extensively studied and is paramount to AD pathology [2,3]. Hyperphosphorylation of tau especially on Ser214 and Ser262, leads to lose its ability to bind to MTs and may also sequester normal tau, preventing binding to MTs, resulting in disruption of the MT [4]. Hyperphosphorylated tau is also more resistant to proteases and this makes it more prone to aggregate to form PHFs in NFT´s. Neurofibrillary tangles (NFT) (figure 6) are one of the main diagnostic criteria of AD. Each of these lesions contains filamentous aggregates composed of the microtubule-associated protein (MAP) tau [9]. The normal function of tau protein is to stabilize axonal microtubules and regulate intracellular vesicle transport. Hyperphosphorylation of tau associated with AD impairs its ability to regulate microtubule assembly and promotes the protein aggregation into paired helical filaments (PHF). To understand the roles of normal and abnormal tau protein has been important to elucidate the structure and the mechanisms by which self-assembles it. Contains six human tau isoforms that result from splicing process ("splicing") alternative. The C-terminal domain containing 3 or 4 repetitive sequences involved in the binding of tau to microtubules that are key to the ability to promote their assembly One reason why a change in the functionality of tau is phosphorylation significant abnormal sites in their structure, essentially residues Ser/Thr Pro followed: Ser202, Thr205, Ser396 and Ser404 (22). Such phosphorylations are catalyzed by two protein kinases: the cdk5 / p35 and GSK3b system (32). In the cytoplasm, there is normally phosphorylated tau and it is postulated that these post-translational modifications regulate tau's ability to associate with microtubules and other cytoskeletal filaments. In AD, tau is hyperphosphorylated in these key sites, which changes the dynamics of action in regulating the interaction patterns within the cytoskeleton causing their self-association and training, progressively, PHF

No tau mutations have been reported to cause AD, but differences in tau haplotype and mutations may be the cause of other neurodegenerative disorders such as progressive supranuclear palsy [10]. NFT pathology in the brain occurs in a sequential manner. The altered protein Tau is less able to bind to other cytoskeletal proteins and added in lethal NFT seen in degenerating neurons of AD patients. The total length of p35 is normally regulated and has a very short half-life; degradation is usually carried out by its association with Cdk35, which the hyperphosphorylated. Moreover, p25 is completely stable, it accumulates in large amounts in EA (10 to 40 times and in the same regions where present NFT; levels Cdk5 and p35 have to remain stable in EA), maintains a permanent activation of Cdk5 and seems to precede the formation of NFTs. The connection between p25 and the formation of amyloid plaques is unknown. These findings provide several future therapeutic strategies: altered level of cut (cleavage) of p35, inhibition/blocking Cdk5 (necessary for day to day neuronal enzymes), blocking p25 or protease that produces it. Other proteins (protein associated with the cytoskeleton, focal adhesion kinase, glutaredoxin, utropina) have been implicated as mediators in the formation of NFTs or degeneration of neurons affected. The presence of few neurofibrillary tangles in the hippocampus and in the parahippocampal gyrus (in AD their presence is most notable in the entorhinal cortex) and senile plaques.

The possible role of Tau in dementia took center stage in AD with the discovery of mutations in the tau gene on chromosome 17; frontotemporal call Ademencia with Parkinsonism linked to chromosome 17 "(FTDP-17) includes a large number of mutations, which can result in a variety of currently known. These include fronto-temporal dementia (characterized by frontal and anterior temporal atrophy), Pick's disease (characterized by intra-neuronal inclusions called Pick bodies, Alternative Predominant in Clew of AD (AD @ AVPO-characterized by the lack of plates. presence of tangles predominantly in limbic and paralimbic cortical areas), progressive supranuclear palsy and corticobasal degeneration The shape of the Tau inclusions (including PH-Tau) depends partly on the causative mutation thereof; and those related to the PH-Tau inclusions produced in one or more anatomical sites from the cerebral cortex to the spinal cord, also Tau deposits can be found in neurons, tangles, Pick bodies or glial cells. The absence of plates, particularly of compact manifold, in many of the tauopathies suggests that Tau abnormalities are responsible for dementing disorder, including some variations of AD (e.g., AD-VPO). Known mutations occur in a reduced protein Tau Tau ability to interact with microtubules on production or Tau isoforms with four repeated microtubules together. These lead to the assembly of the Tau in similar or identical to those found in AD filaments. Several missense mutations also have a stimulating effect on filament formation heparin-induced Tau. The assembly of tau into filaments may be a gain of toxic function believed to be the underlying cause of death of nerve cells affected.[8].

### 4.5. Apo-E

Apolipoprotein E (ApoE) is the major apolipoprotein present in high-density lipoproteins (HDL) and is synthesized in the brain, primarily by astrocytes and to a lesser degree by microglia. ApoE is a 299 amino acid glycoprotein which organize into 2 functional domains; residues 1-191 form the amino-terminal (ApoE NT) "receptor binding domain" and residues 216-299 form the carboxyl-terminal (ApoE CT) "lipid binding domain". Both domains have been reported to be involved in the interaction between ApoE and Aβ. Three common isoforms of apoE exist in humans and result from amino acid interchanges at positions 112 and 158. ApoE2 has cysteines while apoE4 has arginines at both sites. ApoE3 has a cysteine and an arginine at positions 112 and 158, respectively. The most common form of apoE is apoE3, which is present in 77% of the general population; ~15% of the population have apoE4, and ~8% have the apoE2 [27]. The APOE ε4 allele markedly increases AD risk and decreases age of onset, likely through its strong effect on the accumulation of amyloid-β (Aβ) peptide. In contrast, the APOE ε2 allele appears to decrease AD risk [28]. ApoE4 is associated with an early age of AD onset. [29].

ApoE isoform differentially affect the apoE:lipid ratio of glia-secreted particles where apoE4 exhibits a higher apoE:lipid ratio compared to apoE3. ApoE mediates transport of glia-secreted particles to neurons for development, axon myelination, synaptogenesis and maintenance. Additionally, apoE redistributes cholesterol released after neuron injury or degeneration for membrane repair and remyelination [30]. The higher apoE:lipid ratio in apoE4 suggests that at similar apoE protein concentration, apoE4 may deliver less cholesterol to neurons, compared to apoE3. ApoE4 particles were also shown to be less efficient at inducing cholesterol efflux from neuronal cells compared to apoE3 [3l]. Brain apoE particles exhibit differing binding affinities to the amyloid-β peptide in a manner that is apoE isoform-dependent, therefore,

ApoE isoform may influence AD pathogenesis via direct or indirect interactions with Aβ. Furhermore, ApoE plays essential role in facilitating the proteolytic clearance of soluble Aβ. E4 apolipoprotein E isoform has been considered a risk factor for developing Alzheimer's disease. The exact mechanism by which the presence ApoE affects Alzheimer's is still unknown; appears to promote the formation and stabilizes the aggregation of beta amyloid fibril in plaques that appear in Alzheimer's disease. Aβ protein is considered the major component of these plates and is a proteolytic product of the precursor protein of Aβ peptide. The gene encoding apolipoprotein E (ApoE) is known as allelic variants APOEε2, and APOEε4 APOEε3 and a rare allelic variant known as APOEε3r APOEε3. In studies in populations of individuals with Alzheimer's disease and race from different geographical origins, it has been shown that APOEε4 allele is a risk factor that influences age of onset of symptoms. The APOEε4 allele is 50% of individuals with Alzheimer's disease and delayed onset of the presence of a copy of the allele increases the risk of late onset and three times in two copies in 12 times. Individuals with late onset carrying one or two copies of allele APOEε4 develop symptoms of disease 10 to 20 years earlier, compared with individuals not carrying this allele. The APOEε2, much less common in individuals with Alzheimer's disease and in the general population, allele appears to act as a protective factor for the onset of disease. The APOE-4 contributes to the accumulation of Aβ by slowing evacuation of the brain, which may explain why some people accumulate more Aβ, which other, increasing the risk of Alzheimer's. Individuals with APOE-e4 have much more protein Aβ in the brain, that individuals with the APOE-e2 and APOE-e3 (the other two common forms of protein gene) forms these data are obtained using the methodology of the microdialysis ; that involves the implantation of a dialysis membrane in a brain region to monitor chemical processes in the tissues of a living organism. [32-34].

## 5. Molecular markers for early Alzheimer´s Disease

The rational approach of neurodegenerative diseases associated with dementia, particularly Alzheimer's disease, has led researchers around the world to think this entity as a systemic process that involves changes not only in the brain but also peripherally, so that has begun to seek so-called "peripheral biomarkers". These biomarkers can be found in platelets, lymphocytes, cultured fibroblasts and cerebrospinal fluid samples of patients affected [35]. Since AD has a long preclinical stage of the disease, the biomarker should also be predictive and. In AD, naturally, the biomarker should be relevantly linked to either amyloid- or tau pathology.

The hypothesis that the AD is systemic, has led to the search for peripherals markers, which can manifest biochemical changes related to the disease markers. Studies of the incidence and transmission patterns in families of patients with AD show that relatives of affected individuals have an increased risk of developing AD when compared with members of the general population. Concordance rates between monozygotic twins pro sides with EA are 40-60%, suggesting a strong but not absolute genetic influence of disease. Another significant problem is that some cognitively healthy subjects exhibit substantial AD type neuropathology [36]. On the other hand, some patients with severe cognitive impairment display very little neuropathology. It is also common that patients with other dementias, for example vascular dementia or dementia with Lewy bodies, have concomitant AD neuropathology or AD patients have vascular or LB pathology [37].

It has been hypothesized that the AD associated changes in CSF biomarkers would be evident before the clinical diagnosis of AD and could be used to predict the development of AD in MCI patients. For example, CSF Aβ42 levels were decreased and CSF tau and phospho tau levels were increased in those MCI patients who received a diagnosis of AD during a follow-up period of approximately four years [38].

Numerous different proteins and molecules that are present in CSF have been studied as potential biomarkers for AD, such as glycosylated acetylcholinesterase [39], transglutaminase [40], 24S-hydroxycholesterol [41], isoprostane [42]. It is also possible that the most accurate diagnosis of early AD can be achieved by using a panel of several different biomarkers [43]. Even though the above mentioned and numerous other molecules including neurofilament proteins, neuromodulin and neuronal thread protein have been studied [44], at the present, the only usable biomarkers are the CSF Aβ42, tau and phospho-tau levels in CSF.

Since platelets contain the amyloid precursor protein and secrete β-amyloid peptide, express neurotransmitters and some neuron-related proteins, such as NMDA receptors [45], in our group of work we are analyzing platelets from AD patients and subjects controls. Western blotting experiments of APP showed one protein of about 130 Kd and several proteins of about 106 to 110 Kd. The 130 Kd protein is the mature APP. The other proteins of lower molecular weights are the APP immature isoforms [46]. A high mature APP to immature APP isoform ratio (O.6 or higher) it has been related to a normal APP processing. Conversely, a lower ratio (< 0.6) it has been related to an altered APP processing [47]. We previously showed mature APP to immature APP isoform ratio in platelet samples of AD Mexican subjects was similar to the reported in previous studies [48]. This means that an increased degradation of this precursor protein is being performed in peripheral tissues. In addition, we found no statistical differences were detected for gender, age, and any specific ApoE allele in AD patients. Furthermore, statistical analysis between EOAD patients and LOAD suggests that no statistical differences among both groups in neither the APP isoforms nor any of the ApoE genotypes [46]. These data are in consonance with previous studies suggesting that ApoE genotyping is not sufficient as a diagnostic test for AD [49].

We have assessed the role of oxidative stress markers (lipoperoxides, nitric oxide metabolites) and membrane properties such as membrane fluidity in AD patients. We found a reduced fluidity in the platelet inner mitochondrial membrane in AD patients compared with healthy controls of similar age. It has been suggested that oxidative stress could be partially responsible for the diminution of membrane fluidity [50]. This change in membrane fluidity can modify the activities of the membrane-bound proteins such as transport or receptor proteins. At this regard, it has been hypothesized that a reduced fluidity of the inner mitochondrial membrane may diminish significantly the rate of mitochondrial ATP synthesis. Oxidative stress and mitochondrial failure has been associated to Alzheimer's pathology [51]. We measured the rate of mitochondrial ATP hydrolysis catalyzed by the F0F1-ATPase and we found that this activity increases significantly in patients with probable AD as compared to the control subjects. However, the transmembrane pH gradient driven by ATP hydrolysis was lower in

AD samples as compared to the controls (0.5 ± 0.1 pH units). This suggests a functional alteration of the F0F1-ATPase [45].

The fluidity of plasma membrane of erythrocytes were not modified significantly in samples of Mexican AD patients compared to healthy controls, regardless of increased lipid oxidation in erythrocytes AD patients. These data were similar to the previously reported [52] This suggests that inner mitochondrial membranes are more sensitive to oxidative stress than erythrocytes. it has been reported an increase in fluidity in whole membranes from platelets of AD patients [53]. This increase is due to a functionally abnormal membrane compartment resembling endoplasmic reticulum [54]. It is worth noting that platelets contain a few mitochondria, therefore, the contribution of mitochondrial membranes to the whole cell membranes is minimal [55]. Additionally, we found a significant decrease of membrane fluidity in hippocampal neurons from AD patients compared with membranes from elderly non demented controls. Lower membrane fluidity in AD patients was correlated with abnormal APP processing and cognitive decline [56].

The human cytochrome c oxidase is the terminal enzyme complex of the respiratory chain; it is located in the inner mitochondrial membrane where it catalyzes the transfer of electrons from reduced cytochrome c to molecular oxygen. Mitochondrial cytochrome c oxidase (MTCO) is made up of 13 subunits; its catalytic core is made up from the protein products of the MTCO I, II, and III genes that are encoded in mitochondrial DNA. Diminished cytochrome c oxidase activity has been described in AD postmortem cerebral cortex [57-60] and platelets [61]. Kish et al. [62] reported a reduced level of this protein complex in AD brain. These data could suggest that brain cytochrome oxidase is kinetically abnormal; thus, this dysfunction must arise from a catalytic defect rather than an underproduction [61]. However, mutations of the mitochondrial genome are widely recognized as important causes of disease [63]. Analysis of mitochondrial cytochrome c oxidase II gene obtained from blood samples of Mexican patients with AD revealed that 4 nonrelated patients with probable AD harbored the polymorphism A8027G (three of them were diagnosed with LOAD, with familial history of the disease and one of them with EOAD.This polymorphism shows a frequency of 12% in the analyzed sample. Four patients with EOAD harbored only one of thefollowing point mutations: A8003C, T8082C, C8201T, andG7933A, respectively. The A8003C transversion converts a polar neutral asparagine residue to a basic histidine. The T8082C transition converts proline to a leucine. C8201T transition converts a nonpolar aromatic phenylalanine to a nonpolar leucine. G7603A transversion converts a basic arginine to a basic histidine. From the 33 patients that were enrolled for this study only 8 of them presented a nucleotide variation in MTCO II gene, representing the 24% of the total of the patients. Three of the eight patients (37.5%) showed nucleotide variation and were diagnosed with LOAD. While, five of the eight patients (62.5%) were EOAD [64].

## 6. Histopathology of EOAD

Definitive diagnosis of AD late/onset is based on examination of brain tissue obtained at autopsy. The histopathology of EOAD is a neurodegenerative process characterized by selective and progressive death of neuronal cells in specific brain areas, primarily in the neocortex and hippocampus, which is clinically reflected by a dementia state. The clinical picture of dementia AD is accompanied by a massive buildup of insoluble filaments having ß-folded conformation which define two main types of lesions: neuritic plaques (NP) and neurofibrillary tangles (NFT) (figures 6-8). The major protein component of the NP fibrils is the beta-amyloid peptide and the NFT, tau. In general, it should be noted that both the formation of fibrils ß amyloid as the PNs of NFT.

The NP are composed of two main components: a core of extracellular amyloid ß and an arrangement of nerve terminals degenerate, uniquely shaped, dystrophic neurites, which may be intracellular or extracellular nature depending on their state of degeneration. These neurites surround the core board. Characteristically NP in EOAD are surrounded by numerous glial cells which, in encapsulate way. NP density correlates with the degree of the EOAD. In the case of Alzheimer's, as well as in healthy older adults can be found in the brain amyloid deposits without neuritic ß component. Unlike NP, this type of injury, called senile plaque, not correlated with EA. These findings have suggested that senile plaques are a risk factor for the development of the disease, that is, its presence is necessary but not sufficient for the onset.

The number of NFT observed in post-mortem histology of Alzheimer's cases correlate with the severity and duration of dementia. The NFT can be of two types: intracellular and extracellular depending if they are within the neuron or in the extracellular space with the death of the same. There are ways to evolve as the NFT changes from one state to another. It is clear that the dystrophic neurites are also part of the fibrillary degeneration of neuronal cells. Neurites are formed from the accumulation of abnormal filaments at the terminals of the cell axons and dendrites.

In OEAD the evolution of neurofibrillary formation in the hippocampus is very fast, the NFT appear in greater numbers in the transition zone (trans-enthorinal) and its adjacent layer II of the enthorinal cortex, which are located in the parahippocampal, temporal lobe. This information is key to understanding the pathophysiology of EOAD and its rapid development as well as its clinical correlation, since neuronal cells of layer II (enthorinal) on cortex relay zone where axons of associative neocortical areas arrive. The axons from layer II reach the hippocampus through a defined path via piercing call, and then synapse hippocampal pyramidal neuron. Once the information is processed, hippocampal axons synapse with output layer IV of the entorhinal cortex and hence the information to the entire neocortex is shipped. In other words the synaptic connections of the neocortex and the hippocampus is limited to the entorhinal cortex. In EOAD, to be destroyed these two layers also very fast; "off"... these two important areas of the brain, concomitant destruction of the hippocampus creates a complete disconnect with the associative areas of the neocortex

In Los Altos de Jalisco (Mexican region), there are many affected, even compare this (region) with others in the country, and in the world (the epidemiological analysis) exhibited a high prevalence. In autopsies members of these families show the basics of pathological diagnosis: a) neuritic plaques; b) neurofibrillary tangles; c) granulo-vacuolar degeneration; d) congophilic degeneration and Hirano body´s (these also observed in others pathologies).

The autopsy of a member family (3 affected) exhibited the typical diagnostic markers mentioned above; even using routine stains (H/E). Figure 6 exhibited degeneration and neuronal death (arrows); in the center of picture you can see the arrow labeled occupy the space surrounded by tangles neuron and glia.

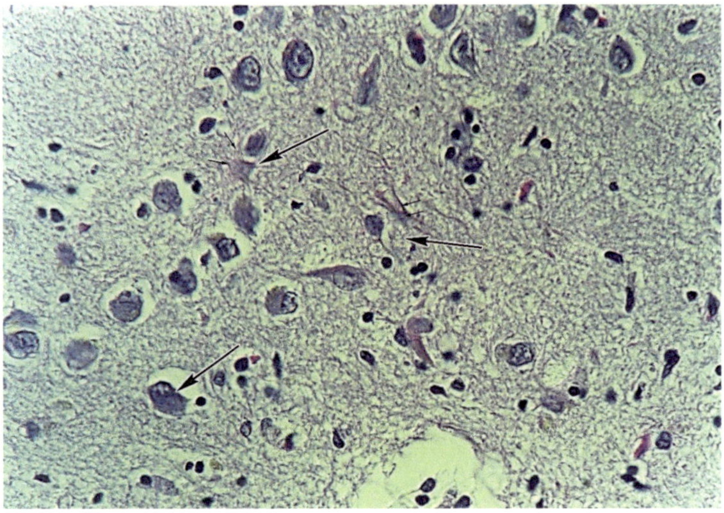

**Figure 6.** Exhibited the typical image of a neuritic plaques surrounded of gliosis (arrows).

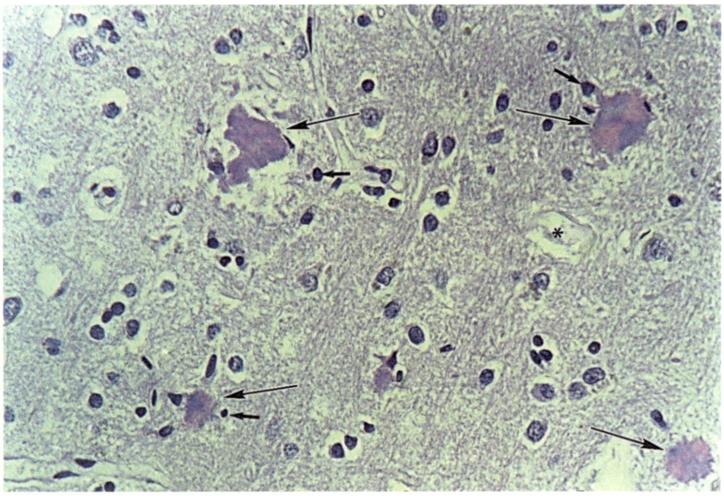

**Figure 7.** Exhibited in the center (arrows) a neuritic plaque, and marked with asterisks neurons showing intra/extra cellular tangles.

Neuritic plaques in EOAD are more complex; they consist of extracellular insoluble deposits formed by various compounds, the most abundant Aβ protein. This protein, as discussed above, is derived by proteolytic processing of a larger protein APP. The plates can be described as diffuse or classical. Diffuse are added amorphous Aβ are not associated with dystrophic neurites or abnormal neurons. Neuritic plaques are composed classical extracellular insoluble deposits formed by various compounds, the most abundant is the Aβ protein. This protein, as discussed above, is derived by proteolytic processing attic of a larger protein APP. The plates can be described as diffuse or classical. Diffuse are added amorphous Aβ, and are not associated with dystrophic neurites or abnormal neurons. Classical neuritic plaques contain fibrillar aggregates of dense insoluble Aβ surrounded dystrophic neurites, astrocytes and activated microglia assets which are associated with neuronal degeneration and loss. Containing dense fibrillar aggregates of amyloid β insoluble surrounded dystrophic neurites, astrocytes and activated microglia assets which are associated with neuronal degeneration and loss. In the vessels of the hippocampus and cortex, the existence of numerous neuritic plaques is observed. Neuritic plaques consist of clusters of axons degenerate dendritic spines and with a core containing extracellular linear filaments formed by the β-amyloid peptide. Amyloid deposits in senile plaques and in blood vessels of the cerebral cortex amyloid β fragment, whose amino acid sequence provided the basis for cloning the gene expressing the β amyloid was found. This gene encodes the APP protein, fragments that originates from proteolysis from 38 to 42 amino acids, the Aβ. In families with early disease has come to identify a place on the long arm of chromosome 21; duplicated in Down syndrome region near the gene encoding APP.

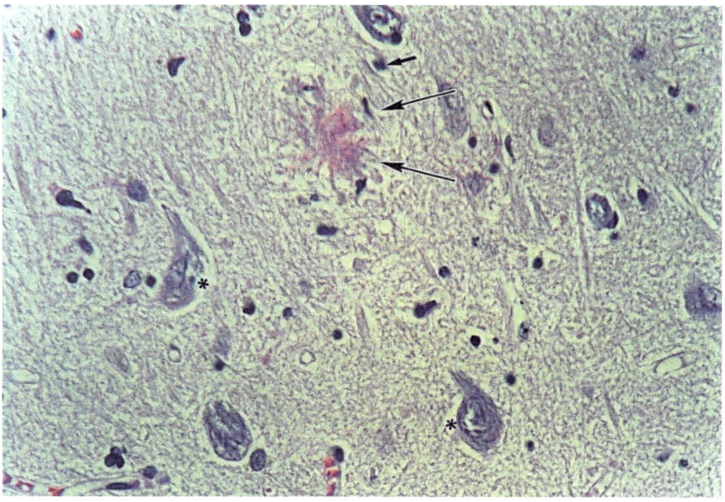

## 7. Neurofibrillary tangles in EOAD

Constitute one of the main lesions associated with the disease, and its presence is essential for diagnosis, Consist of abnormal fibrous inclusions in the perinuclear cytoplasm of neurons. The bulk density of neurofibrillary tangles in EOAD cases found in the neurons of the entorhinal cortex and CA1 region of the hippocampus and subiculum (layers III, V and VI of the neocortex). Several studies have shown a correlation between the load of neurofibrillary tangles and the degree of cognitive impairment, which has been correlated to these lesions have a direct effect on neuronal function. Despite being one of the cardinal lesions of AD is not pathognomonic of it. You can find (in addition to normal people) in other diseases such as: posttraumatic and pugilistic dementia or parkinsonism-dementia complex.

Finally the figure 9 exhibited the typical image of the granulo-vacuolar degeneration (arrows), and we appreciate the fine neuropil granulation, and fuzzy presence of tangles.

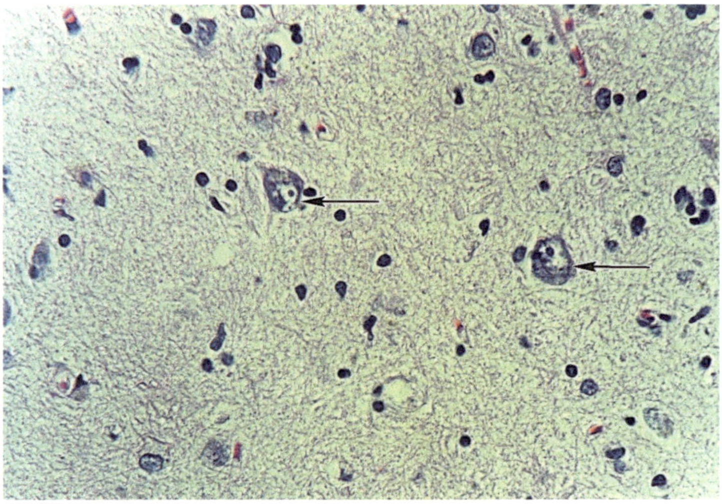

## 8. Granulovacuolar Degeneration in EOAD

Consists of an alteration of neurons in which the presence is observed in the cytoplasm of clustered small vacuoles, each of which contains a basophil granule inside, we observed this degeneration in all the hippocampus (also the enthorinal area). This granule appears to consist of several different proteins, such as neurofilament, tubulin, tau and ubiquitin among others. Little is known about the nature and significance of these alterations. Although you can find in elderly otherwise healthy brains, their presence in large numbers at the junction between the CA1 and CA2 regions of the hippocampus is strongly associated with AD.

Today it is a challenge the diagnosis of Alzheimer's... More interdisciplinary research is needed

## Acknowledgements

Dr Raúl Mena-López *(in memoriam)*

## Author details

Genaro Gabriel Ortiz[1*], Fermín P. Pacheco-Moisés[2], Erika D. González-Renovato[1], Luis Figuera[3], Miguel A. Macías-Islas[4], Mario Mireles-Ramírez[5], L. Javier Flores-Alvarado[4], Angélica Sánchez-López[1], Dhea G. Nuño-Penilla[1], Irma E. Velázquez- Brizuela[4], Juan P. Sánchez-Luna[1] and Alfredo Célis de la Rosa[4]

*Address all correspondence to: genarogabriel@yahoo.com

1 División de Neurociencias. Centro de Investigación Biomédica de Occidente (CIBO), Instituto Mexicano del Seguro Social (IMSS). Guadalajara, Jalisco, México

2 Departamento de Química, Centro Universitario de Ciencias Exactas e Ingenierías. Universidad de Guadalajara. Guadalajara, Jalisco, México

3 División de Genética. Centro de Investigación Biomédica de Occidente, Instituto Mexicano del Seguro Social. Guadalajara, Jalisco, México

4 Centro Universitario de Ciencias de la Salud. Universidad de Guadalajara. Guadalajara, Guadalajara, Jalisco, México

5 Departamento de Neurología. Unidad Médica de Alta Especialidad (UMAE)- Hospital de Especialidades; Centro Médico Nacional de Occidente. Instituto Mexicano del Seguro Social (IMSS). Guadalajara, Jalisco, México

## References

[1] Goedert M, Spillantini MG. (2006), A century of Alzheimer's disease. Science. 2006; 314:777-781.

[2] Goeder t M, Klug A, Crowther RA. Tau protein, the paired helical filament and Alzheimer's disease. Journal of Alzheimer's Disease. 2006; 9:195-207.

[3] Gong C-X, Liu F, Grundke-Iqbal I, Iqbal K. Dysregulation of protein phosphorylation/dephosphorylation in Alzheimer's disease: a therapeutic target. Journal of Biomedicine & Biotechnology. 2006;(article ID 31825):1-11.

[4] Zhou L-X, Zeng Z-Y, Du J-T, Zhao Y-F, Li Y-M. (2006), The self-assembly ability of the first microtubule-binding repeat from tau and its modulation by phosphorylation. Biochemical & Biophysical Research Communication. 2006; 348:637-642.

[5] Cruts, M. (2009). Alzheimer Disease & Frontotemporal Dementia Mutation Database. http://www.molgen.ua.ac.be/ADMutations/

[6] Farrall AJ, Wardlaw JM. Blood-brain barrier: ageing and microvascular disease systematic review and meta-analysis. Neurobiol Aging. 2009; 30: 337–52.

[7] Popescu BO, Toescu EC, Popescu LM. Blood-brain barrier alterations in ageing and dementia. J Neurol Sci. 2009; 283: 99–106.

[8] Cacabelos R, Fernandez-Novoa L, Lombardi V, Kubota Y, Takeda M. Molecular genetics of Alzheimer's disease and aging. Methods Find Exp Clin Pharmacol 27, Suppl A: 1–573, 2005.

[9] Turner RS. Alzheimer's Disease. Seminars in Neurology. 2006; 26(5):499-506.

[10] Price JL, Morris JC. Tangles and plaques in nondemented aging and "preclinical" Alzheimer's disease. Ann Neurol 1999;45:358-368.

[11] Delabio R, Rasmussen L, Mizumoto I, Viani GA, Chen E, Villares J, Costa IB, Turecki G, Linde SA, Smith MC, Payão SL.PSEN1 and PSEN2 Gene Expression in Alzheimer's Disease Brain: A New Approach. J Alzheimers Dis. 2014 Jan 1;42(3):757-60.

[12] Kim DH, Yeo SH, Park JM, Choi JY, Lee TH, Park SY, Ock MS, Eo J, Kim HS, Cha HJ.Gene. 2014 Jul 25;545(2):185-93.

[13] Jiao B, Tang B, Liu X, Xu J, Wang Y, Zhou L, Zhang F, Yan X, Zhou Y, Shen L. Mutational analysis in early-onset familial Alzheimer's disease in Mainland China. Neurobiol Aging. 2014 Aug;35(8):1957.e1-6. doi: 10.1016/j.neurobiolaging.2014.02.014.

[14] Wu L, Rosa-Neto P, Hsiung GY, Sadovnick AD, Masellis M, Black SE, Jia J, Gauthier S. Early-onset familial Alzheimer's disease (EOFAD). Can J Neurol Sci. 2012 Jul;39(4): 436-45.

[15] Kim DH, Yeo SH, Park JM, Choi JY, Lee TH, Park SY, Ock MS, Eo J, Kim HS, Cha HJGenetic markers for diagnosis and pathogenesis of Alzheimer's disease. Gene. 2014 Jul 25;545(2):185-93. doi: 10.1016/j.gene.2014.05.031.

[16] Pilotto A, Padovani A, Borroni B. Clinical, biological, and imaging features of monogenic Alzheimer's Disease. Biomed Res Int. 2013;2013:689591.

[17] El Kadmiri N, Hamzi K, El Moutawakil B, Slassi I, Nadifi S. Genetic aspects of Alzheimer's disease. Pathol Biol (Paris). 2013 Dec;61(6):228-38.

[18] Michikawa M. Role of apolipoprotein E in the molecular pathomechanism of Alzheimer disease. Nihon Shinkei Seishin Yakurigaku Zasshi. 2014 Feb;34(1):5-9. Review. Japanese. PMID: 2506926

[19] Nicolas M, Hassan BA. Amyloid precursor protein and neural development. Development. 2014 Jul;141(13):2543-8. doi: 10.1242/dev.108712.

[20] Jiang T, Yu JT, Tian Y, Tan L. Epidemiology and etiology of Alzheimer's disease: from genetic to non-genetic factors. Curr Alzheimer Res. 2013 Oct;10(8):852-67.

[21] Rahman B, Meiser B, Sachdev P, Barlow-Stewart K, Otlowski M, Zilliacus E, Schofield P. To know or not to know: an update of the literature on the psychological and

behavioral impact of genetic testing for Alzheimer disease risk. Genet Test Mol Biomarkers. 2012 Aug;16(8):935-42.

[22] Wain KE, Uhlmann WR, Heidebrink J, Roberts JS. Living at risk: the sibling's perspective of early-onset Alzheimer's disease. J Genet Couns. 2009 Jun;18(3):239-51.

[23] Ringman JM, C, Diaz-Olavarrieta Y, Rodriguez M, Chavez F, Paz, J, Murrell M,Macias-Islas M, Hil Kawas. Female preclinical presenilin-1 mutation carriers unaware of their genetic status have higher levels of depression than their non-mutation carrying kin. J Neurol Neurosurg Psychiatry 2004; 75 :500–502. doi: 10.1136/jnnp.2002.005025

[24] Ringman JM, Diaz-Olavarrieta,Y, Rodriguez, Chavez M,. Fairbanks F, Paz A, Varpetian HC, Maldonado M,. Macias-Islas M, J. Murrell JB, Ghetti l, Kawas C. Neuropsychological function in nondemented carriers of presenilin-1 mutations. NEUROLOGY 2005;65:552–558

[25] Ringman JM, Rodriguez Y, Diaz-Olavarrieta C, Michael T, Fairbanks L, Paz F, Varpetian, Chaparro H, Macias-Islas M, Murrell J, Bernardino Ghetti B, Kawas C. Performance on MMSE sub-items and education level in presenilin-1mutation carriers without dementia International Psychogeriatric Association 2006;2-10 doi:10.1017/S10416102060037

[26] Murrell J, Ghetti B, Cochran E, Macias-Islas M, Medina L, Varpetian A, Jeffrey L. Cummings LJ, Mario, Mendez MF, Claudia Kawas C, Helena Chui, Ringman JM. The A431E mutation in PSEN1 causing Familial Alzheimer's Disease originating in Jalisco State, Mexico: an additional fifteen families. Neurogenetics DOI 10.1007/s10048-006-0053-1

[27] Corder EH. Gene dose of apolipoprotein E type 4 allele and the risk of Alzheimer's disease in late onset families. Science, 1993; 261(5123): 921-3.

[28] Fagan AM. Unique lipoproteins secreted by primary astrocytes from wild type, apoE (-/-), and human apoE transgenic mice. J Biol Chem. 1999; 274(42): 30001-7.

[29] Gong JS. Apolipoprotein E (apoE) isoform-dependent lipid release from astrocytes prepared from human-apoE3- and apoE4-knock-in mice. J Biol Chem, 2002; 31: 31.

[30] Vance JE, Hayashi H. Formation and function of apolipoprotein E-containing lipoproteins in the nervous system. Biochim Biophys Acta. 2010; 1801(8): 806-18.

[31] Boyles JK. A role for apolipoprotein E, apolipoprotein A-I, and low density lipoprotein receptors in cholesterol transport during regeneration and remyelination of the rat sciatic nerve. J. Clin. Invest., 1989; 83: 1015-1031.

[32] Gong JS. Novel action of apolipoprotein E (ApoE): ApoE isoform specifically inhibits lipid-particle-mediated cholesterol release from neurons. Mol Neurodegener, 2007; 2: 9.LaDu MJ. Association of human, rat, and rabbit apolipoprotein E with beta amyloid. J Neurosci Res. 1997;. 49(1): 9-18.

[33] Golabek AA, Kida, E, Walus M, Perez C, Wisniewski, T, Soto C. Sodium dodecyl sulfate-resistant complexes of Alzheimer's amyloid beta-peptide with the N-terminal, receptor binding domain of apolipoprotein E. Biophys J. 2000; 79, 1008-1015.

[34] Tamamizu-Kato S, Cohen JK, Drake CB, Kosaraju MG, Drury J, Narayanaswami V. Interaction with Amyloid beta Peptide Compromises the Lipid Binding Function of Apolipoprotein E. Biochemistry; 2008.

[35] Consensus report of the Working Group on: "Molecular and Biochemical Markers of Alzheimer's Disease". The Ronald and Nancy Reagan Research Institute of the Alzheimer's Association and the National Institute on Aging Working Group. Neurobiol Aging. 1998; 19:109-116.

[36] Price JL and Morris JC. Tangles and plaques in nondemented aging and "preclinical" Alzheimer's disease. Ann Neurol 1999;45:358-368.

[37] Neuropathology Group. Medical Research Council Cognitive Function and Aging Study. Pathological correlates of late-onset dementia in a multicentre, community-based population in England and Wales. Neuropathology Group of the Medical Research Council Cognitive Function and Ageing Study (MRC CFAS). Lancet. 2001; 357:169-175.

[38] Herukka S-K, Hallikainen M, Soininen H, Pirttilä T. CSF Aβ42 and Tau or phosphorylated Tau and prediction of progressive mild cognitive impairment. Neurology. 2005; 64, 1294-1297

[39] Saez-Valero J, Barquero MS, Marcos A, McLean GA, Small DH. Altered glycosylation of acetylcholinesterase in lumbar cerebrospinal fluid of patients with Alzheimer's disease. J Neurol Neurosurg Psychiatry. 2000; 69:664-667.

[40] Bonelli RM, Aschoff A, Niederwieser G, Heuberger C, Jirikowski G. Cerebrospinal fluid tissue transglutaminase as a biochemical marker for Alzheimer's disease. Neurobiol Dis 2002;11:106-110.

[41] Leoni V, Shafaati M, Salomon A, Kivipelto M, Bjorkhem I, Wahlund LO. Are the CSF levels of 24S-hydroxycholesterol a sensitive biomarker for mild cognitive impairment?. Neurosci Lett. 2006; 397:83-87.

[42] Montine TJ, Kaye JA, Montine KS, McFarland L, Morrow JD, Quinn JF. Cerebrospinal fluid Aβ42, tau and F2-isoprostane concentrations in patients with Alzheimer's disease, other dementias, and in age.matched controls. Arch Pathol Lab Med. 2001;125:510-512.

[43] Simonsen AH, McGuire J, Hansson O, Zetterberg H, Podust VN, Davies HA, et al. Novel panel of Cerebrospinal fluid biomarkers for the prediction of progression to Alzheimer dementia in patients with mild cognitive impairment. Arch Neurol. 2007; 64:366-370.

[44] Blennow K. Cerebrospinal fluid protein biomarkers for Alzheimer's disease. NeuroRx. 2004; 1:213-225-

[45] Martínez-Cano, E., Pacheco-Moisés, F.P., Ortiz, G.G., Macías-Islas, M.A., Sánchez-Nieto, S., and Rosales-Corral, S.A. 2004, Rev. Neurol., 39, 1

[46] Sánchez-González, V.J., Ortiz, G.G., Gallegos-Arreola, P., Macías-Islas, M.A., et al., Altered β-amyloid precursor protein isoforms in Mexican Alzheimer's Disease patients J.J. 2006, Dis. Markers, 22, 119.

[47] Mecocci, P., Cherubinia, A., Flint Beal, M. et al., 1996, Neurosc Lett., 207,129, 132.

[48] Borroni B., F. Colciaghi, C. Caltagirone et al., Platelet amyloid precursor protein abnormalities in Mild Cognitive Impairment predict conversion to dementia of Alzhemier type, Arch Neurol 60 (2003), 1740–1744.

[49] Mayeux R., A. Saunders, S. Shea et al., Utility of the apolipoprotein E genotype in the diagnosis of Alzheimer's disease, NEJM 338 (1998), 506–511.

[50] Ortiz G.G., F. Pacheco-Moises, M. El Hafidi, A. Jimenez-Delgado, M.A. Macias-Islas,S.A. et al. Detection of membrane fluidity in submitochondrial particles of platelets and erythrocyte membranes from Mexican patients with Alzheimer disease by intramolecular excimer formation of 1,3 dipyrenylpropane. Dis Markers 2008:(24) 151-156.

[51] Bonilla E, K. Tanji, M. Hirano, T.H. Vu, S. DiMauro, E.A. Schon, Mitochondrial involvement in Alzheimer's disease. Biochim Biophys Acta 1999:(1410) 171-182.

[52] Hajimohammadreza I, Brammer MJ, Eagger S, Burns A, Levy R. Platelet and erythrocyte membrane changes in Alzheimer's disease. Biochim Biophys Acta. 1990; (1025): 208-214.

[53] Zubenko GS, Kopp U, Seto T, Firestone LL. Platelet membrane fluidity individuals at risk for Alzheimer's disease: a comparison of results from fluorescence spectroscopy and electron spin resonance spectroscopy. Psychopharmacology. 1999; (145): 175-180.

[54] Zubenko GS, Malinakova I, Chojnacki B. Proliferation of internal membranes in platelets from patients with Alzheimer's disease.. J Neuropathol Exp Neurol. 1987; (46): 407-418.

[55] Fukami MH, Salganicoff L. Isolation and properties of human platelet mitochondria. Blood. 1973; (42): 913-918.

[56] Zainaghi IA, Forlenza OV, Gattaz WF. Abnormal APP processing in platelets of patients with Alzheimer's disease: correlations with membrane fluidity and cognitive decline. Psychopharmacology (Berl). 2007; (192): 547-553.

[57] Kish SJ, Bergeron C, Rajput A. Brain cytochrome oxidase in Alzheimer's disease. Journal of Neurochemistry. 1992; 59 (2):. 776–779.

[58] Mutisya EM, Bowling AC, Beal MF. Cortical cytochrome oxidase activity is reduced in Alzheimer's disease. Journal of Neurochemistry. 1994; 63(6):.2179–2184.

[59] Parker WD Jr, Parks J, Filley CM, Kleinschmidt BK. Electron transport chain defects in Alzheimer's disease brain. Neurology. 1994; 44(6): 1090–1096.

[60] Valla J, Berndt JD, Lima FG. Energy hypometabolism in posterior cingulate cortex of Alzheimer's patients: superficial laminar cytochrome oxidase associated with disease duration. Journal of Neuroscience. 2001; 21(13): 4923–4930.

[61] Cardoso SM, Proenca MT, Santos S, Santana I, Oliveira CR. Cytochrome c oxidase is decreased in Alzheimer's disease platelets. Neurobiology of Aging. 2004; 25(1): 105–110.

[62] Kish S. J., C. Bergeron, A. Rajput et al., "Brain cytochrome oxidase in Alzheimer's disease," Journal of Neurochemistry, vol. 59, no. 2, pp. 776–779, 1992.

[63] Hirano M, A. Shtilbans, R. Mayeux et al., "Apparent mtDNA heteroplasmy in Alzheimer's disease patients and in normals due to PCR amplification of nucleus-embedded mtDNA pseudogenes," Proceedings of the National Academy of Sciences of the United States of America, vol. 94, no. 26, pp. 14894–14899, 1997

[64] Loera-Castañeda V, Lucila Sandoval-Ramírez, Fermín Paul PachecoMoisés, Miguel Ángel Macías-Islas et al. Novel Point Mutations and A8027G Polymorphism in Mitochondrial-DNA-Encoded Cytochrome c Oxidase II Gene in Mexican Patients with Probable Alzheimer Disease. International Journal of Alzheimer's Disease Volume 2014, Article ID 794530, 5 pages

Chapter 11

# Gait Pathway in Subcortical Vascular Dementia and in Alzheimer's Disease

Rita Moretti, Arianna Sartori, Beatrice Baso and
Silvia Gazzin

Additional information is available at the end of the chapter

http://dx.doi.org/10.5772/59834

## 1. Introduction

Gait impairment, worse equilibrium scores and falls are associated with leukoaraiosis, as widely recognised [1-6]. In Binswanger's disease with a severe leukoaraiosis gait disorders are clearly evident while patients with mild periventricular changes may present subclinical forms of gait disorders, as proposed by some authors (see data in [7]).

Gait disorders in the elderly are particularly relevant, since they can influence the loss of functional independence and death [8]. As anticipated, cerebral small vessel disease (both white matter lesions and lacunar infarcts) correlates with gait parameters: stride length and a lower gait velocity [8]. Most importantly, subcortical vascular lesions seem to increase the possibility of falls, even if clear evidences are still lacking [9-11].

Walking difficulties in Alzheimer's disease are well described [12]: patients show slow and irregular steps, difficulties in turning and avoiding obstacles [13, 14]. These disturbances have been described also in patients free from extrapyramidal, ataxic, paretic signs, and clinically relevant musculoskeletal impairments [12, 14]. Moreover, Alzheimer's disease patients have a worse balance [12, 14, 15] and a higher risk of falls compared with matched controls [16, 17]. The prevalence of gait abnormalities varies widely across the studies (from 8.7% [18] to over 90% [19]); this can be explained because of different inclusion criteria and/or assessment procedures.

These observations have been confirmed by studies demonstrating that patients with Alzheimer's disease walk more slowly compared to healthy controls [12] and these gait problems have been interpreted as manifestations of the extrapyramidal deficits (well-known to affect

12–28% of Alzheimer patients), or as side effects of drug treatment (e.g. neuroleptic agents) [20]. Since a overt walking problems and trunk movement alterations can be seen also in absence of extrapyramidal signs, it has been proposed that some Alzheimer's disease patients may present "frontal gait disorder", a syndrome coterminous with gait apraxia [21, 15]. The lack of a standardised instrument to assess gait has been implicated as a possible cause for the low frequency of reports on the topic.

Since the walking assessment cannot discriminate between walking disorders caused by gait apraxia and other neurological causes of walking difficulty, there has been the necessity to exclude alternative causes of walking abnormalities in Alzheimer's disease (overt extrapyramidal impairments or other concurrent neurological diseases); in order to assess gait capacity, a new test has been proposed and a large proportion of the sample (40%) scored below cut off, even if the percentage of severely impaired was smaller. Although the possibility of right–left confusion, working memory deficits, and problems with verbal comprehension was minimised by demonstrating the items, the complexity of some of them might have contributed to inflating the proportion of patients performing poorly. Even though, the presence of associated vascular pathology in a few patients also cannot account for the outcome. Neuroradiological signs of white matter changes were reported in three of the 24 patients (22.5%) in the Della Sala *et al.*'s study [12], who scored below cut off in the assessment of walking skills.

Therefore, in a well-defined population suffering from subcortical vascular dementia and Alzheimer's disease (standing from a neurological, clinical, and radiological criteria), we tried to explore gait, balance and equilibrium alterations, and a behavioral complex symptom, such as apathy, even considering precipitant factors, such as concomitant pathologies and consequent therapies. We now present an extension of the work, with a speculation on what we observed for a two-year follow-up.

## 2. Subjects and methods

### 2.1. Patients

From June 1st 2010 to June 1st 2013, 155 patients diagnosed with Alzheimer's disease (AD), according to NINDCS-ADRDA criteria [22], and 673 patients with subcortical vascular dementia (according the NINDS-AIREN criteria for probable VaD [23]) (age 65–94 years) have been examined in Cognitive Disorder Unit Evaluation of the University of Trieste and enrolled in the present study.

The inclusion criteria were a Mini-Mental State Examination (MMSE) scores of at least 14 and satisfying the fourth edition of the Diagnostic and Statistical Manual of Mental Disorders (DSM-IV) criteria for dementia. As far as neuroimaging is concerned, subcortical VaD (sVAD) was diagnosed when the CT/MRI scan showed moderate to severe ischemic white matter changes [24] and at least one lacunar infarct. In order to be enrolled into the study, Alzheimer's subjects had to show on brain MRI the classical pattern of atrophy of AD (hippocampal atrophy) and display hypoperfusion in temporoparietal and precuneus regions (AD) on HMPAO-SPECT. The neurologist (RM) assessed independently, after the radiologist's opinion, brain CT and/or MRI images and all the diagnoses have been confirmed after a long term clinical follow-up (12 and 36 months).

Exclusion criteria were: normal pressure hydrocephalus, diagnoses of major stroke or brain haemorrhage, previous brain tumours, white matter lesions due to specific aetiologies (e.g. multiple sclerosis, vasculitis, brain irradiation, and genetic forms of vascular dementia such as CADASIL or CARASIL). Finally, also major psychiatric illness (e.g.. schizophrenia, bipolar disorders, psychosis, compulsive-obsessive disorders, etc) or central nervous system disorders and alcoholism were excluded. Also absence of an informed caregiver, unavailability of neuroradiological examination, and/or the use of psychotropic drugs within two months prior to the clinical assessment implied patient's exclusion from the study. According to these exclusion criteria, 27 AD patients and 70 sVAD patients were excluded. We did not consider a discriminant/exclusion criteria depression, referring to different studies (such as [25]), according to the potential correlation to vascular dementia predisposing factor.

### 2.2. Study design

This was a prospective cohort study, designed to investigate behavioural alterations, and in particular apathy of a AD and of a sVAD population. Study subjects underwent the following evaluations. The standardized baseline assessment implied a detailed history, physical examination (pulse rate and rhythm, blood pressure, heart size and sounds, peripheral pulses, retinal vessel and carotid artery evaluation), EKG, chest X-ray, laboratory tests and psychiatric evaluation. All patients were followed with neurological examinations scheduled every four months, while the complete neuropsychological examination was conducted at baseline and at 36 months. We conducted the study in accordance with the Declaration of Helsinki and with the Ethics Guidelines of the Institute.

### 2.3. Outcome measures

All patients were studied, with complete neurological and neuropsychological examinations. Main outcomes of the study were: global performance, which was assessed using the Mini Mental State Examination [26], Frontal Assessment Battery (FAB) [27]; global behavioral symptoms, assessed by the Neuro Psychiatric Inventory, NPI [28]; the caregiver stress, assessed by the Relative Stress Scale, RSS [29]. In addition to these main outcome measures, the Clinical Insight Rating Scale (CIR) [30] (which provides a measure of its four comprising items – awareness, cognitive deficit, disease progression and functional deficit) was performed. The Barthel index (BI) [31] and the Instrumental activity of Daily living (IADL) [32] have been used to assess functional activities and complex activities of daily living, respectively. Mobility problems were evaluated by the Tinetti scale for equilibrium/balance and gait [33]: in particular, a semiquantitative assessment was used, consisting of the modified Tinetti test with 17 items, 9 for body balance (0-16), 8 for gait (0-12). Patients were registered for their medical intake.

## 3. Statistical analysis

Statistical analyses were performed using the Statistical Package for the Social Sciences (SPSS, version 16.0). Wilcoxon Signed Ranks test was used to analyze the Within-group changes, from baseline to 24 months, of the overall scores for each efficacy variable.

Behavioral outcome measures, cognition, Tinetti scale, global, balance and equilibrium, and BI correlations were analyzed applying the Spearman's rank correlation analyses.

## 4. Results

The study subjects were 128 AD patients and 603 sVAD patients. All the patients could be fully studied (mean age 72.3 ± 7.3 years, range= 62-94 years). 1 AD patient and 5 sVAD patients died during the two-year follow-up. As anticipated, the diagnosis based on clinical history, neuropsychological assessment and neuroimaging was reinforced by subsequent follow-up in all cases.

All the selected patients underwent neuroimaging: 128 AD patients did MRI studies; 603 sVAD patients did CT scans; moreover, 201 of the latter completed the diagnostic pathway with MRI images, in case of not adequate imaging acquisition or not convincing data. Therefore, the patients who did CT/MRI were homogeneously recruited and no demographical/social/cultural/clinical difference distinguished from each other.

A neurologist (RM) revised all the imaging, employing the Blennow *et al.* [34] scale for CT scans and the Scheltens *et al.* [35] scale for MRI imaging in sVAD patients and Wahlund *et al.* [36], Kantarci *et al.* [37] and den Heijer *et al.* [38] criteria for AD MRI imaging. There was 95.8% inter-rater agreement for the independent assessment of the scans (kappa=0.8).

Patients were allowed to continue any previous therapy (e.g. antihypertensive, antidyslipidemic, antidiabetic drugs). During the follow-up, the patients were prescribed neuroleptics and/or benzodiazepines.

A synopsis of the cognitive performances obtained by the two groups has been reported in Table 1-2-3-4.

| **Baseline** | **sVAD** | **AD** | **P value (between groups)** |
|---|---|---|---|
| **MMSE** | 25.8 (2.4) | 19.9 (1.9) | <0.01 |
| Arithmetic calculations (WAIS) § | 6.3 (1.6) | 8.6 (1.2) | <0.05 |
| Digit span forward (WAIS) | 5.8 (1.5) | 5.1 (0.6) | <0.05 |
| Digit span backward (WAIS) | 4.4 (2.5) | 2.6 (0.8) | <0.05 |
| **FAB total score** | 9.2 (2.1) | 11.8 (1.2) | <0.05 |

**Table 1.** Cognitive synoptical results obtained by the two groups studied. Values are mean (SD); ns = not significant. § number of mistakes.

| 24-month follow-up | sVAD within group (24 months vs baseline) | AD within group (24 months vs baseline) | P value (between groups) |
|---|---|---|---|
| **MMSE** | 20.2 (2.2)<br>(-5.2 (.0.3); p<0.01) | 15.1 (1.7)<br>(-4.85 (0.2); p<0.01) | <0.01 |
| **Arithmetic calculations (WAIS) §** | 5.4 (1.1)<br>(-0.9 (0.5); ns) | 3.4 (1.7)<br>(-5.2 (0.5); p<0.01) | <0.05 |
| **Digit span forward (WAIS)** | 4.1 (1.4)<br>(-1.7 (0.1); p<0.05) | 3.2 (0.2)<br>(-1.9 (0.4); p<0.05) | <0.05 |
| **Digit span backward (WAIS)** | 3.6 (0.3)<br>(-0.8 (2.2); ns) | 1.9 (0.1)<br>(-0.5 (0.7); p<0.05) | <0.01 |
| **FAB total score** | 4.7 (1.5)<br>(-4.5 (0.6); p<0.01) | 7.5 (0.2)<br>(-3.3 (1.0); p<0.05) | <0.01 |

**Table 2.** Cognitive synoptical results obtained by the two groups studied, at 12 months. Values are mean (SD); ns = not significant. § Number of mistakes. In brackets, in each column, comparison within group, 24 months *vs* baseline, reported as mean, SD, and p.

| Tests | Baseline sVAD | Baseline AD |
|---|---|---|
| **Barthel Index** | 87.41 ± 11.3 | 92.14 ± 0.11 |
| **Instrumental Activity of Daily Living** | 6.8 ± 0.34 | 5.84 ± 1.3 |

**Table 3.** TESTs results in the patients observed during follow-up.

| Tests at 24 months | sVAD | AD | Between groups (sVAD vs AD) |
|---|---|---|---|
| **Barthel Index** | -25.17± 3.4 p<0.01 | -13.57 ± 3.4 p<0.05 | p<0.01 |
| **Instrumental Activity of Daily Living** | -1.7 ± 0.3 p<0.05 | -3.4 ± 3.4<br>p<0.01 | p<0.01 |

**Table 4.** Results at 24 months: a comparison over baseline.

In summary, there are some important cognitive differences in the two groups: AD patients did worse in MMSE, in arithmetic calculation and in digit tasks of WAIS, IADL; sVAD patients did generally worse in FAB tests, Barthel Index.

From the behavioral perspective (Table 5-6), at baseline, the AD group had a worse score of NPI and BEHAVE-AD, and their caregivers did have a heavier stress (RSS). On the contrary, sVAD patients, at baseline did feel much more depressed (as stated by NPI partial scores, not purposely evaluated in this topic) and did have a better insight in their situation. After 24 months, AD patients showed higher NPI and Behave scores; sVAD patients did show more insight. Surprisingly, the stress levels of the caregivers were not significantly different in the two groups. sVAD patients did manifest more overt apathy, which increase during follow-up and remained a major key point in behavior disturbances of these patients.

Moreover, there was a dramatic decrease, either in gait and equilibrium control, either in the combined synoptical measure (of total score) in both groups, with sVAD patients showing a constantly worse performance, compared to AD patients (Table 7-8).

| baseline | sVAD | AD | P value |
|---|---|---|---|
| RSS | 24.7 (8.7) | 36.1 (8.5) | (p<0.01) |
| NPI | 16.9 (0.3) | 24.4 (5.2) | (p<0.01) |
| CIR | 3 (0.2) | 2 (0.5) | (p<0.05) |

**Table 5.** Behavioral synoptical results. Values are mean (SD); ns = not significant.

| 24-month follow-up | sVAD | AD | P value |
|---|---|---|---|
| RSS | 47.5 (1.3)<br>(+22.8 (5.9), <0.01) | 45.2 (2.1)<br>(+9.1 (6.8), <0.05) | ns |
| NPI | 34.1 (0.8)<br>(+17.2 (0.5), <0.01) | 56.3 (4.5)<br>(+31.9 (1.1), <0.01) | (p<0.01) |
| CIR | 2.2 (0.3)<br>(-0.8 (0.1), ns) | 1.0 (0.3)<br>(-1.0 (0.3), <0.05) | (p<0.01) |

**Table 6.** Behavioral synoptical results. Values are mean (SD); ns = not significant; in brackets, in each column, comparison within group, 24 months *vs* baseline, reported as mean, SD, and p.

| Tests | sVAD | AD | P value |
|---|---|---|---|
| TINETTI equilibrium | 10.1 ± 0.1 | 14.3 ± 1.1 | <0.001 |
| TINETTI gait | 10.2 ± 1.1 | 11.4 ± 0.3 | <0.05 |
| TINETTI tot. score | 20.3 ± 1.2 | 25.7 ± 1.4 | <0.001 |

**Table 7.** Gait TESTs results in the patients observed at baseline.

| Tests at 24 months | Over baseline<br>sVAD | Over baseline<br>AD | Between groups<br>(sVAD vs AD) |
|---|---|---|---|
| TINETTI equilibrium | -5 ± 0.6 p<0.01 | -3.4 ± 0.6 p<0.01 | P<0.001 |
| TINETTI gait | -7.9 ± 1.1 p<0.01 | -3.1± 1.1 p<0.01 | P<0.001 |
| TINETTI tot. score | -12.9 ± 0.2 p<0.01 | -6.5 ± 0.2 p<0.01 | P<0.001 |

**Table 8.** Results at 24 months: a comparison over baseline at 24 months.

Spearman's rank correlation analyses indicated that there was a significant correlation between Gait scores (total and separately, gait and equilibrium) and FAB scores (**total Tinetti score/FAB**: r=0.81, $p < 0.05$ baseline; r=0.83, p < 0.01 over 24 months); **gait Tinetti score/FAB:** r=0.82, $p < 0.01$ over baseline; r=0.87, p < 0.01 over 24 months); **equilibrium Tinetti score/FAB:** r=0.81, $p < 0.05$ over baseline; r=0.83, p < 0.01 over 24 months) in sVAD.

Spearman's rank correlation analyses indicated that there was a significant correlation between Tinetti total, and equilibrium and gait score and BI over baseline, and 24 months (**total Tinetti score/BI**: r=0.81, $p < 0.05$ over baseline; r=0.89, p < 0.01 over 24 months); **gait Tinetti score/BI:** r=0.82, $p < 0.01$ over baseline; r=0.89, p < 0.01 over 24 months; **equilibrium Tinetti score/BI:** r=0.84, $p < 0.01$ over baseline; r=0.89, p < 0.01 over 24 months) in sVAD.

Furthermore, we have found a correlation between Tinetti equilibrium score and NPI over 24, months (equilibrium Tinetti/NPI: r=0.78, p<0.05 in sVAD; r=0.87, p<0.01 in AD), and Tinetti gait score and NPI over 24 months (**gait Tinetti /NPI**: r= 0.78, p<0.05 in sVAD; r=0.86, p<0.01 in AD), and Tinetti total score and NPI over 24 months (**Tinetti total score/NPI**: r= 0.78, p<0.05, in sVAD; r= 0.93, p<0.01 in AD).

Spearman's rank correlation analyses indicated that there was a significant correlation between Gait scores (total scores and separately, gait and equilibrium) and MMSE (**total Tinetti score/MMSE**: r=0.81, $p < 0.05$ over 24 months in AD).

Surprisingly, we have found only a correlation between benzodiazepines intake and Tinetti equilibrium score at 24 months (respectively r=0.77, p<0.05 in sVAD; r=0.84, p<0.01 in AD).

We distinguished typical from atypical neuroleptic intake (Table 9). Moreover, since quetiapine, as an atypical neuroleptic, has a lower dopamine affinity compared to olanzapine, we considered separately the compounds, concluding as follows:

- Typical neuroleptics: a significant correlation between haloperidol intake and Tinetti equilibrium score at baseline and at 24 months (respectively: r=0.61, p<0.05, at baseline and r=0.81, p<0.01 in AD patients; r=0.72, p<0.05 at 24 months in sVAD); between haloperidol intake and Tinetti total score at baseline and 24 months (respectively: r=0.81, p<0.01 and r=0.86, p<0.01 in AD; only at 24 months r=0.71, p<0.01 in sVAD); not significant correlation between promazine chloridate intake and Tinetti sub-scores at baseline and at 24 months in AD; we have found a positive correlation between the equilibrium score of Tinetti test and promazine intake at 24 months in sVAD, not in AD group (r=0.74, p<0.05).

- Atypical neuroleptics: we have found a significant correlation between olanzapine intake and Tinetti equilibrium score at 24 months in AD groups (none of sVAD took olanzapine in our study) (r=0.74, p<0.05) and between olanzapine intake and Tinetti total score at 24 months (r=0.71, p<0.05); we have found a positive correlation between the equilibrium score of Tinetti test and quetiapine intake at 24 months (respectively: r=0.79, p<0.05 in AD group; r=0.82, p<0.01 in sVAD). The mean dose of olanzapine remained stable during the 24-month follow-up (5.2-5.4 mg/day); on the contrary, quetiapine dosage increased up to 24-month follow-up (56.3-89.6 mg/day).

| Drug utilization | Baseline sVAD | 24 months sVAD | Baseline AD | 24 months sVAD |
|---|---|---|---|---|
| **Benzodiazepines** | 144 patients | 289 patients | 298 patients | 304 patients |
| lorazepam, mean (±SD) dose | 1.27± 0.3 mg/day | 2.56 ± 0.65 mg/day | 3.94 ± 1.5 mg/day | 4.56 ± 1.65 mg/day |
| delorazepam, mean (±SD) dose | 1.21 ± 0.8 mg/day | 2.61 ± 1.29 mg/day | 3.1 ± 1.54 mg/day | 4.1 ± 1.89 mg/day |
| bromazepam, mean (±SD) dose | 2.11 ± 1.1 mg/day | 3.41 ± 0.8 mg/day | 4.6 ± 1.4 mg/day | 5.41 ± 1.8 mg/day |
| **Typical neuroleptics** | 88 patients | 356 patients | 88 patients | 127 patients |
| haloperidol, mean (±SD) dose | 1.56 ± 0.54 mg/day | 2.34 ± 0.67 mg/day | 2.87 ± 1.54 mg/day | 3.56 ± 0.54 mg/day |
| promazine chloridrate, mean (±SD) dose | 53.12 ± 12.23 mg/day | 59.12 ± 16.91 mg/day | 63.12 ± 7.2 mg/day | 67.12 ± 1.56 mg/day |
| **Atypical neuroleptics** | 4 patients | 23 patients | 63 patients | 83 patients |
| olanzapine, mean (±SD) dose | 0.0 ± 0 mg/day | 0 ± 0 mg/day | 5.6 ± 1.6 mg/day | 5.9 ± 2.94 mg/day |
| quetiapine, mean (±SD) dose | 37.5 ± 5.21 mg/day | 56.9 ± 3.5 mg/day | 66.8 ± 3.5 mg/day | 89.9 ± 3.5 mg/day |

**Table 9.** A synopsis of the CNS drugs employed by the patients.

## 5. Discussion

Walking is a complex mechanism, based on motor control, step rhythm, muscular activation and dys-activation, motor adjustment, attention, perception and so on. Spinal and brainstem activation, which seems to be fundamental for quadrupeds, is not so dominant in humans, where gait depends more on cortical and subcortical inputs [39].

The motor cortex, represented by distinct areas in the frontal lobes, receives a variety of inputs: sensory areas, motor control structures, and modulatory pathways including the thalamus and basal ganglia (BG). Movement planning and performance are strictly dependent from this cluster of architectonically distinct frontal fields [40]. In particular, SMA activates immediately before gait ignition in normal walking, suggesting a preparatory activity for each sub-component of a movement sequence [41]. It has been suggested that this activity may reflect sub-movement program selection, subsequently sent to the M1. On the other hand, BG generate a phasic activity, which switches off SMA output and which is probably involved in providing a non-specific cue both to trigger the sub-movement and to instruct the SMA to prepare for the next, finally generating an "automatic" movement sequence [42, 7]. In conclusion, internal cues give rise to automatic movement sequences, as a result of the cooperation of BG and SMA [7].

Gait control and in particular gait variability are deeply influenced by BG compensatory activity [43]. Rosano and colleagues reported that subclinical brain vascular abnormalities (WM infarcts and hyperintensities in MRI) were more frequent and severe in patients with a greater variability of step length, independently from age, gender, and cognitive function [43]. Moreover, older people and patients with leukoaraiosis show higher-level gait alterations, supporting the previous observations [39]. These data have been clinically confirmed by other works by the LADIS group [11], by Srikanth *et al.* [44] and by Masdeu and Wolfson [45].

Though, there are quite real differences among the few other studies on this point. It has been established by Della Sala *et al.* [12] that even AD, in a sizeable proportion (40% of their population) scored as having gait alteration. Though, it must be pointed out that the presence of associated vascular pathology, declared by the writers themselves is a not indifferent proportion (22.5%), even if they asserted that this could not account for the outcome. The Authors declared that their patients showed the gait apraxia phenomenon, referring to deficits of a relatively unitary function, with the reference to a theoretical model. Within the dichotomy, proposed by Benke [46], between a conceptual system of motor acts and a system which controls sensorimotor and spatial-temporal features of movement, gait apraxia would arise from the impairment of the latter system. Gait apraxia suggested Della Sala *et al.* [12] should also be distinguished from ideomotor apraxia, which hampers individual movements and meaningless gestures. What we observed in our study was the dramatically significant overcome of gait disturbances, either considering balance, either gait by itself, in pure sVAD rather than in pure AD pathology. Gait imbalance in AD relates with progressive and dramatic worsening of global cognitive functions (MMSE), with behavioural deterioration (NPI) and with consequent drugs intake.

On the contrary gait and balance in sVAD is a very precocious symptom, which relates, from the very beginning with frontal executive functions (FAB) and Barthel Index (BI) (Table 10).

| Gait disturbances | sVAD | AD |
|---|---|---|
| | Peculiar | Unspecific |
| Characteristics | Early | Late |
| | Frequent | Less frequent |
| | Frontal executive functions (FAB) | Global cognitive functions (MMSE) |
| Relate to | Barthel Index (BI) | Behavioral performance (NPI) |
| | | Drugs intake |

**Table 10.** Summary: characteristics of gait disturbances in sVAD and AD patients.

Insofar, we hypothesize that even though gait apraxia is one of the symptoms declared in AD, affecting highly routinized synergistic actions, it relates to AD cognitive worsening. On the contrary, it is a key, precocious and very peculiar aspect of sVAD. Therefore, considering this point, it can be found a good explanation of the phenomenon, in Liston *et al.* [7] work; they suggested that microvascular alteration affecting the SMA, its connections in the periventricular WM, or the BG can cause a higher-level gait disorders (HLGDs), a hypothesis that seems to agree with the concept of gait apraxia caused by any mesial frontal lesion (SMA anatomical location) purposed by Meyer [47]. A further clinical confirmation is provided by current evidence of gait abnormities in early vascular dementia, in particular when WM alterations affect strategic pathways (linking the BG to the ventro-lateral nucleus of the thalamus and to the SMA and frontal areas) [48, 49]; these critical locations compromise the timing cues from the BG; the analogy to PD disconnections may suggest similar gait abnormalities. It is well known and widely accepted that leukoaraiosis is associated with gait impairment, falls, and worse equilibrium scores [1, 3-6, 8, 50]. Some authors suggest a spectrum of severity in gait disorders associated with WM abnormalities: on one side, severe gait disorder observed in Binswanger's disease with massive leukoaraiosis [7], on the other subclinical forms of gait disorders can occur in patients with mild periventricular changes.

However, it has been demonstrated that many patients with vascular-HLGDs present with disequilibrium as primary complaint rather than timing and movement ignition problems [4, 51, 7]. To explain this phenomenon it has been purposed that an alteration of the sensory/PMA pathways, compromising the contribute to sub-movements initiation and control of sensory input (proprioceptive, auditory, vestibular and visual information), may represent their primary disorder [7]. The preservation of BG/SMA pathways guarantees the generation of automatic, internally cued movements,

A clear point should be made in our study to the extremely strict exclusion criteria in AD and in sVAD recruitment, basically founded on clinical signs and neuroimaging world-wide accepted criteria. For example, in order to eliminate any confounding, we excluded patients with brainstem lesions, which ischemic lesions could cause specific gait and equilibrium abnormalities. Similarly, we considered also concurrent medications and co-morbidities, in order to ensure that the gait and balance alterations observed should be considered as an exclusive result of subcortical WM widespread damage. During the follow-up, a general worsening, decrease of behavioural control, and consequent pharmacologic intake (neuroleptics and benzodiazepines) stressed but did not cause directly the described gait abnormalities. In conclusion, it might be stated that subcortical lesions cause "per se" the interruption of long loop reflexes of deep white motor tracts and descending motor fibers arising from medial cortical areas (see data and literature in: Guerini *et al.* [10], Moretti *et al.* [52]), translating in gait alteration and imbalance. Moreover, subcortical vascular lesions involve fibres connecting frontal cortex and subcortical structures, which are responsible for motivation, executive function, planning and attention too (see in particular frontal eye fields). It has been suggested (see data and Literature in Moretti *et al.* [52]) that the basal ganglia maintains cortically selected motor set in the supplementary motor area and provides internal cues to the supplementary motor area in order to enable each sub movement to be correctly linked together [53-56].

## Author details

Rita Moretti[1*], Arianna Sartori[2], Beatrice Baso[2] and Silvia Gazzin[3]

*Address all correspondence to: moretti@univ.trieste.it

1 Clinica Neurologica, Responsabile Ambulatorio Complicanze Internistiche Cerebrali, Dipartimento Universitario Clinico di Scienze Mediche, Chirurgiche e della Salute, Università degli Studi di Trieste, Italy

2 Clinica Neurologica, Dipartimento Universitario Clinico di Scienze Mediche, Chirurgiche e della Salute, Università degli Studi di Trieste, Italy

3 Area Science Park, FIF, Basovizza, Ospedale di Cattinara, Trieste, Italy

## References

[1] Steingert A, Hachinski VC, Lau C, et al. Cognitive and neurologic findings in subjects with diffuse white matter lucencies on computed tomographic scan (leuko-araiosis). Arch Neurol. 1987;44(1):32–5.

[2] Junqué C, Pujol J, Vendrell P, et al. Leuko-araiosis on magnetic resonance imaging and speed of mental processing. Arch Neurol. 1990;47(2):151–6.

[3] Masdeu JC, Wolfson L, Lantos G, et al. Brain white matter changes in the elderly prone to falling. Arch Neurol. 1989;46 (12):1292–6.

[4] Baloh RW, Yue Q, Socotch TM, et al. White matter lesions and disequilibrium in older people. I. Case-control comparison. Arch Neurol. 1995;52(10):970–4.

[5] Mirsen TR, Lee DH, Wong CJ et al. Clinical correlates of white-matter changes on magnetic resonance imaging scans of the brain. Arch Neurol. 1991;48(10):1015–21.

[6] Inzitari D, Cadelo M, Marranci ML, et al. Vascular deaths in elderly neurological patients with leukoaraiosis. J Neurol Neurosurg Psychiatry 1997;62(2):177–81.

[7] Liston R, Mickelborough J, Bene J, et al. A new classification of higher level gait disorders in patients with cerebral multi-infarct states. Age Ageing. 2003;32(3):252–8.

[8] de Laat KF, van Norden AG, Gons RA, et al. Gait in elderly with cerebral small vessel disease. Stroke. 2010;41(8):1652-8.

[9] Guttmann CR, Benson R, Warfield SK, et al. White matter abnormalities in mobility impaired older persons. Neurology. 2000; 54(6):1277-83.

[10] Guerini F, Frisoni GB, Marrè A, et al. Subcortical vascular lesions predict falls at 12 months in elderly aptients discharged from a rehabilitation ward. Arch Phys Med Rehabil. 2008;89(8):1522-7.

[11] Baezner H, Blahak C, Poggesi A, et al. Association of gait and balance disorders with age-related white matter changes. Neurology. 2008;70(12):935-42.

[12] Della Sala S, Spinnler H, Venneri A. Walking difficulties in patients with Alzheimer's disease might originate from gait apraxia. J Neurol Neurosurg Psychiatry 2004;75(2): 196-201.

[13] Ala TA, Frey WH. Validation of the NINCDS-ADRDA criteria regarding gait in the clinical diagnosis of Alzheimer disease. A clinicopathologic study. Alzheimer Dis Assoc Disord. 1995;9(3):152–9.

[14] Alexander NB, Mollo JM, Giordani B, et al. Maintenance of balance, gait patterns, and obstacle clearance in Alzheimer's disease. Neurology. 1995;45(5):908–14.

[15] Visser H. Gait and balance in senile dementia of Alzheimer's type. Age Ageing. 1983;12(4):296–301.

[16] Buchner DM, Larson EB. Falls and fractures in patients with Alzheimer-type dementia. JAMA.1987;257(11):1492–5.

[17] van Dijk PT, Meulenberg OG, van de Sande HJ, et al. Falls in dementia patients. Gerontologist. 1993;33(2):200–4.

[18] Koller WC, Wilson RS, Glatt SL, et al. Motor signs are infrequent in dementia of the Alzheimer type. Ann Neurol. 1984;16(4):514–16.

[19] Fransenn EH, Kluger A, Torossian CL, et al. The neurologic syndrome of severe Alzheimer's disease. Relationship to functional decline. Arch Neurol 1993;50:1029–39.

[20] Burns A, Jacoby R, Levy R. Neurological signs in Alzheimer's disease. Age Ageing. 1991;20(1):45–51.

[21] Kurlan R, Richard IH, Papka M, et al. Movement disorders in Alzheimer's disease: More rigidity of definition is needed. Mov Disord 2000;15(1):24–9.

[22] McKhann G, Drachman D, Folstein M, et al. Clinical diagnosis of Alzheimer's disease: report of the NINCDS-ADRDA Work Group under the auspices of Department of Health and Human Services Task Force on Alzheimer's Disease. Neurology. 34(7): 939–44.

[23] Román GC, Tatemichi TK, Erkinjuntti T et al. Vascular dementia: diagnostic criteria for research studies. Report of the NINDS-AIREN International Workshop. Neurology. 1993;43(2):250- 60.

[24] Erkinjuntti T. Vascular dementia: challenge of clinical diagnosis. Int Psychogeriatr. 1997;9:77–83.

[25] Bus BA, Marijnissen RM, Holewjin S, et al. Depressive symptom clusters are differentialy associated with atherosclerotic disease. Psychol Med. 2011;41(7):1419-28.

[26] Folstein MF, Folstein SE, McHugh PR. "Mini-Mental state". A practical method for grading the cognitive state of patients for the clinician. J Psychiatr Res. 1975;12(3): 189–98.

[27] Dubois B, Slachevsky A, Litvan I, et al. The FAB: a Frontal Assessment Battery at bedside. Neurology. 2000;55(11):1621-6.

[28] Cummings JL, Mega M, Gray K, et al. The Neuropsychiatric Inventory: comprehensive assessment of psychopathology in dementia. Neurology. 1994;44(12):2308–14.

[29] Greene JG, Smith R, Gardiner M, et al. Measuring behavioural disturbance of elderly demented in patients in the community and its effects on relatives: a factor analytic study. Age Ageing. 1982;11(2):121–6.

[30] Ott BR, Lafleche G, Whelihan WM, et al. Impaired awareness of deficits in Alzheimer Disease. Alzheimer Dis Assoc Disord. 1996;10(2):68-76.

[31] Mahoney FI, Barthel DW. Functional evaluation: the Barthel Index. Md State Med J. 1965;14:61-65.

[32] Lawton MP, Brody EM. Assessment of older people: self-maintaining and instrumental activities of daily living. Gerontologist. 1969;9(3):179-86.

[33] Tinetti ME. Performance-oriented assessment of mobilty problems in elderly patients. J Am Ger Soc. 1986;34(2):119-26.

[34] Blennow K, Wallin A, Uhlemann C, et al. White-matter lesions on CT in Alzheimer patients: relation to clinical symptomatology and vascular factors. Acta Neurol Scand. 1991;83(3):187-93.

[35] Scheltens P, Barkhof F, Leys D, et al. A semiquantative rating scale for the assessment of signal hyperintensities on magnetic resonance imaging. J Neurol Sci. 1993;114(1): 7-12.

[36] Wahlund LO, Almkvist O, Blennow K, et al. Evidence-based evaluation of magnetic resonance imaging as a diagnostic tool in dementia workup. Top Magn Reson Imaging. 2005;16(6):427-37.

[37] Kantarci K, Jack CR Jr. Neuroimaging in Alzheimer disease: an evidence-based review. Neuroimaging Clin N Am. 2003;13(2):197-209.

[38] den Heijer T, Geerlings M, Hoebeek F, et al. Use of hippocampal and amygdalar volumes on MRI to predict dementia in cognitively intact elderly. Arch Gen Psychiatry 2006;63(1):57-62.

[39] Carboncini MC, Volterrani D, Bonfiglio L, et al. Higher level gait disorders in subcortical chronic vascular encephalopathy: a single photon emission computed tomography study. Age Ageing. 2009;38(3):302-7.

[40] Donoghue JP, Sanes JN. Motor areas of the motor cortex. J Clin Neurophysiol. 1994;11(4):382-96.

[41] Georgiou N, Iansek R, Bradshaw JL, et al. An evaluation of the role of internal cues in the pathogenesis of parkinsonian hypokinesia. Brain. 1993;116(Pt 6):1575–87.

[42] Phillips JG, Martin KE, Bradshaw JL, et al. Could bradykinesia in Parkinson's disease simply be overcompensation? J Neurol. 1994;241(7):439–47.

[43] Rosano C, Brach J, Studenski S, et al. Gait variability is associated with subclinical brain vascular abnormalities in high-functioning older adults. Neuroepidemiology. 2007;29(3-4):193-200.

[44] Srikanth V, Beare R, Blizzard L, et al. Cerebral white matter lesions, gait and risk of incident falls: a prospective population based study. Stroke. 2009;40(1):175-80.

[45] Masdeu JC, Wolfson L. White matter lesions predispose to falls in older people. Stroke. 2009;40(9):e546.

[46] Benke T. Two forms of apraxia in Alzheimer's disease. Cortex. 1993; 29(4):715-29.

[47] Meyer JS, Barron DW. Apraxia of gait: a clinico-physiological study. Brain.1960;83(2): 261–84.

[48] Hennerici MG, Oster M, Cohen S, et al. Are gait disturbances and white matter degeneration early indicators of vascular dementia? Dementia. 1994;5(3-4):197–202.

[49] Moretti R, Torre P, Antonello RM, et al. The on-freezing phenomenon: cognitive and behavioural aspects. Parkinsons Dis. 2011; Article id:746303;1-7.

[50] Junque C, Pujol J, Vendrell P et al. Leuko-araiosis on magnetic resonance imaging and speed of mental processing. Arch Neurol. 1990;47(2):151–6.

[51] Waite LM, Broe GA, Creasey H, et al. Neurological signs, aging, and the neurodegenerative syndromes. Arch Neurol. 1996;53(6):498–502.

[52] Moretti R, Torre P, Antonello RMA. Basal ganglia: functional and organic roles in behavior and cognition. Nova Science Publishers Inc, New York; 2009.

[53] Iansek R, Bradshaw JL, Phillips JG, et al. Interaction of the basal ganglia and supplementary motor area in the elaboration of movement. In: Glencross DJ, Piek JP (ed.) Motor control and sensorimotor integration. Amsterdam: Elsevier Science; 1995. p37–59.

[54] Lee AC, Harris JP. Problems with perception of space in Parkinson's disease: a questionnaire study. Neuro-Ophthalmology 1999;22(1):1-15.

[55] Almeida QJ, Frank JS, Roy EA, et al. An evaluation of sensorimotor integration during locomotion toward a target in Parkinson's disease. Neuroscience. 2005;134(1): 283-93.

[56] Gurvich C, Georgiou-Karistianis N, Fitzgerald PB, et al. Inhibitory control and spatial working memory in Parkinson's disease. Mov Disord 2007;22(10):1444-50.

Chapter 12

# The Alzheimer's Patient in the Emergency Department — Specificities of Care

De Breucker Sandra, Pepersack Thierry and
Bier Jean-Christophe

Additional information is available at the end of the chapter

http://dx.doi.org/10.5772/59326

## 1. Introduction

In Belgium, like in almost all other European countries, Alzheimer's disease affects a growing number of people as our western population is growing older and the life expectancy is expanding.

We estimate the prevalence of AD to 800.000 people in France and 420.000 people in Benelux (Belgium, Netherlands, Luxemburg).

Although the prevalence is very low before age of 70, it exceeds 20 % of men and 30 % of women after 90 years old [1].

Alzheimer's disease has a heavy impact on physical, psychological and social equilibrium of the patient and his family. Alzheimer's disease has still a bad image in the society, because it is described like a slowly progressive but inexorable illness, affecting not only intellectual abilities, but also physical integrity.

Beyond the basic care, the Alzheimer patients need from professionals a specific support, which implies a better knowledge of the illness and listening skills of the patient and his family.

Alzheimer's disease patients need regularly to be hospitalized, and the emergency room is their main way to be admitted to the hospital. However, the lack of knowledge of professionals on Alzheimer's disease induces suffering for the patient and his family, as they are too often considered as heavy and non-cooperating patients.

The purpose of this article is to give some useful bases to inhospital caregivers who are confronted to Alzheimer's disease patients, especially in emergency unit.

## 2. Alzheimer's disease

Alzheimer's disease is the most frequent cause of dementia, accounting for 50% to 60% of all cases. It is a neurodegenerative disease, which affects cognitive functions, psychological and behavioural balance. Alzheimer's disease is a neurodegenerative disorder in which two proteins (amyloid-β and Tau) undergo pathological changes, consisting in brain accumulation of an insoluble form of amyloid-β, and in hyperphosphorylation of the tau protein with modifications of the stereotactic configuration. Although the exact chronology and interaction between these proteins is still debated, it is generally accepted that these alterations arise years and probably decades before the appearance of any clinical symptoms [2].Thus, physiopathology associated an accumulation of beta amyloid peptides in senile plaques and tangles (induced by tau protein abnormalities) in the neurofibrils with lipid oxidation and peroxidation, glutamatergic toxicity, and on inflammation, leading to neuronal apoptosis. Another physiopathological change concerns

Other physiopathological change concerns possible heavy metals accumulation, vascular or infectious processes... Finally, there is an increasing evidence that vascular dysfunction plays an important role in the clinical decompensating Alzheimer's disease [3].

Its course is slow, insidious and lasts for years.

Psychological and Behavioral Symptoms of Dementia (BPSD) may appear at any time of the disease but usually appear later in its course. They can represent loss of initiative to manage daily activities (apathy), changes in the personality (irritability, paranoiac thoughts, delusions) or changes in the mood and the behaviour (anxiety, depression, aggressiveness, appetite disorders, wandering). Noteworthy, sleep disorders, depression and anxiety or even apathy may all emerge before the onset of cognitive symptoms in many cases.

Finally, the neuronal loss is high and more physical neurological syndromes emerge (epilepsy, walking disorders, higher risk of falls, immobilization, swallowing disturbances, malnutrition and dehydration).

As for many syndromes, the clinical diagnosis is based on different criteria [4,5].

First, the patient's and family 's anamnesis informs the clinician when and how the disease began, how it evolves and if it has a negative impact on daily activities.

The personal and familial history, socio-educational and co-morbid features will complete the history.

Biological tests can be restricted to those allowing to exclude pathologies interfering with cognition, for example folic acid or vitamin B12 deficiency, dysthyroidism, ionic and metabolic disorders. When the clinical features or history suggest syphilis, HIV or borreliosis, specific serologies should be performed.

Cognitive assessment should be completed with a validated screening test, such as a Mini Mental State Examination (MMSE) [4]. Space-time orientation and immediate memory represent 16 points of the total 30 points. In case of doubt, a total score equal or over 24/30 should be followed by a comprehensive cognitive assessment performed by a neuropsychologist. It emphasizes multiple cognitive disorders and helps the clinician to define the diagnosis as best as possible.

Brain neuroimaging (CT scan, magnetic resonance imaging) completes the workup. It detects potentially treatable cerebral lesions (tumors, hematoma, hydrocephaly,...), and associated causes (vascular lesions). It also gives anatomic indices to describe specific Alzheimer features (ie hippocampic atrophy).

Functional neuroimaging (Pet Scan, SPECT) explores topographic hypometabolic zones, helping to approach the diagnosis when clinical features are unusual.

Finally, lumbar puncture is a complementary diagnostic tool, it allows to confirm the diagnosis if the clinical presentation is more atypical: low levels of b-amyloid 42 and high levels of tau and phosphotau protein seem highly sensitive and specific (80%) to Alzheimer's disease.

When the diagnosis is defined, the Alzheimer's disease management should begin with the announcement of the diagnosis to the patient and his family. It is important to take into account the patient's anxiety related to the delay of the disease announcement itself to find the good moment to announce it. Most of Alzheimer patients wish to be informed of their diagnosis (72 to 96% from one study to another) and 7% of caregivers wish their parents to be informed from what they suffer, to respect his/her autonomy of decision [6,7].

The information on the disease must be clear, concise and should focus on the course of illness, its main comorbidities, the need to provide more help for daily activities...

It is also important to talk about medicolegal issues, such as the ability to drive a car, to set up a personal property manager.

The caregiver approach should consist in a specific education on the illness, whether for the basics or a true course called « psychoeducation ». A study demonstrated that a caregiver's specific training delays the time of institutionnalization until 500 days [8], and decreases the risk of caregiver's mood disorders [9]. An American study showed that a daily home caregiver to help the main caregiver lowered the number of hospitalizations, the length of stay of demented patients [10].

The treatment consists in a global approach; pharmacological and non-pharmacological approaches should always coexist.

Two drug classes are currently available; cholinesterase inhibitors (donepezil, rivastigmine, galantamine) and N Methyl D Aspartate receptor antagonists (memantine). Although they have only a minor effect on the course of the illness, cholinesterase inhibitors are actually recommended in mild to moderate Alzheimer's disease.

A French study showed that Alzheimer patients treated by cholinesterase inhibitors are later institutionalized than those not treated [11]. Memantine has a greater protective effect on memory in later stages of the disease, and it seems to have a positive impact on some behavioural disturbances [12,13]. The combination of the two classes is probably promising, further studies are expected to confirm it clearly.

The treatment of behavioural and psychological and social disorders needs to first identify the triggering and/or worsening factors (environmental factors, organic causes such as pain, constipation, infections; iatrogenic causes and depression).

Non-pharmacological approach includes different therapies: aromatherapy, musical therapy, physical exercises... Until now, none of these therapies have been shown effective, due to the lack of reproducible methodology from one study to another [14].

If necessary, neuroleptics can help to manage BPSD, following the rule « the lowest dose, the shortest time » as possible, to avoid adverse reactions (drowsiness, falls, extrapyramidal syndromes) and its bad impact on quality of life, wellness feeling, and the risk to worsen cognitive disorders [15,16].

## 3. The caregiver's burden

Formal caregivers, (spouses or children), informal caregivers (neighbours, friends, home care nurses) suffer from the « collateral distress » of Alzheimer's disease. This is influenced by the lack of knowledge on the illness, its course and its prognosis. Moreover, caregivers are often the first who refer their proxy to the memory clinic, because they suffer, without knowing why: the feel « abnormally exhausted ». Studies show that caregivers suffer more from anxiety, depression, and alcohol abuse and have a higher risk of mortality [4].

At the diagnosis announcement, different kinds of reactions are observed.

Some of them deny it. Some others tend to be more protective with the patient, and are usually hyperinvesting in the care of their parent.

Sometimes conflicts appear between the patient, his family and the institution of care. It is particularly true if the family feels guilty and ambivalent toward their parent and because they refer the heavy task on care people.

Before the patient will be referred to a nursing home, the main caregiver must be psychologically and physically sustained by a trained team, and he must be informed on the possibilities to have periods of rest during the course of the illness.

Home care should be strictly organised and adapted from the beginning until the end of the course of the disease. Even after the institutionalization, the family should be followed specifically.

Advanced directives for the patient could also be discussed with them.

Though defined as a chronic disease, the disease progression to terminal illness is rarely recognized as a « palliative process ». An American study followed 300 institutionalized Alzheimer's patients and their proxies during 18 months. 55% of the patients died during this period; 41% had pneumonia, 52% had fever episode, 85% had problems to eat alone. In emergencies, 46% had dyspnea, 39% experienced pain. In the last 3 months of life, 40% had experienced « aggressive therapies »: they were hospitalized; they were referred to an emergency department, or even underwent artificial nutrition.

When patients and their proxies had been well informed on the prognosis and the course of the disease, patients had a more worthy end-of-life experience [17]. It emphasizes the importance to educate the care staff, whether for home care, hospital care or nursing home care [18].

## 4. The patient with dementia at the emergency department

Among patients older than 60 years old admitted in emergency department, 13% have cognitive disorders. When they are admitted at hospital by another way, only 8% have cognitive problems [19].

Most of time, the urgent admission of a demented patient is more justified by the lack of structural or human support than the acute illness itself: the emergency room becomes the only « wipe out » for burden families, sometimes also for burden professionals in nursing homes.

More, literature reports that proxies express very few their wish to find an alternative structure to take care of their parents [20].

The reason of admission is most often a somatic problem.

In a prospective study conducted by B Vellas et al, the two first causes of admission of demented patients in emergency wards were behavioural disorders (26,3%) and falls (18,6%) [21].

A retrospective study in United Kingdom, between 2002 and 2007, showed that demented patients (20% Alzheimer, 11% vascular dementia, 69% not defined in the medical file) were more frequently admitted via the emergency room than non-demented patients. The diagnosis of dementia is rarely evoked in the file (6-10%). Most are hospitalized for somatic problems (syncope, pneumonia, urinary tract infection, dehydration) and more significantly than non-demented patients [22].

In a French study (REAL.FR), investigators followed 516 patients with light to moderate Alzheimer disease during one year. 27% of them were hospitalized at least once. Predictive factors of hospitalization were: caregiver's burden (the most frequent), loss of autonomy in one or more basic daily activities (Katz scale) or in two or more instrumental daily activities, the presence of at least 2 current illnesses, depressive disorders, polypharmacy, disinhibition, delirium, score > 5 on Reisberg's illness rating scale (moderate dementia or severe cognitive decline) and the need for external help for housekeeping [23]. After 2 years of follow-up, predictive factors of rehospitalisation were need for basic daily activities, caregiver's burden and high level of BPSD based on NPI scale (Neuropsychiatric Inventory) [24].

In case of real emergency, the GP should refer the patient with a detailed file containing medical and dementia history, current medications, and a brief summary of home care providers' journal, to distinguish chronic and new symptoms. For example, alteration of vigilance is a challenging situation with a broad differential diagnosis: an underlying acute medical illness, epilepsy, drug intoxication, delirium should always be excluded.

It is important to note that most of common pathologies associated with advancing dementia have an underlying illness that needs a specific causal treatment.

Bradshaw et al studied 250 patients aged over 70 with a co-morbid mental health problem and followed them up for 180 days. Twenty-seven per cent did not return to their original place of residence after the hospital admission, and 31% had died after 180 days. Significant predictors for poor outcomes were co-morbidity, nutrition, *cognitive function, behavioural and psychiatric problems and depression* [25].

Medical doctors working in the emergency unit should avoid the use of neuroleptics, or other sedative drugs to treat delirium and BPSD, and a non-pharmacological approach should always be proposed. This implies that any new problematic symptom, including agitation, delirium, paranoia, hallucination, and anxiety ... should preferably be managed in collaboration with the physicians who know the patient and the course of the disease. A conservative and comprehensive management of the probable cause of the problem (loss of senses such as sight or hearing; changing habits or care behaviour,..) is the most appropriate.

When drug will be offered, causal effect treatment with the fewest side effects is preferred. It is particularly important to pay attention to any anticholinergic effects and to possible interactions with other medications.

In all cases, we should also exclude organic cause (metabolic disorder, including urinary infections, subdural hematoma in case of fall or even the occurrence of new epilepsy...) before considering the appropriate treatment.

### 4.1. Delirium and dementia

Delirium is very common in elderly patients admitted in the emergency unit. Risk of delirium is higher for demented patients. It is sometimes the first symptom leading to the diagnosis of dementia.

Most of the time, causes of delirium are not purely neurological and toxic, metabolic causes (hypoglycemia, anemia, heart failure), drugs interactions, current infections or pain have all to be tracked.

Features of delirium are characterized by altered vigilance status, cognitive disorders not related to previous cognitive state, symptoms of rapid onset and fluctuation and a strong evidence of underlying organic disease (DSM IV-TR) [26]. Demented patients with delirium are less able to explain their symptoms than non-demented patients and than demented patients without delirium. They have more difficulties to understand explanations and diagnosis delivered by professionals in the emergency ward [27]. Moreover, delirium in urgent situations is a prognostic factor for loss of autonomy: according to a study of Vida, delirious patients loose more autonomy than non-delirious patients [28]. Finally, delirium is an independent prognostic factor for length of stay and risk of mortality at 6 months [29,30]. In the absence of altered mental status, this syndrome might be missed unless it is actively looked for using a validated delirium assessment.

The environment of the emergency room is seldom adapted to patients with delirium: people have to wait several hours to be managed, rooms have no windows, there is no time markers in the rooms (no clocks, diaries), meals are served at every hours night and day.

It is therefore important to screen for delirium: the most used screening is CAM (Confusion Assessment Method) [31]. Health care providers in emergency units have often not enough time to assess completely the situation, to communicate efficiently with the patients and to take care of their needs.

In front of patient with acute or subacute delirium; fluent aphasia has to be excluded. It could be interpreted as confusion. If the onset of aphasia was sudden, brain imagery and electroencephalogram should always be done.

Management of delirium involves ensuring safety, improving functioning, identifying and treating the illness underlying the delirium, and use of antipsychotics or benzodiazepines to control behavioural symptoms and prevent mortality. Haloperidol, an old typical neuroleptic is the most commonly used antipsychotic in delirium. Atypical antipsychotics may be as efficacious as haloperidol in the treatment of delirium, but have less side effects [32]. In addition, to restore good quality of sleep and normal circadian rhythm, the use of melatonin can sometimes help. Anticholinesterases or memantine have few impacts on delirium in emergency cases [33]. However, their chronic prescription could decrease the risk of delirium and BPSD in dementia especially in case of Alzheimer disease.

Non pharmacological approach in emergency units would consist in faster management of the patient in quiet rooms with windows, clocks and calendars should be implemented. Beds with barriers, with comfortable mattress should be proposed.

### 4.2. Paranoia and dementia

Paranoia is a manifestation induced by excess of dopaminergic metabolites. As for other delirious ideas, it can also results from errors of interpretation or of reasoning, especially in dementia (objects lost interpreted as stolen...) [34].

In combination with a decrease of dopaminergic drugs, a conservative treatment has first to be considered. Anticholinesterase and memantine have both a top-grade places to avoid as far as possible the use of neuroleptics in terms of side effects, particularly in case of dementia [35-37]. Sometimes, trazodone 50 to 200 mg/day can help [38].

However, in emergency and only during the acute phase, haloperidol 1 to 4 mg could be proposed. But, in case of chronic use, new generation of neuroleptics (quetiapine for example) should be preferred with the necessity to track any extrapyramidal signs and to adapt the treatment very regularly.

### 4.3. Depression and dementia

Depression is frequently associated with dementia either as a triggering factor of the disease or as its consequence. However, depression is rarely the cause of emergency admission in case of dementia. If suicidal risk should be systematically screened, its arisen is exceptional perhaps as a consequence of memory disturbances, mood and cognitive fluctuations. Planning and executive difficulties could also explain the low rate of suicide in demented patients. Impulsive suicidal acts are nevertheless possible. Depression influences cognitive and functional capacities of all individuals, demented or not. This is of particular importance in case of minor and major neurocognitive deterioration, and it should be systematically screened and treated, in order to improve the quality of life of the patient and its caregivers, and to preserve the patient's residual functional and cognitive capacities. The preferential choice will then consider a drug with as least as possible interactions with other concomitant medications (often a selective serotonin reuptake inhibitor), taking into account the impact on appetite and sleep of the patient. A recent meta-analysis showed that psychological interventions associated with antidépressive drugs can reduce symptoms of depression and clinician-rated anxiety for people with dementia [39].

On the other hand, any caregiver's depression should be aggressively pursued and handled in view of its great incidence and of its heavy impact.

Nevertheless, we can't underestimate the ability of emergency caregivers to communicate with demented patients: Eder points out their need of knowledge of dementia, ie the different kinds of dementia, its progression, its symptoms, in order to communicate and manage adequately these patients [40].

Restraint is also a frequent ethical problem in emergency units. It raises ethical questions to all of us but especially to caregivers: « Should I respect the patient's autonomy, if he is in danger for himself or for others? How to justify it? » [41].

Finally, the length of stay in emergency unit depends on the downstream bed availability. Time spent by caregivers to find a bed is also wasted time to communicate with the patient.

Therefore, the management of these patients must be lead by an interdisciplinary approach. Nevertheless, in some countries like France, only 20% of hospitals have a geriatric unit. There is then an urgent need to sensitize medical hospital managers and policy makers to improve the geriatric offer in terms of acute settings.

At a medical level, the emergency physician should work together with geriatricians to understand how to integrate the acute illness into the patient's geriatric syndromes.

It is therefore useful to define a care pathway for the demented patient, from home care to hospital management.

We could imagine to apply to emergency units what already exists in terms of technological innovation for home care of elderly (demented) patients: for example, the European HOPE project (Smart Home for Elderly People) aimed to improve communication and information

http://dx.doi.org/10.5772/59326

to proxies to take care of their elderly demented parent; this system helped to maintain quality of life, and to improve health care, security and communication with the patient [42].

## 5. Proposition of a care pathway of demented patients

The general practitioner (GP) is the first health care provider involved [20]. He should be trained to inform families of the dementia's symptoms, their expected evolution and their potential complications. This is first, to prevent crisis and proxy's burden.

A crisis is an episode of acute disorganization with symptoms that lead patients and their caregivers to call an emergency care help. It refers to a sudden change in the course of the patient's and family's habits, while it is very important to maintain them stable for dementia's stability [43].

It happens too often that patients are admitted to emergency units on the request of GP, without evident urgent situation. When the problem is not urgent, the GP should refer the demented patient to geriatric or neurological consultation, or to the geriatric day hospital.

We developed in Belgium a specific care program for the geriatric patient which could offer alternative approach for the demented patient: since 2007, Belgian hospitals had to develop pilot projects for geriatric day hospitals, internal liaison (mobile team for geriatric patients hospitalized in other units than geriatric departments) and external liaison with home care and nursing home care providers. The referring GP contacts the coordinator of the geriatric care program and they decide together when and how to admit the patient at hospital, in order to avoid the mandatory passage to the emergency department if the patient doesn't require urgent care. It allows also providing counselling on how to adapt transiently home care.

## 6. Conclusion

Alzheimer's disease is a frequent pathology. It would be considered as a pandemic illness in the future 20 years. As the demented patient is often admitted at hospital by the emergency unit, it is crucial that emergency caregivers have the best knowledge of the disease, to offer the best adapted care, to support family and to avoid unnecessary admissions.

## Acknowledgements

The authors report no conflict of interest for this manuscript.

In addition to the authors, we thank Mrs Micheline Burg and Mrs Christel Cleutinx for their careful review of the English version of the manuscript.

## Author details

De Breucker Sandra[1*], Pepersack Thierry[1] and Bier Jean-Christophe[2]

*Address all correspondence to: Sandra.De.Breucker@erasme.ulb.ac.be

1 Erasme University Hospital– Free University of Brussels, Department of Geriatrics, Brussels, Belgium

2 Erasme University Hospital– Free University of Brussels, Department of Neurology, Brussels

## References

[1] Lobo A, Launer LJ, Fratiglioni L, Andersen K, Di Carlo A, Breteler MM, Copeland JR, Dartigues JF, Jagger C, Martinez-Lage J, Soininen H, Hofman A. Prevalence of dementia and major subtypes in Europe: A collaborative study of population-based cohorts. Neurologic Diseases in the Elderly Research Group. Neurology. 2000;54(11 Suppl 5):S4-9.

[2] Jack CR Jr, Albert MS, Knopman DS *et al* (2011). Introduction to the recommendations from the National Institute on Aging–Alzheimer's Association workgroups on diagnostic guidelines for Alzheimer's disease. Alzheimers Dement; 7: 257–62

[3] Iadecola C. The overlap between neurodegenerative and vascular factors in the pathogenesis of dementia. Acta Neuropathol. 2010 Sep;120(3):287-96.

[4] Hort J, O'Brien JT, Gainotti G, Pirttila T, Popescu BO, Rektorova I, Sorbi S, Scheltens P; on Behalf of the EFNS Scientist Panel on Dementia. EFNS guidelines for the diagnosis and management of Alzheimer's disease. Eur J Neurol. 2010 ; 17:1236-1248.

[5] American Psychiatric Association-DSM IV. Manuel diagnostique et statistique des troubles mentaux. Paris : Masson, 1996.

[6] Johnson, H. & Bouman, W. P. & Pinner, G. (2000) On disclosing the diagnosis in Alzheimer's disease: a pilot study of current attitudes and practice. International Psychogeriatrics 2000 ; 2(2) : 221-9.

[7] Pinner G. Truth-telling and the diagnosis of dementia. British Journal of Psychiatry 2000 ; 176 : 514-515.

[8] Mittelman MS, Haley WE, Clay OJ, Roth DL. Improving caregiver well-being delays nursing home placement of patients with Alzheimer disease. Neurology 2006; 67: 1592–1599.

[9] Mittelman MS, Brodaty H, Wallen AS, Burns A. A three-country randomized controlled trial of a psycho-social intervention for caregivers combined with pharmacologi-

http://dx.doi.org/10.5772/59326

cal treatment for patients with Alzheimer disease: effects on caregiver depression. Am J Geriatr Psychiatry 2008; 16: 893–904.

[10] Shelton P, Schraeder C, Dworak D, Fraser C, Sager MA. Caregivers' utilization of health services: results from the Medicare Alzheimer's Disease Demonstration, Illinois site. J Am Geriatr Soc. 2001;49(12):1600-5.

[11] Gillette-Guyonnet S, Andrieu S, Cortes F, Nourhashemi F, Cantet C, Ousset PJ, Reynish E, Grandjean H, Vellas B. Outcome of Alzheimer's disease: potential impact of cholinesterase inhibitors. J Gerontol A Biol Sci Med Sci. 2006;61(5):516-20.

[12] Becker M, Andel R, Rohrer L, Banks SM. The effect of cholinesterase inhibitors on risk of nursing home placement among medicaid beneficiaries with dementia. Alzheimer Dis Assoc Disord. 2006 Jul-Sep;20(3):147-52.

[13] Gauthier S, Loft H, Cummings J. Improvement in behavioural symptoms in patients with moderate to severe Alzheimer's disease by memantine: a pooled data analysis. Int J Geriatr Psychiatry 2008; 23: 537–545.

[14] Douglas S, James I, Ballard C. Non-pharmacological interventions in dementia. Advances in Psychiatric Treatment 2004 ;10: 171-179.

[15] Ballard, C. G., O'Brien, J., James, I., et al. Dementia: Management of Behavioural and Psychological Symptoms. Oxford: Oxford University Press ; 2001.

[16] McShane, R., Keene, J., Gedling, K., et al. Do neuroleptic drugs hasten cognitive decline in dementia? Prospective study with necropsy follow-up. BMJ 1997 ; 314 : 211–212.

[17] Mitchell SL, Teno JM, Kiely DK, Shaffer ML, Jones RN, Prigerson HG, Volicer L, Givens JL, Hamel MB. The clinical course of advanced dementia. N Engl J Med. 2009 Oct 15;361(16):1529-38.

[18] Villars H, Oustric S, Andrieu S, Baeyens JP, Bernabei R, Brodaty H, Brummel-Smith K, Celafu C, Chappell N, Fitten J, Frisoni G, Froelich L, Guerin O, Gold G, Holmerova I, Iliffe S, Lukas A, Melis R, Morley JE, Nies H, Nourhashemi F, Petermans J, Ribera Casado J, Rubenstein L, Salva A, Sieber C, Sinclair A, Schindler R, Stephan E, Wong RY, Vellas B. The primary care physician and Alzheimer's disease: an international position paper. J Nutr Health Aging. 2010 ;14(2):110-20.

[19] Shah MN, Jones CM, Richardson TM, Conwell Y, Katz P, Schneider SM. Prevalence of depression and cognitive impairment in older adult emergency medical services patients. Prehosp Emerg Care. 2011;15(1):4-11.

[20] Moulias R, Hervy MP, Ollivet C, Emmanuelli X. Alzheimer et maladies apparentées : traiter, soigner et accompagner au quotidien. Paris : Elsevier Masson ; 2005.

[21] Nourhashémi F, Andrieu S, Sastres N, Ducassé JL, Lauque D, Sinclair AJ, Albarède JL, Vellas BJ. Descriptive analysis of emergency hospital admissions of patients with Alzheimer disease. Alzheimer Dis Assoc Disord. 2001;15(1):21-5.

[22] Natalwala A, Potluri R, Uppal H, Heun R. Reasons for hospital admissions in dementia patients in Birmingham, UK, during 2002-2007. Dement Geriatr Cogn Disord. 2008;26(6):499-505.

[23] Balardy L, Voisin T, Cantet C, Vellas B. Predictive factors of emergency hospitalisation in Alzheimer's patients: results of one-year follow-up in the REAL.FR Cohort. J Nutr Health Aging. 2005;9(2):112-6.

[24] Voisin T, Andrieu S, Cantet C, Vellas. Predictive factors of hospitalizations in Alzheimer's disease: a two-year prospective study in 686 patients of the REAL.FR study. BJ Nutr Health Aging. 2010;14(4):288-91.

[25] Bradshaw LE1, Goldberg SE, Lewis SA, Whittamore K, Gladman JR, Jones RG, Harwood RH. Six-month outcomes following an emergency hospital admission for older adults with co-morbid mental health problems indicate complexity of care needs. Age Ageing. 2013 Sep;42(5):582-8.

[26] American Psychiatric Association. Diagnostic and Statistical Manual of Mental Disorders (IV-TR). 4th-Text Revised. Washington, D.C. : Arlington ; 2000.

[27] Han JH, Bryce SN, Ely EW, Kripalani S, Morandi A, Shintani A, Jackson JC, Storrow AB, Dittus RS, Schnelle J. The effect of cognitive impairment on the accuracy of the presenting complaint and discharge instruction comprehension in older emergency department patients. Ann Emerg Med. 2011 Jun;57(6):662-671.

[28] Vida S, Galbaud du Fort G, Kakuma R, Arsenault L, Platt RW, Wolfson CM. An 18-month prospective cohort study of functional outcome of delirium in elderly patients: activities of daily living. Int Psychogeriatr. 2006;18(4):681-700.

[29] Han JH, Shintani A, Eden S, Morandi A, Solberg LM, Schnelle J, Dittus RS, Storrow AB, Ely EW. Delirium in the emergency department: an independent predictor of death within 6 months. Ann Emerg Med. 2010 Sep;56(3):244-252.

[30] Han JH, Eden S, Shintani A, Morandi A, Schnelle J, Dittus RS, Storrow AB, Ely EW. Delirium in older emergency department patients is an independent predictor of hospital length of stay. Acad Emerg Med 2011 ; 18 : 451-7.

[31] Monette J, Galbaud du Fort G, Fung SH, Massoud F, Moride Y, Arsenault L, Afilalo M. Evaluation of the Confusion Assessment Method (CAM) as a screening tool for delirium in the emergency room. MGen Hosp Psychiatry. 2001;23(1):20-5.

[32] Grover S, Matoo SK, Gupta N. Usefulness of atypical antipsychotics and choline esterase inhibitors in delirium: a review. Pharmacopsychiatry. 2011;44(2):43-54.

[33] Overshott R, Karim S, Burns A. Cholinesterase inhibitors for delirium. Cochrane Database Syst Rev. 2008; (1):CD005317.

[34] Perez-Madriñan G1, Cook SE, Saxton JA, Miyahara S, Lopez OL, Kaufer DI, Aizenstein HJ, DeKosky ST, Sweet RA. Alzheimer disease with psychosis: excess cognitive impairment is restricted to the misidentification subtype. Am J Geriatr Psychiatry. 2004;12(5):449-56.

[35] Campbell N, Ayub A, Boustani MA, Fox C, Farlow M, Maidment I, Howards R. Impact of cholinesterase inhibitors on behavioral and psychological symptoms of Alzheimer's disease: a meta-analysis. Ann Pharmacother. 2008 Jan;42(1):32-8.

[36] Maidment ID, Fox CG, Boustani M, Rodriguez J, Brown RC, Katona CL. Efficacy of memantine on behavioral and psychological symptoms related to dementia: a systematic meta-analysis.Clin Interv Aging. 2008;3(4):719-28.

[37] Daiello LA1, Beier MT, Hoffmann VP, Kennedy JS. Pharmacotherapy of behavioral and psychological symptoms of dementia: a review of atypical antipsychotics. Consult Pharm. 2003 Feb;18(2):138-52, 155-7.

[38] López-Pousa S1, Garre-Olmo J, Vilalta-Franch J, Turon-Estrada A, Pericot-Nierga I. Trazodone for Alzheimer's disease: a naturalistic follow-up study. Arch Gerontol Geriatr. 2008 Sep-Oct;47(2):207-15.

[39] Orgeta V1, Qazi A, Spector AE, Orrell M. Psychological treatments for depression and anxiety in dementia and mild cognitive impairment. Cochrane Database Syst Rev. 2014; 22;1:CD009125.

[40] Eder S. The Alzheimer's challenge. Emerg Med Serv. 2005;34(6):99-103.

[41] McBrien B. Exercising restraint: clinical, legal and ethical considerations for the patient with Alzheimer's disease. Accid Emerg Nurs. 2007;15(2):94-100.

[42] Pilotto A, D'Onofrio G, Benelli E, Zanesco A, Cabello A, Margelí MC, Wanche-Politis S, Seferis K, Sancarlo D, Kilias D. Information and communication technology systems to improve quality of life and safety of Alzheimer's disease patients: a multicenter international survey. J Alzheimers Dis. 2011;23(1):131-41.

[43] Michon A. Crisis intervention in dementia. Psychol Neuropsychiatr Vieil. 2006;4(2): 121-5.

# Chapter 13

# Uncontrolled Sexual Behaviour in Dementia

Susan van Hooren and Wim Waterink

Additional information is available at the end of the chapter

http://dx.doi.org/10.5772/59979

## 1. Introduction

Uncontrolled sexual behaviour in dementia is considered as a symptom of the behavioural disturbances seen in dementia, such as agitation, disinhibition, apathy, depression, and psychotic behaviour. The combination of these behavioural problems and progressive cognitive dysfunctions are the main characteristics of dementia. The behavioural problems, are present in 80-95% of the patients with dementia [1]. These symptoms decrease the quality of life of patients, increase the likelihood of institutionalization, and contribute most to caregivers burden. Although less common than most other behavioural problems, uncontrolled sexual behaviour is often more disruptive and upsetting to a spouse, institutional staff and other residents [2-4]. Therefore, these sexual behaviours are a tremendous challenge for health care providers in institutional care settings. However, a literature search utilizing Pubmed showed that only 0,5% of the literature addressing dementia concerns sexual functioning, and even less focuses on uncontrolled sexual behaviour. Thus, uncontrolled sexual behaviour is a serious neglected area in this field, while the majority of health care providers agree that more information and institutional training is needed [2, 5, 6].

## 2. Uncontrolled sexual behaviour

Uncontrolled sexual behaviour is labelled and defined in many ways in the literature. Synonyms used are 'Disinhibited sexual behaviour' [7], 'Inappropriate sexual behaviour' [8, 9], 'Inappropriate sexual expression' [2], 'Increased sexual activity' [10], and 'Hypersexuality' [11]. All phrases imply that this behaviour is a sexual act (verbal or physical) which is unacceptable, inappropriate, disinhibited, or uncontrolled within the (social) context in which it is carried out. Examples are sexual comments, masturbation in public, grabbing at the genitals and/or breasts of other persons, chasing other residents for sexual purposes, and exposing one's genitals in public. Some of these behaviours may be inappropriate only because they are performed in public and therefore should not be confused with sexual appetite and behaviour in older people due to a normal sex drive. There is no widely agreed definition of when this behaviour becomes inappropriate and so it is subject to subjective interpretation of the observer. In this chapter, 'uncontrolled' is used reflecting a reduced capacity to manage an impulsive response to a situation.

There are several types of behaviours identified in the literature to cluster uncontrolled sexual behaviour. In some reviews of the literature, three types were suggested, i.e. sex talk, sexual acts, and implied sexual acts [11-13]. Sex talk is regarded as the most common form and involves inappropriate language, that is not in line with the patient's premorbid personality. Sexual acts include touching grabbing, exposing or masturbating in public or in private settings. Implied sexual acts involve reading pornographic material in public or requesting unnecessary genital care. In an observational study that included 40 patients with dementia living in a nursing home [14], research assistants scored whether exposed sexual behaviour was appropriate, ambiguous or inappropriate. The patients were systematically observed on nine separate five minute occasions in the nursing home during different situations, such as at meals, being groomed or dressed, in their rooms. Most sexual behaviour was coded as inappropriate or ambiguous. Overall, this scoring leaves substantial gaps for individual interpretation of the observer. Besides, the three types of sexual behaviour were not based on empirical evidence.

More recently, two observational studies shed more light on the definition and measurement of uncontrolled sexual behaviour. In the first study [15], sexual behaviours were observed and afterwards clustered in several types. Based on an observational study which included 12 patients with dementia, aged between 53 and 84 years of age, nineteen sexual behaviours were obtained from observations and interviews with their caregivers and categorised by the authors in three types, i.e. 'sexual acts with contact with others', 'sexual acts with non-contact with others', and 'verbal sexual behaviour'. The most frequently observed sexual behaviours consisted of patients stroking their own genitals in private, touching areas of another person and verbal provocation. In the second study [16], 68 health professionals were questioned, working in institutions with patients with progressive neurological disease or patients with acquired brain injury, which resulted in 145 examples of uncontrolled sexual behaviours. Incidents of touching others inappropriately was the most common uncontrolled sexual behaviour.

Based on the abovementioned study in which an observation instrument was developed [16, 17], items were identified for the development of a questionnaire regarding sexual behaviour in dementia (SBDQ; [6]). The questionnaire consisted of four discrete behaviour categories: verbal comments, non-contact behaviour, exposure, and touching others. 115 health professionals were asked to rank the behavioural descriptors in terms of severity. This resulted in four levels of severity for each behaviour category. The rankings resulted in categorisations of uncontrolled sexual behaviours that are more evidence based and initiated a methodological tool that may have value for clinical use and research purposes. The validity and reliability of this scale was investigated and established (see also, [6]).

## 3. Uncontrolled sexual behaviour in dementia

Because of the limited coverage of uncontrolled sexual behaviour within the literature and the use of different definitions and categorisations, it is difficult to obtain a robust view of prevalence of these behaviours in dementia. Nevertheless, there are some studies which offer an insight in the frequency of uncontrolled sexual behaviour in dementia. For example, Burns et al. (1990) found that 7% of 178 patients with Alzheimer's disease showed sexual inappropriate behaviour (i.e. exposure, obscene sex language, masturbation, propositioning others). A more recent study [19] showed nearly a similar prevalence rate (8%) of references to sexual behaviour in medical records of 165 older people with dementia living in a residential care facility. The prevalence is substantially lower in a mixed cohort with patient living in nursing homes and patients living in the community. Of the 2278 participants only 41 (i.e. 1,8%) had a documentation of verbal or physical aberrant sexual behaviour [8]. In an observational study, there was a clear difference in prevalence rates between types of dementia, such as Alzheimer's disease, vascular dementia, pick's disease [14]. Patients with Alzheimer's disease expressed less uncontrolled sexual behaviour compared to patients diagnosed with other types of dementia (i.e. 9% versus 28%). This difference was also seen in other studies. For example, Alagiakrishnan (2005) demonstrated that 53,6% of the patients expressing uncontrolled sexual behaviour were diagnosed with vascular dementia, while 22% was diagnosed with Alzheimer. And even in the sample of twenty patients expressing uncontrolled sexual behaviour of De Medeiros et al. (2008), this difference was significant ($p<0.01$). The higher percentages of uncontrolled sexual behaviour in non-Alzheimer's types of dementia may be explained by a relatively higher likelihood of brain pathology that is associated with hyper sexuality (e.g. striatum, frontal lobes, temporo-limbic system and hypothalamus (e.g. [12]).

It not clear whether uncontrolled sexual behaviour is more prevalent in men than women or in patient with more severe dementia. Most studies only included men and dementia severity was often not investigated with regard to uncontrolled sexual behaviour. In studies that focused on uncontrolled sexual behaviour and included severity of dementia, the results were inconclusive. Burns et al. (1990) found a positive association with severity of dementia, while De Medeiros et al. (2008] concluded that half of the subjects with uncontrolled sexual behaviour had mild dementia, whereas most subjects with non-sexual behaviours had severe dementia. However, this difference did not reached significance. In both studies the frequency of sexual behaviour was equal for men and women, while two other studies have shown that sexual behaviour was more prevalent in men [5, 8].

In sum, based on these cross-sectional studies, prevalence rates of uncontrolled sexual behaviour in dementia vary between 1,8%-28%, which depends on type of dementia.

## 4. Etiology

The etiology of uncontrolled sexual behaviour is rather complex and must be considered within a biopsychosocial perspective [20]. Generally, the literature attributes this behaviour to biological changes associated with dementia, such as changes in brain structures and/or neurotransmitters. Case studies demonstrated that dysfunction of interconnected brain structures may cause uncontrolled sexual behaviour. Four major brain systems have been suggested [12, 13], i.e. the frontal lobes, the temporo-limbic system, the striatum, and the hypothalamus. Head trauma to the frontal and temporal lobes may decrease inhibitory impulses often needed to keep sexual feeling in control and therefore result in uncontrolled sexual behaviour. Pick's disease and Kluver-Bucy syndrome is associated with frontal and temporal pathology. These patients are characterized by social inappropriate behaviour, including uncontrolled sexual behaviour. Injury to the striatal region, as in Huntingtons and Parkinson disease, may result in obsessive-compulsive sexual behaviour [21]. Lesions to the right hypothalamus can cause manic symptoms, including increased sexual desire.

Psychological factors may also contribute to uncontrolled sexual behaviour or maintain this behaviour. First, some behavioural problems, including depression, hyperactivity, or mania, may increase sexual interest and result in uncontrolled sexual behaviour [19]. Other diagnoses, such as delirium, epileptic seizures and alcohol abuse may also cause uncontrolled sexual behaviour [7, 21]. Second, the amount of sexual interest is also determined by premorbid patterns of sexual activity [20]. Third, uncontrolled sexual behaviour may be due to disorientation, which is often seen in the patient with dementia. For example, because of the cognitive impairments, the patient with dementia may not be aware of his or her surroundings, and display behaviour considered normal in private but not in public. Similarly, a patient may misidentify another person as their spouse, and display behaviour appropriate for a married couple [9].

Psychosocial factors that may be associated with uncontrolled sexual behaviour are lack of a usual partner, lack of privacy, or an under stimulating environments. Older adults in residents may lack physical closeness, especially when they don't have a partner. Physical closeness might reduce loneliness and anxiety of the patient with dementia. When this need is not met, it is possible that this may take the form of physical aggression in persons not knowing how to appropriately meet their needs for closeness and intimacy. In nursing homes, there is often a lack of privacy and less opportunities for patients to be intimate with their partner. This may even be aggravated by the relatively passive and conservative attitude in some health professionals toward older people sex issues [2, 5]. In addition, an under stimulating environment may increase boredom and loneliness, which may result in disruptive sexual behaviour. In conclusion, the etiology of uncontrolled sexual behaviour is rather complex and there are many factors that could cause or maintain uncontrolled sexual behaviour.

Empirical studies addressing the etiological factors of uncontrolled sexual behaviour in dementia are very sparse. Since uncontrolled sexual behaviour may have an immense impact on patients and their relationship with others, family, caregivers, and institutional staff, it is important to gain more information on uncontrolled sexual behaviour and its etiology. More insight in uncontrolled sexual behaviour in dementia and the etiology, would be useful in diagnosing symptoms of uncontrolled sexual behaviour and could provide directions for interventions in order to help the patient, health professionals, and families to deal with this behaviour.

## 5. Management

The management of uncontrolled sexual behaviour is often a challenge. Less is known about the best way to act, while the need for evidence based guidelines is growing. Overall, management of uncontrolled sexual behaviour can be divided in behavioural strategies and

pharmacological treatment. Because many of the drugs carry significant risk of adverse side effects, it is important to start with a solid assessment of the situation (including the degree of risk to others) and appropriate behavioural treatment.

### 5.1. Assessment

First of all, the exact target behaviour, context and involved factors need to be defined; what form? In what context? Frequency? What factors contribute? What is known from the (sexual) history? Is it a desire for closeness, comfort, or lack of privacy? Is it a problem and to whom? Are there any risks and to whom? Do the patient have insight? What is the mental/cognitive status? [12, 20]. These questions may be answered by direct observation of the patient, in an open discussion with main staff and significant others, and/or a standardised measurement, like the SBDQ [6]. In addition, it is important to rule out delirium and consider mood disorders or psychosis. These disorders need other management than uncontrolled sexual behaviour. Examining physical status and current medications is needed to determine (bio)medical causes. Different classes of medications have shown to induce uncontrolled sexual behaviour, in clinical settings [22]. For example, atypical antipsychotics can induce uncontrolled sexual behaviour by blocking the effects of selective serotonin reuptake inhibitors [23]. The reason for this is, that selective serotonin reuptake inhibitors typically suppresses sexual drive [7, 24-26]. In sum, a careful assessment provides information to choose an appropriate treatment (strategy) and a good baseline to properly evaluate the process and the effects of treatments.

### 5.2. Behavioural treatment

After a careful assessment, it is possible to develop a care plan with the involved care professionals and it is recommended to involve significant others. A care plan may include elements that are directed to the patient, significant others, other residents, and the staff. To the patient, many behavioural strategies may be initiated depending on the form of behaviour, the contributing factors, and the patients cognitive functioning (possibilities for new learning). Examples of behavioural strategies are distraction during presence of uncontrolled sexual behaviour via substitution of other activities, redirecting via conversation or humour, ignore unwanted behaviour and encourage appropriate behaviour, modification of social cues that are being misinterpreted, removing 'triggers' of the behaviour, substitute caregivers to the sex that does not match their sexual preference, avoidance of external cues such as over stimulating television or radio programs, trousers that open in the back or with zippers in case of exposing behaviour, providing single rooms, "not disturb" signs, and/or allowing doors to remain shut to provide privacy to let the patient satisfy their sexual needs [9, 12, 27-29]. To the significant others or spouses it is useful to give additional information to reframe the behaviour and reassurance that these behaviours are not a reflection of their relationship.

Providing staff supervision and additional education may be extremely helpful, because care professionals report that it is often difficult to cope with these behaviours or it is distressing for them [2, 30]. There should be a good balance between openness to the patients need for normal sexual expression while preventing uncontrolled sexual behaviour [12]. It is also critical to prepare students for uncontrolled sexual behaviour. In a study in which a young student introduced herself to several residents, she was confronted with uncontrolled sexual behaviour and responded with guilt, confusion, and distress [30]. More reflection on own behaviour and small changes in the appearance, like another manner of dressing, may help in provoking less uncontrolled sexual behaviour. In addition, providing more information on the etiology of the behaviour may aid to reduce guilt and confusion of the student or care professional. Because students and care professionals may be uncomfortable discussing uncontrolled sexual behaviour, it is important that the supervisor initiates the topic and provide coping strategies to them. Specific methods, like role playing, may be quite helpful to prepare the student for uncontrolled sexual behaviour [30].

After all, it is important that evidence based guidelines will be developed in addition to a policy and procedures within an organisation.

### 5.3. Pharmacological treatment

Different classes of medication (e.g. antidepressant, antiandrogen, antipsychotic, and anticonvulsant medications) have been proposed in the treatment of uncontrolled sexual behaviour [31]. The basis for medication treatment comes from the similarities of paraphilias with sexual behaviour [32]. Paraphilias and hypersexual behaviour, both involve uncontrolled sexual behaviour. Hence, pharmacological treatment of uncontrolled sexual behaviour is focused on pharmacological agents that affect monoamine neurotransmitters and that enhance central serotonergic function in particular (see also, [33]). However, there is not yet convincing data supporting the use of a particular medication. Most evidence is in the form of case reports and data are also lacking with regard to the advantage of any medication over placebo or in comparison with other medications [31, 34].

## Author details

Susan van Hooren[1,2*] and Wim Waterink[1]

*Address all correspondence to: Susan.vanhooren@ou.nl or susan.vanhooren@zuyd.nl

1 Faculty of Psychology and Educational Sciences, Open University of the Netherlands, The Netherlands

2 Zuyd University of Applied Sciences, Heerlen, The Netherlands

## References

[1] Aalten P, De Vugt ME, Jaspers N, Jolles J, Verhey FR. The course of neuropsychiatric symptoms in dementia. Part II: relationships among behavioural sub-syndromes and the influence of clinical variables. Int J Geriatr Psychiatry. 2005;20(6):531-6.

[2] Holmes D, Reingold J, Teresi J. Sexual expression and dementia. Views of caregivers: A pilot study. Int J Geriatr Psychiatry. 1997;12(7):695-701.

[3] Mayers KS. Sexuality and the patient with dementia. Sexuality and disability. 1994;12(3):213-9.

[4] Mayers KS, McBride DC. Sexualized components of verbally abusive statements by residents with dementia diagnoses. Sexuality and disability. 1996;14(2):109-16.

[5] Archibald C. Sexuality, dementia and residential care: managers report and response. Health Soc Care Community. 1998;6(2):95-101.

[6] Bartelet M, Waterink W, Van Hooren S. Extreme sexual behavior in dementia as a specific manifestation of disinhibition. Journal of Alzheimer's Disease. 2014;42:S119-S24.

[7] Alkhalil C, Tanvir F, Alkhalil B, Lowenthal DT. Treatment of Sexual Disinhibition in Dementia: Case Reports and Review of the Literature. American Journal of Therapeutics. 2004;11(3):231-5.

[8] Alagiakrishnan K, Lim D, Brahim A, Wong A, Wood A, Senthilselvan A, et al.. Sexually inappropriate behaviour in demented elderly people. Postgrad Med J. 2005;81(957):463-6.

[9] Kamel HK, Hajjar RR. Sexuality in the nursing home, part 2: Managing abnormal behavior-legal and ethical issues. J Am Med Dir Assoc. 2003;4(4):203-6.

[10] Haussermann P, Goecker D, Beier K, Schroeder S. Low-dose cyproterone acetate treatment of sexual acting out in men with dementia. Int Psychogeriatr. 2003;15(2):181-6.

[11] Wallace M, Safer M. Hypersexuality among cognitively impaired older adults. Geriatr Nurs. 2009;30(4):230-7.

[12] Black B, Muralee S, Tampi RR. Inappropriate Sexual Behaviors in Dementia. Journal of Geriatric Psychiatry and Neurology. 2005;18(3):155-62.

[13] Ozkan B, Wilkins K, Muralee S, Tampi RR. Pharmacotherapy for inappropriate sexual behaviors in dementia: a systematic review of literature. Am J Alzheimers Dis Other Demen. 2008;23(4):344-54.

[14] Zeiss AM, Davies HD, Tinklenberg JR. An observational study of sexual behavior in demented male patients. Journal of Gerontology. 1996;51:M325-M9.

[15] Tzeng Y, Lin L, Shyr YL, Wen J. Sexual behaviour of institutionalised residents with dementia – a qualitative study. J Clin Nurs. 2009;18(7):991-1001.

[16] Knight C, Alderman N, Johnson C, Green S, Birkett-Swan L, Yorstan G. The St Andrew's Sexual Behaviour Assessment (SASBA): development of a standardised recording instrument for the measurement and assessment of challenging sexual behaviour in people with progressive and acquired neurological impairment. Neuropsychol Rehabil. 2008;18(2):129-59.

[17] Johnson C, Knight C, Alderman N. Challenges associated with the definition and assessment of inappropriate sexual behaviour amongst individuals with an acquired neurological impairment. Brain Injury. 2006;20(7):687-93.

[18] Burns A, Jacoby R, Levy R. Psychiatric phenomena in Alzheimer's disease. IV: Disorders of behaviour. British Journal of Psychiatry. 1990;157:86-94.

[19] De Medeiros K, Rosenberg PB, Baker AS, Onyike CU. Improper sexual behaviors in elders with dementia living in residential care. Dement Geriatr Cogn Disord. 2008;26(4):370-7.

[20] Series H, Degano P. Hypersexuality in dementia. Advances in psyciatric treatment. 2005;11:424-31.

[21] Guay DR. Inappropriate sexual behaviors in cognitively impaired older individuals. Am J Geriatr Pharmacother. 2008;6(5):269-88.

[22] Bardell A, Laus T, Fedoroff JP. Inappropriate sexual behaviour in a geriatric population. International Psychogeriatrics. 2011;23(7):1182-8.

[23] Lam MHB, Fong SYY, Wing Y-K. Sexual disinhibition in schizophrenia possible induces by risperidone an quetiapine. Psychiatry and Clinical Neuroscience. 2007;61(333).

[24] Baldwin DS. Sexual dysfunction associated with antidepressant drugs. Exp Opin Drug Safety. 2004;4/3:457-70.

[25] Jacobsen FM. Fluoxetine-induced sexual dysfunction and an open trial of yolimbine. Journal of Clinical Psychiatry. 1992;53:119-22.

[26] Levinsky AM, Owen NJ. Pharmacological treatment of sexual inhibition in dementia. Case reports and review of the literature. American Journal of Geriatric Soc 1999;47:231-4.

[27] Lesser JM, Hughes SV, Jemelka JR, Griffith J. Sexually inappropriate behaviors. Assessment necessitates careful edical and psychological evaluation and sensitivity. Geriatrics. 2005;60(1):34-7.

[28] Buhr GT, White HK. Difficult behaviors in long-term care patients with dementia. J Am Med Dir Assoc. 2006;7:180-92.

[29] Tsatali MS, Tsolaki MN, Christodoulou TP, Papaliagkas VT. The Complex Nature of Inappropriate Sexual Behaviors in Patients with Dementia: Can We Put it into a Frame? Sexuality and disability. 2011;29(2):143-56.

[30] Mayers KS. Inappropriate social and sexual responses to a female student by male patients with dementia and organic brain disorder. Sexuality and disability. 2000;18(2):143-7.

[31] Joller P, Gupta N, Seitz DP, 'Frank C, Gibson M, Gill SS. Approach to inappropriate sexual behaviour in people with dementia. Can Fam Physician. 2013;59(3):255-60.

[32] Krueger RB, Kaplan MS. The paraphilic and hypersexual disorders. An overview. Journal of Psychiatric Practice. 2001;7(391-403).

[33] Kafka MP. The monoamine hypothesis of the pathophysiology of paraphilic disorders: An update. In: Prentky RA, Janus ES, Seto MC, editors. Sexually coercive behaviour Understanding and management. New York: New York Academy of Sciences.; 2003. p. 86-94.

[34] Mania I, Evcimen H, Mathews M. Citalopram Treatment for Inappropriate Sexual Behavior in a Cognitively Impaired Patient. Prim Care Companion J Clin Psychiatry. 2006;8(2):106.